Tropical Medicine: Clinical Studies

Tropical Medicine: Clinical Studies

Editor: Cyrus Hank

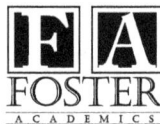

FA
FOSTER
ACADEMICS

www.fosteracademics.com

www.fosteracademics.com

FA **FOSTER**
ACADEMICS

Cataloging-in-Publication Data

Tropical medicine : clinical studies / edited by Cyrus Hank.
   p. cm.
Includes bibliographical references and index.
ISBN 978-1-63242-820-2
1. Tropical medicine. 2. Medical climatology. 3. Medicine. 4. Clinical medicine. I. Hank, Cyrus.
RC961 .T76 2019
616.988 3--dc23

Foster Academics,
118-35 Queens Blvd., Suite 400,
Forest Hills, NY 11375, USA

ISBN 978-1-63242-820-2 (Hardback)

Contents

Preface

The field of medicine that deals with the health issues that are unique, or are more widespread, in tropical and subtropical regions is known as tropical medicine. Some common diseases in the tropical and subtropical regions include malaria, tuberculosis and HIV/AIDS. However, there are several non-communicable diseases and neglected tropical diseases which affect the health of people living in the tropical and subtropical regions. Lack of preventive medicine, education and proper diet have led to a significant mortality due to non-communicable diseases, such as cancer, respiratory diseases and cardiovascular diseases. Chagas disease, dengue, leprosy, rabies and eumycetoma are some common examples of neglected tropical diseases. This book unfolds the innovative aspects of tropical medicine which will be crucial for the progress of this field in the future. It is compiled in such a manner, that it will provide in-depth knowledge about the theory and practice of tropical medicine. This book includes contributions of experts and scientists which will provide innovative insights into this field.

After months of intensive research and writing, this book is the end result of all who devoted their time and efforts in the initiation and progress of this book. It will surely be a source of reference in enhancing the required knowledge of the new developments in the area. During the course of developing this book, certain measures such as accuracy, authenticity and research focused analytical studies were given preference in order to produce a comprehensive book in the area of study.

This book would not have been possible without the efforts of the authors and the publisher. I extend my sincere thanks to them. Secondly, I express my gratitude to my family and well-wishers. And most importantly, I thank my students for constantly expressing their willingness and curiosity in enhancing their knowledge in the field, which encourages me to take up further research projects for the advancement of the area.

Editor

Poverty-related diseases (PRDs): unravelling complexities in disease responses in Cameroon

Valerie Makoge[1,3]* , Harro Maat[2], Lenneke Vaandrager[1] and Maria Koelen[1]

Abstract

Background: In Cameroon, poverty-related diseases (PRDs) are a major public health concern. Research and policies addressing PRDs are based on a particular understanding of the interaction between poverty and disease, usually an association between poverty indicators and health indicators for a specific country or region. Such indicators are useful but fail to explain the nature of the linkages between poverty and disease or poverty and health. This paper presents results of a study among university students, unravelling how they perceive diseases, the linkages with poverty, their responses to diseases and the motivations behind reported responses.

Based on the health belief model, this cross-sectional study was carried out among 272 students at the universities of Buea and Yaoundé in Cameroon. Data were collected using questionnaires containing items matching the research objectives. The questionnaires were self-completed.

Results: Malaria was considered as the most common disease perceived and also a major PRD. Contrary to official rankings of HIV/AIDS and TB, cholera and diarrhoea were considered as other major PRDs. Also, typhoid fever was perceived to be more common and a PRD than HIV/AIDS and TB combined. The most prominently attributed cause for disease was (lack of) hygiene. In response, students deployed formal and/or informal healthcare strategies, depending on factors like available money, perceived severity of the disease and disease type. Discrepancies were observed in respondents' response to diseases generally and to malaria in particular. Even though, overall, respondents pre-dominantly reported a formal healthcare response toward diseases in general, for malaria, informal responses dominated. There was an overall strong awareness and (pro)activity among students for dealing with diseases.

Conclusions: Although the high use of informal facilities and medication for malaria may well be a reason why eradication is problematic, this seems to be a deliberate strategy linked to an awareness of the limitations of the formal health system. In any intervention intended to foster health, it is therefore vital to consider people's perceptions toward diseases and their response strategies. Our results give important leads to health promotion interventions to develop group-specific programs.

Keywords: Poverty-related diseases, Disease responses, Health belief model, Malaria, University students, Cameroon

* Correspondence: valmakoge@yahoo.co.uk
[1]Health and Society (HSO) group, Wageningen University, P.O. Box 8130, 6700 EW Wageningen, The Netherlands
[3]Institute of Medical Research and Medicinal Plant studies (IMPM), P.O. Box 13033, Yaoundé, Cameroon
Full list of author information is available at the end of the article

Background

The eventual success of health-promoting interventions for infectious diseases in developing countries depends on a prior understanding of the complexities surrounding people's efforts to respond to illnesses. Poverty makes such efforts more complicated. The recognition of linkages between poverty and health has led to the term poverty-related diseases (PRDs). PRDs are diseases whereby poverty is a factor that increases the chances of getting the disease and hinders proper treatment and cure [1, 2]. According to the World Health Organization (WHO), the major PRDs are malaria, human immuno-deficiency virus (HIV)/AIDS and tuberculosis [3]. Cameroon, located in Central Africa, is one of those nations in which PRDs are a significant public health concern. In Cameroon, for instance, everyone is at risk of malaria but the burden is felt more by the poor. Malaria accounts for most hospitalisations, and up to 40% of family income is reportedly spent on its prevention and treatment [4]. The prevalence of HIV in Cameroon is the highest in the sub-region of West and Central Africa, standing at 5.1% [5]. Also, about 33,000 tuberculosis infections are recorded each year, with over 2000 annual deaths [6] mostly in association with HIV [7, 8].

Research and policies addressing PRDs are based on a particular understanding of the interaction between poverty and disease, measured as an association between poverty indicators and health indicators for a specific country or region. Such indicators provide an adequate picture of the diseases most prevalent among the poor but do not further explain the nature of the linkages between poverty and disease or poverty and health [1, 9]. Besides disease prevalence and income levels, living conditions influence vulnerability towards certain diseases and are thus also important for understanding PRDs [10].

Rather than approaching PRDs from statistics, we study people's own perspective on the connections between poverty and health. We investigated perceptions and responses to health issues among university students in Cameroon, a group that is well-educated but has an income level that on average is close to the official poverty line of US$1.25 a day (see Table 1). Common diseases in this group are similar to those in other groups in Cameroon, although some studies have reported a high prevalence of sexually transmitted infections (STIs) among students (e.g. 31% for gonorrhoea) due to a reduced awareness of preventive strategies [11]. Malaria has been reported to account for up to 65% of absences from schools [4, 12]. Many factors influence a person's selective response to illness. The options available to acquire treatment or medication in Cameroon include government hospitals and healthcare centres, church-related hospitals and clinics, private doctors, private pharmacies (big and small), community health workers and street vendors [13]. The use of informal healthcare providers in Cameroon is common [14, 15]. Acquiring care from formal healthcare services is not always an obvious first step in Cameroon where most healthcare is an out-of-pocket expense [16, 17].

The aim of our study was to get a deeper understanding of the complexities surrounding responses towards diseases among university students in Cameroon. Such understanding is essential for the design and assessment of interventions geared at promoting health [18, 19] among poor groups in society.

We used the health belief model (HBM) [20] to understand students' response to diseases. The health belief model is a model commonly used in health education and health promotion that aims to predict and understand health behaviours of people in terms of belief patterns they may have [20–23]. According to the HBM, people's response to diseases is guided by two main beliefs: a belief in a health threat (presence of disease) and a belief in the effectiveness of deploying a response strategy [20, 22]. Because PRDs are primarily infectious

Table 1 Background characteristics of student respondents from UB and UNIYAO

		UB (N = 161)	UNIYAO (N = 111)	p value
		%	%	
Sex	Male	43.5	32.4	0.66
	Female	56.5	67.6	
Participants' age in ranges	<25	77.4	52.3	<0.05
	25 or older	22.6	47.7	
Single people (vs married)	Married	0.6	1.8	0.363
	Single	99.4	98.2	
Participants' income level (per month)	<20,000 FCFA	42.5	44.0	0.820
	20–50,000 FCFA	36.6	39.4	
	50–100,000 FCFA	11.8	10.1	
	>100,000 FCFA	9.2	6.4	

diseases, the first belief implies a perceived susceptibility to infection and a perception that this infection could be harmful. The second belief in the context of our study implies a belief that both formal and informal health facilities and medication can be used to respond to diseases and that these actions will be effective [22]. Figure 1 shows how we operationalise disease responses in the HBM.

The specific objectives of our study were to assess the perceptions of university students in Cameroon about common diseases and diseases related to poverty, to find out how they respond to diseases, to ascertain the motivations for their responses and finally, to identify the determinants (perceived benefits and barriers) for the participants' use of the healthcare services.

Methods

Survey design and respondents

Our study was part of a larger project that had as objective to create an understanding of the social and material dynamics that enable the capacity to preserve health, anticipate health risks and mitigate or recover from stressors such as PRDs in Cameroon. This study took place between 2013 and 2014 and was carried out in the Southwest and Centre regions of Cameroon.

Respondents were selected among students at the University of Buea (UB), located in the Southwest region, 4.1537° N, 9.2920° E, and the University of Yaoundé (UNIYAO), located in the Centre region 3.8574° N, 11.5014° E of Cameroon. UB, founded in 1995, has a population of about 12,000 students [24]. UNIYAO, the oldest university in Cameroon, was founded in 1962 and has a population of about 33,000 students [25]. Every year, over 1000 students seek entry into the universities of Buea or Yaoundé. Potential students originate from different regions of Cameroon and have either an anglophone or a francophone culture and settle into these settings for studies. Entry into UB

is on a competitive basis following results of the general certificate examination (GCE A'L), whereas entry into UNIYAO is not based on competition. Both universities are state-owned and are top-ranked universities in Cameroon. University students were selected for this study because, despite having education and career opportunities that are better than for most people, during their study, most students live in deprived conditions and face financial challenges. Their experiences and disease response strategies are important for understanding the complexities that exist between poverty and health.

University students reside in what we refer to as campus settings. Most university students live in rented rooms in neighbourhoods close to the university because on-campus rooms are too few to cater for the high demand. Student residences vary in size and can have as few as five rooms, whereas others have up to 40 rooms. For our study, the neighbourhoods visited were the Ngoa-Ekelle in Yaoundé and the Molyko in Buea situated within a few hundred metres of the university and each housing hundreds of students. These neighbourhoods are quite similar, both bustling with commercial activities that centre around students' needs such as photocopying and printing stalls, small restaurants, bars, small pharmacies and cyber cafés. Respondents were following various study programmes offered by the university. The universities offer no free healthcare services to the students, who therefore have to seek healthcare off-campus at personal expense.

Survey instrument

From initial observations and preliminary conversations with students, we obtained an image of the key issues and conditions affecting students' health, from which we designed a questionnaire in line with the health belief model [20]. The questionnaire was comprised of closed questions with yes/no answer options and questions with pre-defined answer categories, with the possibility for multiple responses in some questions.

Individual perceptions

The construct of a perceived threat of disease is characterised by a perceived vulnerability and a perceived severity of disease. These factors have been shown to influence how people respond to diseases [20, 22]. Perceiving diseases as a threat means recognising their presence and their ability to affect a person. This factor was included to pinpoint specific diseases affecting the health and well-being of university students and was measured by asking students to identify what diseases they perceive as common and what diseases they associate with poverty. In addition to the WHO-listed top three PRDs, other diseases such as cholera, diarrhoea, typhoid fever and meningitis were included in this question.

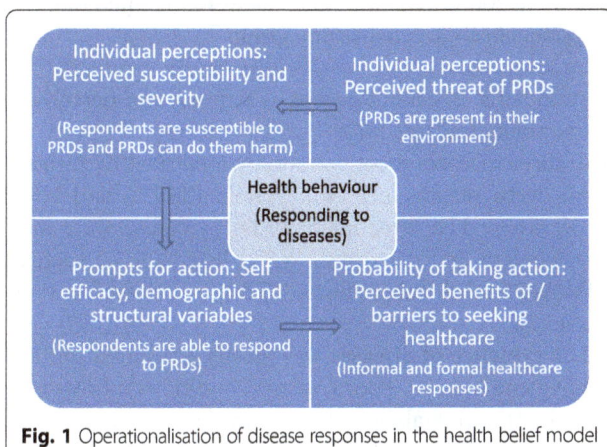

Fig. 1 Operationalisation of disease responses in the health belief model

Perceived vulnerability was constructed as the perception of the risk of contracting diseases. Questions focused on factors reported in the literature as having a direct impact on health and increasing vulnerability to diseases, such as food availability, balanced diet, good and permanent water, and sanitation challenges [26, 27].

Perceived severity, which implies the perception that PRDs could cause harm to respondents, was not specified in the questionnaire because other studies have established this aspect with regard to malaria and HIV in Cameroon [4, 28–30].

Prompts to action

A prompt to action refers to the recognition that actions can be taken to respond to diseases faced by university students. Questions asked included "How would you normally respond to diseases in general?" and "How would you normally respond to malaria?" The additional question about malaria gives further insights into students' responses to PRDs. Because prevalence, morbidity and mortality due to malaria are high in Cameroon [31, 32], all students are likely to have experience in dealing with it.

Probability of taking action

Converting prompts to action into real action depends on the perceived benefits and barriers relating to the effectiveness of the intended action [20]. We included several options for action in the questionnaire, covering both formal and informal medical facilities. An example of a question asked is "What determines whether you seek formal or hospital healthcare?"

Socio-demographic variables like age, sex and other variables shown to influence how people respond to diseases [33] were also obtained in this study.

Procedure

The questionnaires were pre-tested among students at the Catholic University in the Southwest region to ensure that the questions were understandable. Consequent to the pre-test, minor amendments were made relating to the comprehensibility of the questions.

The questionnaires were self-administered. The respondent sampling method followed that previously described by Moyou-Somo et al. [32] whereby, for a population of less than 1000 inhabitants, one out of every two houses is selected for the research. The first building selected was the one closest to the main road, and from this, we moved inwards into the neighbourhood. In our study, we considered the student's room as a house. The first author and trained assistants went into each student building, explained the study and requested participation. The questionnaires were left with the students and picked up later in the day. In total, 300

questionnaires were distributed, and 272 respondents completed and returned the questionnaire, giving a response rate of 90%.

Data analysis

The data were analysed using SPSS Statistics version 22 (SPSS Inc. IBM). Before analysis, data from pre-coded questionnaires were entered into SPSS and checked for errors by the first author and an assistant. Chi-square and ANOVA tests were used to analyse differences between the universities as well as in the factors included in the survey, such as response strategies towards diseases in general and towards malaria in particular. We performed logistic regression analysis to explain trends seen in people's response to malaria. Included in the model were socio-demographic factors (age, sex and income). We also calculated the odds ratio of factors shown to have an influence on people's health, such as food, water and sanitation challenges experienced by people and seeking formal healthcare for malaria; p values <0.05 were considered to be significant.

Ethical clearance for this study was provided by the Wageningen University review board. The aim of the study was carefully explained to all respondents. Respondents signed an informed consent form before participating in the study.

Results

Respondents' characteristics

As shown in Table 1, 272 students (39% males and 61% females) participated in the survey, 98.9% of whom were single. The income of most university students was less than 20,000 FCFA (less than US$34.7) per month. Respondents from the two universities showed no significant differences in background variables such as sex, marital status and income. However, the mean age of students at UB was slightly lower than that of students at UNIYAO (23 and 24.5, respectively; F (1,264), $p < 0.001$). Further analysis revealed that age did not play a significant role in respondents' response to diseases; therefore, all respondents are treated as one group.

Respondents' belief in diseases as a threat and perceived vulnerability towards PRDs

The three diseases most commonly identified by respondents were malaria (91.1%), typhoid (35.7%) and HIV/AIDS (16%). The three major PRDs perceived were malaria, cholera and diarrhoea. WHO-listed PRDs, such as HIV/AIDS and tuberculosis (TB), had lower ratings (Table 2).

The presence of diseases was mostly attributed to (lack of) hygiene (53.2%). Poor hygiene conditions increase respondents' vulnerability to diseases. For example, many respondents had toilets in their rooms for personal use

Table 2 Respondents' classification of common diseases and PRDs

Diseases	Respondents' classification (%)[a]	
	Common diseases	PRDs
Malaria	91.1	36.4
Cholera	6.7	34.4
Diarrhoea	13.8	31.2
Typhoid fever	35.7	28.1
HIV/AIDS	16	20.2
STIs	10.8	9.9
TB	2.6	5.9
Meningitis	1.5	na

na not asked
[a]More than one response was possible

(61.7%), but another group used pit toilets that they shared with neighbours, with a consequent increased infection risk. Other attributed causes were poverty (31.3%), climatic conditions (29.8%) and lack of knowledge (23.8%).

Prompts to action: disease responses

Table 3 shows a picture of the different ways in which students respond to diseases relative to socio-demographic characteristics. It can be seen that, irrespective of socio-demographic characteristics, most people reported that they would use the formal healthcare facilities as their general response to health challenges.

Response to malaria

The picture of using the formal healthcare system as a general response to diseases (70.4%) changes for malaria. Table 4 shows these discrepancies. In the case of malaria, the use of informal treatment and medication was the dominant response (86%), with only about 6% of respondents reporting that they would employ formal healthcare services.

In an effort to explain these discrepancies, we investigated predictors of seeking formal healthcare as well as the odds of water, sanitation and food challenges influencing the way people respond to malaria. Table 5 provides descriptive information regarding the presence or absence of challenges and the selected response to malaria. Logistic analysis regression (results shown in Table 6) did not reveal any socio-demographic factors to be predictors of seeking formal healthcare for malaria. Also, none of those experiencing sanitation, food and water challenges showed increased or decreased odds of seeking formal healthcare in the case of malaria attacks (see Table 7).

Top informal healthcare responses towards malaria

Using small pharmacies (any small shop selling some medication) were reportedly the most common way in which respondents dealt with malaria (52.2%). Self-medication practices (20.6%) were also commonly used. Medicinal plants, usually a combination of different plants, were used for self-medication, with 56.7% of respondents reportedly using a combination of plants to prevent or treat malaria. Common medicinal plants used were fever grass, pawpaw leaves, aloe vera, mango and guava leaves. Using street vendors as informal healthcare providers was the third most commonly reported practice (18.8%).

Probability of taking action: determinants for seeking informal and formal healthcare

Formal healthcare was often sought after self-medication failed (33.2%) or when illness was severe (22.9%). Having money was the most important factor enabling people to make use of official medical facilities. Other important factors were perceived severity of the disease and duration of the illness (Table 8).

Table 3 Variation of health-seeking practices in relation to socio-demographic differences

Socio-demographic variables		Response to diseases in general (N = 272)		
		Formal %	Informal %	Both %
Sex	Male	71.1	23.7	5.2
	Female	70.0	23.8	6.3
Participants' age in ranges	<25	73.1	22.2	4.8
	25 or older	65.5	26.2	8.3
Marital status	Married	100	0.0	0.0
	Single	70.4	24.1	5.5
Participants' income level in thousand FCFA	<20	66.7	30.5	2.9
	20–50	75.0	17.7	7.3
	50–100	65.4	26.9	7.7
	>100	71.4	19.0	9.5

Note: Figures may not add up to exactly 100% because of rounded values

Table 4 Discrepancies in disease responses towards malaria and other diseases

	Formal %	Informal %	Both %
Health-seeking practices in general	70.4	23.7	5.8
Health-seeking practices in the case of malaria	6.4	86.1	7.5

Discussion

The aim of this study was to get a deeper understanding of the complexities regarding the way in which university students respond to diseases present in their environment. Before we delved into how students respond to PRDs, it was important to identify what students consider to be PRDs. Our results show that university students perceive malaria as the top common disease and PRD. Typhoid fever is considered a common disease but was not ranked highly as a PRD, whereas cholera, which was not perceived as very common, was classified as a major PRD. Although our study does not provide a clear explanation for this ranking, it is likely that respondents' ideas of interconnections between hygiene, health and extreme poverty carry a symbolic meaning of the kind of situation they strongly reject [34]. In other words, cholera, and the scare it generates, represents poor social well-being culminating in poor health. This suggests that people's capacity to maintain personal hygiene and ensuring a liveable environment are two sides of the same coin. The fight against PRDs therefore should focus strongly on facilitating good hygiene practices. Overall, official health authorities and international agencies may underestimate people's perception of health and hygiene and their capacity to adapt to changing circumstances such as outbreaks of infectious diseases [35]. We show this in our study by highlighting people's role in responding to diseases that affect them and by underlining the importance of taking this response into account in the design of interventions whose goal is to foster health.

It is noteworthy that respondents' classification of major PRDs differed from that used by health bodies such as the United Nations, WHO, the European Commission [36] and Cameroon's Ministry of Public Health [5]. The United Nations, for instance, listed the major PRDs as malaria, HIV/AIDS and TB in millennium development goal 6 to be eradicated in an allocated 15-year time span. This was not achieved and these diseases are now included in the third sustainable development goal (SDG 3), to be achieved by 2030 [37]. Emphasis on achieving such goals highlights the importance of problems faced by people living in conditions of poverty. Studies such as the one presented here provide insights into the complexities of the interactions between poverty and health—insights that are useful for both governmental and non-governmental organisations and international health bodies in the formulation of policy to improve people's health and well-being and provide information needed for the design and implementation of adequate interventions to promote human health.

As expected, the classification of malaria as a major PRD and a public health concern was uncontested by our respondents, and this is confirmed by other studies in Cameroon [31, 38], Nigeria [39], Ethiopia [40], Kenya

Table 5 Variation in sanitation, food and water challenges with respect to malaria responses

Sanitation, food and water challenges		Response to malaria		
		Formal %	Informal %	Both %
Does participant share toilet with other houses?	Yes	3.8	33.2	3.8
	No	2.6	52.3	3.8
Are there water cuts in the neighbourhood?	Yes	5.7	54.0	5.7
	No	0.8	32.1	1.9
Does participant eat or drink herbs and other parts of plants to prevent or cure disease?	Yes	6.0	43.4	7.2
	No	0.4	42.6	0.4
Is food readily available for the participant?	Yes	3.4	35.7	3.8
	No/sometimes	3.0	50.4	3.8
Does participant cook his/her meals?	Yes/sometimes	5.3	74.8	6.8
	No	1.1	11.3	0.8
Does participant consider his/her diet to be balanced?	Yes/sometimes	3.0	49.1	5.2
	No	3.4	37.1	2.2
Are there days when participant misses one or more meals?	Yes	6.4	77.4	6.8
	No	–	8.6	0.8

Note: Values on table may not add up to exactly 100% because of rounded values

Table 6 Logistic regression model with seeking formal healthcare in the event of malaria as dependent variable

Variables	B	S.E.	Sig.	Exp(B)
Age	0.098	0.075	0.191	1.103
Sex	−0.614	0.533	0.249	0.541
Income	−0.161	0.311	0.604	0.851
Nagelkerke R2				0.041

Table 8 Determinants in favour of using formal healthcare facilities

Determinants	% (N)
Money	53.9 (144)
Severity of illness	40.8 (109)
Duration of illness	20.2 (54)
Fear	7.5 (20)
Unavailability of drugs	6.7 (18)
Attitude of hospital staff	4.1 (11)
Time	2.6 (7)
Distance to healthcare service	1.5 (4)

Note: Multiple responses were possible

[41] and Uganda [42]. The other two WHO-listed PRDs differed in importance in our respondents' perspective. HIV/AIDS was perceived as the third most common disease by 16% of respondents, but it was not ranked among the top three PRDs. This is probably because students are at an age and life stage in which they take a more adventurous and active approach to sexuality [43–45] and therefore may not necessarily link HIV/AIDS to poverty. Our study showed that less than 3% of respondents perceived TB as being common and only about 6% perceived it as a PRD. Actually, in the list of diseases given to respondents, TB appeared at the bottom end of both rankings. Apparently, students do not consider TB a common disease and do not associate it with poverty. Typhoid fever on the other hand was perceived as more common and also more a PRD than HIV/AIDS and TB combined (see Table 2). Our results reveal a chasm between world health bodies' official classifications and what people in conditions of poverty themselves perceive. Although people's perceptions are not infallible, health programmes are likely to be more effective if they match people's perception of disease risk with options for improving their health. We suggest that disease risks perceived by people living in conditions of poverty should be the focus of health-promoting agencies' in the fight against PRDs. Further research could look into other groups in society as well and develop in-country differentiated health programmes.

By looking at PRDs from the respondents' viewpoint, we show that PRDs are not only a list of diseases but also entail people's perceptions of the interlinkages

Table 7 Odds ratios and 95% confidence interval for seeking formal healthcare in the presence of threats

Predictor variables (threats)	OR (95% CI)	p value
Toilet sharing	1.076 (0.616–1.879)	0.798
Water cuts	0.818 (0.456–1.466)	0.499
Drink/eat herbs	0.591 (0.334–1.043)	0.068
Food availability	1.135 (0.651–1.979)	0.655
Food cooking	1.714 (0.795–3.699)	0.166
Balanced meal	1.399 (0.808–2.421)	0.230
Food miss day	0.873 (0.334–2.284)	0.782

between poverty and health, a factor that we consider a relevant focus for the successful achievement of SDG 3.

By identifying common diseases and PRDs through the respondents' eyes, we reveal an interesting perspective on the major threats to students' health and well-being. For one thing, we ascertain factors that increase students' vulnerability to diseases. Some of these factors are under the students' control and others are not. On the one hand, poor hygiene conditions were perceived by respondents as the most pronounced reason for disease presence. This was rated even higher than poverty, even though both may be interlinked [1]. These conditions can be partly controlled by the students themselves, when they clean up their own surroundings to partially reduce the risk of malaria infection [46]. On the other hand, other factors, for example poor housing conditions as observed in the neighbourhoods, are beyond the students' control as they have to take what is available due to the shortage of accommodation possibilities.

Our respondents also attributed disease presence to climatic conditions, lack of knowledge and poor education. Other studies carried out in UB confirmed, for example, that the high prevalence of STIs was linked to students' lack of knowledge on ways to protect themselves [11]. This underlines the need for group-specific health education interventions.

Moreover, our study revealed that the way students respond to disease was not always clear-cut; rather, it was influenced by disease genre. The response to malaria differed from the response to diseases in general. The general response to diseases was indicated as being mostly through formal healthcare facilities (70%). Money was reported as an important indicator for deploying this response strategy. However, our results show different strategies in spending scarce money. Even when the costs of hospital consultation, laboratory examination and buying medication from hospitals can be covered, the decision to do so can be postponed, depending on other factors, most prominently the perceived severity of the disease. Other studies have reported a similar strategic use of available resources [47–51]. Perceived severity is an obvious incentive for hospital-based action [22]. However, confounding factors could be the pain caused by the condition, duration of the illness, unavailability of medication at home, the failure of self-medication to alleviate symptoms or fear instilled by the disease condition. These factors stand on the one hand as enablers of hospital-based responses and, on the other hand, as barriers to this route. Furthermore, these factors indicate the other processes that could occur between the onset of symptoms and the use of formal medical facilities.

Interestingly, our study showed that, in the case of malaria, students' response strategy was very different from that promulgated by health agencies and medical experts. Most respondents (86%) reported using informal health services and medicine as a response to malaria. This indicates a belief that the informal health sector is beneficial and effective in the case of malaria. It is noteworthy, though, that malaria is well-perceived as a severe disease in Cameroon [30, 52] and that our respondents indicated that one of the determinants for seeking formal healthcare was the perceived severity of the disease. Students' response to malaria would therefore be expected to align with what they said was their general response to diseases. However, this was not the case. People obviously do not display a clear-cut logical pattern of response whereby they treat all diseases in the same way. Other factors may play a role in their decisions. These could be psychological or financial. Psychologically, perceptions are important. High-perceived severity of disease, for example, is a reason reported for hospital care [53]. Financial factors too were indicated. In the case of malaria, respondents opted to use small pharmacies, self-medication practices (with medicinal plants) and street vendors. It is not clear from our study why informal healthcare options are chosen to respond to malaria. A possible explanation could be that malaria is very common [4, 28] and an integral part of everyday life. Its constant presence may reduce the perception that it is a life-threatening disease and numb people to its deleterious effects. A qualitative study among a sample of respondents living in these same settings under similar conditions indicated that proximity and money-saving characteristics of informal healthcare providers such as small pharmacies and street vendors made them more enticing options [54]. This has also been reported in other studies [55]. It should be noted that the reason for informal healthcare in the case of malaria could not be explained by sociodemographic characteristics, and the odds did not increase or decrease with challenges that people experienced in relation to sanitation, food and water.

The insights revealed in our study are worthy of consideration in the context of health promotion interventions, as they could throw more light on why malaria is persistent and still a number one problem in Cameroon just like in other parts of sub-Saharan Africa. For instance, our respondents have shown strong awareness and (pro)activity in relation to malaria, but this may well be a reason why eradication is problematic. Aspects such as (1) self-diagnoses of malaria by people leading to (2) (im)proper self-medication practices without necessarily following treatment recommendations or appropriate treatment may have unfavourable outcomes. Also, a link may exist between using the informal sector (small pharmacies, street vendors) and the persistence of malaria, as well as the development of resistance to antimalarial drugs. Our findings therefore underline the need for integrated and all-encompassing strategies in the fight against malaria.

Study limitations

Our study was cross-sectional in nature. A cross-sectional study refers to a study in which data are collected from respondents at a specific point in time and over a short period. In this way, a cross-sectional study will give a picture of the study of interest at the time it is carried out [56]. Our study therefore may not have unravelled all the complexities that change with time in the settings. Even though the perceived severity of malaria is already established in Cameroon, it would have been interesting to see how respondents perceive the severity of all WHO-ranked major PRDs as well, especially TB, which they did not perceive as a major PRD. By using the health belief model as a framework for our study, we may have omitted some aspects that also play a role in the way people respond to disease, such as the role of significant others in the decision to respond to diseases in particular ways.

Conclusions

The aim of this study was to acquire a deeper understanding of the interaction between poverty and disease by investigating the health beliefs of university students in Cameroon. Our study showed that students are well aware of what constitutes common diseases and also display strong beliefs about what diseases can be attributed to poverty. Contrary to official rankings, students consider malaria, cholera, diarrhoea and typhoid fever as major PRDs. Moreover, the results revealed that students consider (lack of) hygiene as a more prominent cause of disease than poverty. Respondents also displayed strong beliefs about their capacity to respond to diseases. Our study found that they deploy both formal and informal response strategies towards diseases, depending on factors like having money to afford the services, perceived severity of the disease, disease genre or belief in the effectiveness of an action to bring relief from the burdens imposed by diseases. A remarkable finding of our study was that university students adopt a mostly informal response to malaria. A better understanding of the practices, surrounding beliefs and group-specific responses to malaria is essential for the effective management and control of the disease.

Abbreviations
HBM: Health belief model; HIV: Human immuno-deficiency virus; PRD: Poverty-related disease; SDG: Sustainable development goal; STIs: Sexually transmitted infections; TB: Tuberculosis; UB: University of Buea; UNIYAO: University of Yaounde; WHO: World Health Organization

Acknowledgements
The authors would like to thank all the university students of Buea and Yaoundé who took part in this study. The authors would also like to thank Lette Hogeling for her assistance in the statistical analysis.

Funding
The following study was supported by Wageningen University. The funders had no role in the design, data collection and analysis of this manuscript.

Authors' contributions
VM, HM and MK designed the present study. VM collected the data and analysed the data with input from HM, LV and MK. VM wrote the first draft of the manuscript. VM, HM, LV and MK finalised the manuscript. All authors read and approved the final manuscript.

Competing interests
The authors declare they have no competing interests.

Author details
[1]Health and Society (HSO) group, Wageningen University, P.O. Box 8130, 6700 EW Wageningen, The Netherlands. [2]Knowledge Technology and Innovation (KTI) group, Wageningen University, Hollandseweg 1, 6708 KN Wageningen, The Netherlands. [3]Institute of Medical Research and Medicinal Plant studies (IMPM), P.O. Box 13033, Yaoundé, Cameroon.

References
1. Stevens P. Diseases of poverty and the 10/90 gap. London: International Policy Network; 2004. http://www.who.int/intellectualproperty/submissions/InternationalPolicyNetwork.pdf. Accessed 26 May 2016.
2. Singh AR, Singh SA. Diseases of poverty and lifestyle, well-being and human development. Mens Sana Monographs. 2008;6(1):187–225. doi:10.4103/0973-1229.40567.
3. WHO. Global report for research on infectious diseases of poverty. World Health Organization. 2012. http://apps.who.int/iris/bitstream/10665/44850/1/9789241564489_eng.pdf. Accessed 17 Sept 2015.
4. CCAM. About_malaria: for a malaria free Cameroon. A bilingual publication of the Cameroon Coalition Against Malaria. 2009;2(1):1–28
5. MINSANTE. Profil des Estimations et Projections en Matière de VIH et SIDA au Cameroun 2010–2020. Yaoundé: Ministère de la Santé Publique; 2009. p. 17.
6. WHO. Towards universal access to diagnosis and treatment of multidrug-resistant and extensively drug-resistant tuberculosis by 2015: WHO progress report 2011. Geneva: World Health Organization; 2011. p. 119.
7. Cambanis A, Ramsay A, Yassin MA, Cuevas LE. Duration and associated factors of patient delay during tuberculosis screening in rural Cameroon. Trop Med Int Health. 2007;12(11):1309–14.
8. Pefura-Yone EW, Kengne AP, Kuaban C. Non-conversion of sputum culture among patients with smear positive pulmonary tuberculosis in Cameroon: a prospective cohort study. BMC Infect Dis. 2014;14(1):1–6.
9. Von Philipsborn P, Steinbeis F, Bender ME, Regmi S, Tinnemann P. Poverty-related and neglected diseases—an economic and epidemiological analysis of poverty relatedness and neglect in research and development. Glob Health Action. 2015;8. doi: http://dx.doi.org/10.3402/gha.v8.25818.
10. WHO. Housing and health. 2010. http://www.who.int/hia/housing/en/. Accessed 12 Sept 2016.
11. Nkuo-Akenji T, Nkwesheu A, Nyasa R, Tallah E, Ndip R, Angwafo IF. Knowledge of HIV/AIDS, sexual behaviour and prevalence of sexually transmitted infections among female students of the University of Buea, Cameroon. Afr J AIDS Res. 2007;6(2):157–63.
12. DHS. The DHS program—Cameroon: standard DHS, 2011. Demographic Health Survey. Cameroon: Institut Nationale de la Statistique; 2011. pp. 188–204.
13. Kamgnia B. Use of health care services in Cameroon. Int J Appl Econom Quant Stud. 2006;3–2:53–64.
14. Hughes R, Chandler C, Mangham-Jefferies L, Mbacham W. Medicine sellers' perspectives on their role in providing health care in North-West Cameroon: a qualitative study. Health Pol Plan. 2013;doi: 10.1093/heapol/czs103.
15. Crabbe F, Carsauw H, Buve A, Laga M, Tchupo J, Trebucq A. Why do men with urethritis in Cameroon prefer to seek care in the informal health sector? Genitourin Med. 1996;72(3):220–2.
16. Jaja PT. Health-seeking behaviour of Port Harcourt city residents: a comparison between the upper and lower socio-economic classes. J Public Health Africa. 2013; doi: http://dx.doi.org/10.4081/jphia.2013.e9.
17. Kankeu HT, Ventelou B. Socioeconomic inequalities in informal payments for health care: an assessment of the 'Robin Hood' hypothesis in 33 African countries. Soc Sci Med. 2016;151:173–86.
18. Mackian S, Bedri N, Lovel H. Up the garden path and over the edge: where might health-seeking behaviour take us? Health Pol Plan. 2004; 19(3):137–46.
19. Grundy J, Annear P. Health-seeking behaviour studies: a literature review of study design and methods with a focus on Cambodia. Melbourne: The Nossal Insitute for Global Health; 2010.
20. Janz NK, Becker MH. The health belief model: a decade later. Health Educ Behav. 1984;11(1):1–47.
21. Hochbaum G, Rosenstock I, Kegels S. Health belief model. Washington: United States Public Health Service; 1952.
22. Koelen MA, van den Ban AW. Health education and health promotion. Wageningen: Wageningen Academic Publishers; 2004.
23. Green EC, Murphy E. Health belief model. The Wiley Blackwell encyclopedia of health, illness, behavior, and society. Chichester: Wiley; 2014.
24. University of Buea. About UB: University of Buea. 2014. http://www.ubuea.cm/about/. Accessed 15 Aug 2015.
25. Institut National de la Statistique. Annuaire Statistique du Cameroun. Yaoundé: Institut National de la Statistique; 2010.
26. WHO. Guidelines for drinking-water quality: recommendations. Geneva: World Health Organization; 2004.
27. Mensah P, Yeboah-Manu D, Owusu-Darko K, Ablordey A. Street foods in Accra, Ghana: how safe are they? Bull World Health Organ. 2002;80(7):546–54.
28. MINSANTE. Plan Strategique Nationale de la lutte contre le paludisme au Cameroun 2007–2010. 2007. http://www.africanchildforum.org/clr/policy%20per%20country/cameroun/cameroun_malaria_2001-2006_fr.pdf. Accessed 8 Oct 2016.
29. Makoge V, Maat H, Edward N, Emery J. Knowledge, attitudes and practices towards malaria in Mbonge and Kumba sub-divisions in Cameroon. Int J Trop Dis Health. 2016;15(2):1–13.
30. Kimbi HK, Nkesa SB, Ndamukong-Nyanga JL, Sumbele IU, Atashili J, Atanga MB. Knowledge and perceptions towards malaria prevention among vulnerable groups in the Buea Health District, Cameroon. BMC Public Health. 2014;14(1):1.
31. Ndo C, Menze-Djantio B, Antonio-Nkondjio C. Awareness, attitudes and prevention of malaria in the cities of Douala and Yaounde (Cameroon). Parasit Vectors. 2011; doi: 10.1186/1756-3305-4-181.

32. Moyou-Somo R, Essomba P, Songue E, Tchoubou NN, Ntambo A, Hiol HN, et al. A public private partnership to fight against malaria along the Chad-Cameroon pipeline corridor: I. Baseline data on socio-anthropological aspects, knowledge, attitudes and practices of the population concerning malaria. BMC Public Health. 2013;13(1):1023.

33. Glanz K, Rimer BK, Viswanath K. Health behavior and health education: theory, research, and practice. San Francisco: Jossey-Bass; 2008.

34. Douglas M. Rules and meanings: the anthropology of everyday knowledge. London: Routledge; 2002.

35. Richards P. Ebola: how a people's science helped end an epidemic. London: Zed; 2016.

36. Gryseels B, Zumla A, Troye-Blomberg M, Kieny MP, Quaglio G, Holtel A, et al. European Union conference on poverty-related diseases research. Lancet Infect Dis. 2009;9(6):334–7.

37. Sachs JD. From millennium development goals to sustainable development goals. Lancet. 2012;379(9832):2206–11.

38. Nkuo Akenji TK, Ntonifor NN, Ching JK, Kimbi HK, Ndamukong KN, Anong DN, et al. Evaluating a malaria intervention strategy using knowledge, practices and coverage surveys in rural Bolifamba, southwest Cameroon. Trans R Soc Trop Med Hyg. 2005;99(5):325–32.

39. Audu O, Bako Ara I, Abdullahi Umar A, Nanben Omole V, Avidime S. Sociodemographic correlates of choice of health care services in six rural communities in North Central Nigeria. Adv Public Health. 2014; http://dx.doi.org/10.1155/2014/651086.

40. Jima D, Tesfaye G, Deressa W, Woyessa A, Kebede D, Alamirew D. Baseline survey for the implementation of insecticide treated mosquito nets in Malaria control in Ethiopia. Ethiop J Health Dev. 2005;19(1):16–23.

41. Imbahale SS, Fillinger U, Githeko A, Mukabana WR, Takken W. An exploratory survey of malaria prevalence and people's knowledge, attitudes and practices of mosquito larval source management for malaria control in western Kenya. Acta Trop. 2010;115(3):248–56.

42. Musoke D, Karani G, Ssempebwa JC, Musoke MB. Integrated approach to malaria prevention at household level in rural communities in Uganda: experiences from a pilot project. Malar J. 2013; doi: 10.1186/1475-2875-12-327.

43. Siegel DM, Klein DI, Roghmann KJ. Sexual behavior, contraception, and risk among college students. J Adolesc Health. 1999;25:336–43.

44. Atuyambe LM, Kibira SPS, Bukenya J, Muhumuza C, Apolot RR, Mulogo E. Understanding sexual and reproductive health needs of adolescents: evidence from a formative evaluation in Wakiso district, Uganda Adolescent Health. Reprod Health. 2015; doi: 10.1186/s12978-015-0026-7.

45. Sekirime WK, Tamale J, Lule JC, Wabwire-Mangen F. Knowledge, attitude and practice about sexually transmitted diseases among university students in Kampala. Afr Health Sci. 2001;1(1):16–22.

46. WHO. World malaria report 2013. http://www.who.int/malaria/publications/world_malaria_report_2013/wmr2013_no_profiles.pdf?ua=1. Accessed 3 Sept 2015.

47. Adedokun BO, Morhason-Bello IO, Ojengbede OA, Okonkwo NS, Kolade C. Help-seeking behavior among women currently leaking urine in Nigeria: is it any different from the rest of the world? Patient Prefer Adher. 2012;6:815–9.

48. Abdulraheem IS, Parakoyi DB. Factors affecting mothers' healthcare-seeking behaviour for childhood illnesses in a rural Nigerian setting. Early Child Dev Care. 2009;179(5):671–83.

49. Burtscher D, Burza S. Health-seeking behaviour and community perceptions of childhood undernutrition and a community management of acute malnutrition (CMAM) programme in rural Bihar, India: a qualitative study. Public Health Nutr. 2015; doi: 10.1017/S1368980015000440.

50. Ahmed SM, Adams AM, Chowdhury M, Bhuiya A. Changing health-seeking behaviour in Matlab, Bangladesh: do development interventions matter? Health Pol Plan. 2003;18(3):306–15.

51. Wang Q, Brenner S, Leppert G, Banda TH, Kalmus O, De Allegri M. Health seeking behaviour and the related household out-of-pocket expenditure for chronic non-communicable diseases in rural Malawi. Health Pol Plan. 2015; 30(2):242–52.

52. Sumbele IUN, Samje M, Nkuo-Akenji T. A longitudinal study on anaemia in children with Plasmodium falciparum infection in the Mount Cameroon region: prevalence, risk factors and perceptions by caregivers. BMC Infect Dis. 2013;13(1):1.

53. Biswas P, Kabir ZN, Nilsson J, Zaman S. Dynamics of health care seeking behaviour of elderly people in rural Bangladesh. Inter J Ageing Later Life. 2006;1(1):69–89.

54. Makoge V, Maat H, Vaandrager L, Koelen M. Health seeking behaviour towards poverty-related diseases (PRDs): a qualitative study of people living in camps and on campuses in Cameroon. PLoS Negl Trop Dis. 2017;11(1): e0005218. doi:10.1371/journal.pntd.0005218.

55. Ondicho JM. Factors associated with use of herbal medicine among the residents of Gucha sub-county, Kenya. Thesis for Master of Science in Applied Epidemiology, Jomo Kenyatta University of Agriculture and Technology, Juja, Kenya; 2015.

56. Levin KA. Study design III: cross-sectional studies. Evid Based Dent. 2006;7(1):24–5.

2

Violence against women and mental disorder: a qualitative study in Bangladesh

Md. Manirul Islam[1]*[iD], Nasim Jahan[2] and Md. Delwar Hossain[3]

Abstract

Background: Violence affects 15–75% of women across the globe and has a significant impact on their health, well-being, and rights. While quantitative research links it to poor mental health, there is a lack of qualitative enquiry in how women experience it, and how it is related to the mental disorders in Bangladesh. This information is important in understanding the situation and structuring a locally appropriate and culturally sensitive program.

Methods: We adopted a phenomenological approach and conducted 16 in-depth interviews, three informal interviews, one focus group discussion, and one key informant interview. We also reviewed published reports and documents. We followed criterion sampling in selecting women with mental disorders who experienced violence. We explored their experiences and understanding of the issues and described the phenomenon.

Results: We found that Bangladesh society was largely controlled by men, and marriage was often forced on women. Women often were blamed for any mishap in the family and married women were under social and emotional pressure to keep the marital relationship going even when painful. We found all forms of violence (physical, emotional, sexual etc.) and most of the time found more than one type in women with mental disorders. Sexual violence is a reality for some women but rarely discussed. We found the society very tolerant with mental disorder patients and those who resorted to violence against them.
We identified four theoretical understandings about the role of violence in mental disorders. Sometimes the violence predisposed the mental illness, sometimes it precipitated it, while other times it maintained and was a consequence of it. Sometimes the violence may be unrelated to the mental illness. The relationships were complex and depended on both the type of mental disorder and the nature and intensity of the violence. We found most of the time that more than one type of violence was involved and played more than one role, which varied across different types of mental disorders. Interestingly, not all violence that mentally disordered women faced was because they were women, but because of mental disorders, which brought violence to them as a consequence.

Conclusions: The findings of this first ever qualitative study into the experiences of violence by women with mental disorder in Bangladesh can be used in developing a culturally specific intervention to reduce both violence and mental disorders in women.

Keywords: Violence against women, Mental disorders, Bangladesh, Qualitative study

* Correspondence: ted@icddrb.org; Dr.Munir1962@gmail.com
[1]Training Unit, icddr,b, 68, Shaheed Tajuddin Ahmed Sarani, Mohakhali, Dhaka 1212, Bangladesh
Full list of author information is available at the end of the article

Background

Violence against women means "any act of gender-based violence that results in, or is likely to result in, physical, sexual or psychological harm or suffering to women, including threats of such acts, coercion or arbitrary deprivation of liberty, whether occurring in public or in private life" [1]. It affects 15–75% of women across the globe and is a significant threat to their health, well-being, and rights [2–4]. A multicenter study in 11 countries in the world has found that around 15–71% of women faced physical and sexual violence and 20–75% emotional abuse in their lifetime. In Bangladesh, between 50 and 70% of women face some form of violence, with the prevalence varying across different settings [5, 6].

Violence against women is associated with a number of mental health problems including mood, anxiety, post-traumatic stress, and somatoform disorders [7–10]. World Health Organization (WHO), in a mixed method research, reported violence as an important factor of poor mental health in women across countries including Bangladesh [5]. García-Moreno et al. in the multicenter study referred to earlier mostly focused on intimate partner violence and its impact on mental health, reported as emotional distress as a part of different dimension of health. They did not address violence committed by others nor did they specifically look into its relationship with mental disorders. A quantitative study in nine low- and middle-income countries found a link between violence with suicides [9]; up to 90% of people may have some form of mental disorder at the time of suicide.

Studies across India and Pakistan found an association between domestic or intimate partner violence, and poor mental health including suicidal ideation [11–13]. Like most others, the studies were quantitative and related the symptoms of poor mental health, rather than examining specific mental disorders.

In a quantitative study in Bangladesh, Naved and Akhtar found that suicidal ideation was more common among women facing physical or emotional violence compared to women who were not facing such violence [14]. However, they also did not specifically focus on different types of mental disorders as a consequence of violence against women nor did they explore the experience of women facing such violence and how it was associated with different types of mental disorders.

Mental disorders are multi-factorial. Several factors often interact in a complex way to cause and or maintain mental disorders; some related to gene and environments predispose an individual in early childhood while others may occur before the disease to precipitate it. Some factors may maintain it. A number of researchers underscored the importance of understanding how violence against women affects their mental health [2, 15]. The exploration is important because the nature and

impact of violence against women vary across cultures. For example, two thirds of women physically abused in Bangladesh did not tell anybody about the violence while about 80% in Brazil and Namibia city did so [5]. The lack of sharing may result in a higher magnitude of mental disorders in women in Bangladesh. In a study carried out in an urban community, around half of adult women reported to have mental disorders [16].

Understanding the mental health problems in women is important because of their increasing participation in economy; their essential roles in growth and development of children and welfare of the elderly [7]. If we want to structure any culturally specific and "internationally instructive" interventions aimed at preventing mental health problem associated with violence among women, we need to explore the experience of women who face violence and understand how it is related to their mental disorder [7, 15].

Qualitative research is an appropriate approach in exploring the experience of women facing violence and its association with mental disorder because of the complex nature of mental disorders and the multifaceted role of various factors including violence in predisposing, precipitating, and maintaining it [17–21].

Methods

We adopted a phenomenological approach to understand and describe the experience of women who faced violence and were suffering from mental disorders. We used a modified Bengali version of the Humiliation, Afraid, Rape, and Kick (HARK) questions to identify women who faced violence and were clinically diagnosed by a mental health professional at the National Institute of Mental Health (NIMH) to determine their mental disorders. We adopted criterion sampling to identify the respondents. We included the respondents with mental disorders who answered "yes" to at least one HARK question and agreed to participate in the study. We chose HARK questions because of its high sensitivity of 81% (95%C.I. 69 and 90%) and specificity of 95% (95%C.I. 91 to 98%) with the cut-off score of ≥ 1 [22]. We initially decided to conduct around 10 interviews to understand and describe the experience of women with mental disorders facing violence; with this number considered adequate for a phenomenological approach [23]. However, we eventually continued to 16 in-depth interviews (IDI) and three informal interviews to achieve maximum saturation. We collected data from patients often complemented by caregivers and from guardians only when the subject was not fully communicable. The median interview time was around 56 min; the shortest one was 39 min while the longest one was of 140 min. All interviews were carried out either by qualified or trained female and or male psychiatrists with postgraduate education. All formal interviews and discussion were carried out at different suitable places of NIMH. Table 1 shows the age, occupation, education, and psychiatric diagnosis of 16 patients involved in in-depth interviews and three patients involved in informal interviews.

We also conducted a focus group discussion (FGD) to get a wider view and triangulate our findings from the in-depth interviews. A total of five physicians, (two women and three men) who were involved in the treatment of patients with mental disorder attended the discussions which lasted a little more than 2 h. The corresponding author moderated the discussion. He also conducted one key informant interview (KI) with a leading psychiatrist in Bangladesh with around 20 years experience to triangulate and validate our earlier findings in IDIs, to capture missing information in the development of theoretical understanding. We used separate interview guides for KI and FGD. We used a judgmental sampling technique in selecting KI and participants for FGD. We also reviewed documents such as magazines, news reports, and other local research reports. We then compared them with our data to cross check and validate our understanding, which contributed to the credibility of our research [24]. The richness of the data (including from patients, psychiatrists, document reviews, and our own familiarity with the context and culture and experience in treating mental disorder patients) allowed us to construct and describe "truly" reflected "essence" of the phenomenon of violence against women and its relationship with mental disorders.

We recorded the interviews and discussion. We then listened to the recorded data to have a "sense of whole" [25] and identified units or segments relevant to our study aims. We took notes on our reflection while listening to the data as we understood it. We translated related verbatim quotes into English and wrote them along with the relevant units and notes with the time locator and file name underneath. That allowed us to track down the segment in the audio recording if needed. The segments were the "meaning units" that constituted the various aspects of "the essential structure" of the whole phenomenon [25]. We decided not to transcribe the data verbatim because of our previous experience where we found typing in local language difficult and contracting out the task of transcription to a Bengali typist not involved in research was ineffective. This was because of difference in accent, choice of words used, and educational background of the participants and transcriber's failure to retrieve cue related information [26, 27]. We listened to the data and reread our notes and placed them all under broad categories. The segmentation and categorization of relevant data gave us "meaning units" of our reflection and quotes to describe "essence" of the phenomenon and allowed us to skip formal coding [25, 27]. We constantly compared categories and looked for the patterns and themes as it emerged during analysis. We summarized, revised, and structured our understanding of various thematic areas of the phenomenon through our insights against the context [27]. Finally, we describe the phenomenon as we understood it with text, diagram, and quotes.

Ethical issues

We used a Bengali consent form and informed the respondents of their right to withdraw from the study at any time even after consenting. We specifically mentioned, "You can leave the discussion (interview) at any time. If you do not take part in the study it will not hamper your treatment" to allay "fear, subconscious repression, and concealment" [28]. We informed participants that they can withhold any information they do not want to disclose and assured them of confidentiality. We obtained verbal consent before interviewing an individual and recorded the consenting process for all IDIs, KI and FGD. We secured assent of the participants who were minor (aged less than 18 years) along with the consent of their mothers and in one case foster mother. We maintained confidentiality in every step of the study. We identified all recorded interview files with a unique code, understandable only to the corresponding author. We replaced the real name with a pseudonym in the article and secured data with the investigators. We were either qualified or trained in psychiatry that allowed us to offer necessary treatment and advice to those in need at NIMH.

Table 1 Demographic and type of mental disorders of the patients of interviews

Age in years (f[1])	Occupation (f)	Years of schooling[2] (f)	Diagnosis[3] (f)
15–20 (8[4])	House wife (8)	0–5 (1)	Depression and related (4)
21–25 (1)	Teacher (2)	6–10 (10)	Bipolar mood disorders (4)
26–30 (4)	Student (6)	11–15 (5)	Obsession (1)
31–35 (4)	Legal counsel (1)	16–20 (2)	Acute stress disorder (1)
36–40 (2)	Unemployed (2)		Conversion disorder (3)
			Schizophrenia (5)
			Mental retardation (3)
			Conduct disorders (1)

Notes: [1]Frequency or how many; [2]Information on years of schooling is missing for one respondent; [3]Three respondents had dual diagnosis, [4]Two participants were 15 years old and two 17 years old

We obtained formal ethical clearance from the National Institute of Mental Health, Bangladesh.

Results

It is important to have "rich contextualized descriptions" in a phenomenological approach [29]. We will first describe the context, then the phenomenon of violence against women with mental disorders and finally our understanding of the relationship between violence against women and mental disorders.

The context

The society was male dominated and women often were blamed for any mishap in the family. Marriage in this society was a universal phenomenon. We found that parents were under great social pressure to marry off their daughter even when they were not grown up. Child (aged less than 18 years) marriage or giving dowry (giving cash or other assets by families of brides to grooms and or their families during the event of marriage) [30], although illegal, was practiced widely. We found it very common among the low socioeconomic groups. A family married off a girl when she was studying at sixth grade. Her mother narrated her experience of why they married off their daughter so early:

> Their family was good, they are showing interest in the girl, do not want anything, and said, "we want the bride only". Then [we] thought we are poor people, marrying her off will need money. Because they are saying [they do not want dowry] and have building [economically better of], let's marry [her] off. The place, where we were tenant, the land lady also pursued. Then [we] married [her] off.

We found married women under social, and emotional obligation for keeping up the marital relationship even if it was painful; a divorcee was considered to be a "bad girl" and with "bad character". A professional woman earnestly longing for her husband in spite of his brutal behavior, divorce and sue described her experiences: "That [I] was married to him; I am his wife, just this much; anything else is not needed. He, keeping me with, can marry five more. I'm his wife, I want only this identity.". The pressure might mount up if the social status of the woman was high. She added: "My father was a village arbitrator, still he is. He used to mediate all the conflicts in the village. If such an event [divorce] happens in my father's house, how will he show his face [in the society].".

We found corporal punishment by mom and dad often an acceptable way of disciplining children or adolescent. Women often accepted violence as usual, in particular if it was by their husbands or parents. We found the phenomenon deeply rooted in the tradition. A discussant narrated his experience where he came across a father in law visibly disappointed with the village arbitration meeting for the violence committed by his son:

> The father in law said, "I used to beat my wife but was not subjected to arbitration. Why is so much this arbitration for now?" [Interviewer: It means cultural factor is an issue]. The other thing is [the tradition of beating wives] has been continuing generation after generation, is it right? Father in law says, "I have beaten my wife, my son has beaten daughter in law, what's wrong with this".

In the absence of a social security system, parents in their old age often live with their sons or daughter. That often created a psychological conflict with in laws. The in laws often influenced the relationship between husband and wife and contributed to violence.

We found a transition in life style meant more women were venturing out in career oriented jobs and often spent more time with their colleagues than their husbands. Easily accessible mobile and social networking sites along with career oriented exposure often raised the possibility of pre or extramarital affair and related violence. A discussant narrated how a lady had a physical fight with her husband over her extramarital affair and attempted suicide and was taken to the hospital: "The lady, has children, has a husband, has everything but she is involved in extra marital affair. How has she done it? Through internet [face book].". We found adolescents or youth often were sexually harassed using mobile or face book to develop a relationship. If fail, they did not oblige, men sometime circulate private photographs or distorted images as revenge. Consequently, parents and their daughters underwent tremendous psychological stress. Parents often stopped their daughters' education and married them off early to avoid further unwanted situation. A psychiatrist narrated his experience:

> Some girls, young girls who go to school, in the villages, in urban areas, while going to school, some *bokhate* [derailed] boys eve teases [sexually harassed] on the way to school, do eve teasing, make suggestive comments, force to stop going to school, [and] give proposal for marriage.

The experience of violence and mental disorder

We found different types of violence such as using swear words, pushing, bashing, slapping, kicking, knocking, injuring head, hitting with a stick, throwing objects at, not giving food or family expense, living separately, taking away children, involving in extra marital affair or second marriage, humiliating arbitration, and violent sexual behavior rendered to the patients with mental disorders.

Participants often reported more than one category of violence. A law professional, narrated her experience of violence she faced from her husband:

> Most of the time, he hurled abusive words. [Interviewer: used abusive words, what else?]. Suddenly, he beats. Because of the beating my head struck a wall [showing how her head struck the wall], fell down. After falling down [he] poured water on my head [it is a culturally acceptable home remedy for the sick]. That is what. [he] used to hit my head most of the time.

We found sexual violence a reality but a taboo. No respondents voluntarily shared their experience of sexual violence they faced. An educated woman confessed previous sexual abuse at the last part of the interview when she was in a good rapport with the interviewer. She also shared how her two and half year old daughter was about to be sexually violated when she went to the wash room leaving her alone outside:

> In front of my own eye, I was just coming down[from the wash room], saw that [he] is removing trouser, my kid's trousers. [Interviewer: who?] That employee. This little kid, only two and a half years old. [Interviewer: Is it girl?] Girl. Has removed trouser and his, I was about to have a churn in head. I went [there] quickly. He left away, saying nothing, left with head down cast.

Sexual abuse most of the time was not reported because the perpetrators were often in close relationship with the victims. A little girl could be sexually abused by the nearest ones who were beyond any suspicion such as uncle in law, uncle, and brother in law, or house tutor. The victims and their families often wanted to keep it secret because exposing the incident would defame not only the victims but also erode family honor. This has profound implication on the development of mental disorders even in later life. Our key informant shared his experience:

> Many girls who faced violence in early childhood, sexually abused, when grown up, many shared with me, "I have faced such an event in my life long time ago, after that I have problems, after that the event comes to my brain and mind"

We found the society very tolerant with mental disorder patients and also inactive against the ones who beat, yelled or threw stone or even burning matchstick at them. The following conversation with an intellectually disabled girl with conduct disorder, who was burnt with a matchstick thrown at her by someone, narrated the phenomenon:

> Girl: Then my body was on fire, and my clothes.
>
> Mother: Half of the shirt burnt
>
> Interviewer: When caught on fire, did you not see [the perpetrator]?
>
> Girl: No.
>
> Mother: Thrown [stick] lit with match.
>
> Girl: Thrown [stick lit] with match.
>
> Interviewer: Thrown a matchstick? Were people around, what did they say? Did they say nothing?
>
> Girl: They poured water on my body.
>
> Interviewer: They poured water then, has he been caught? Has he been told anything?
>
> Girl: No.

We also found the society self-centered and not aware about role of violence and its relationship with mental disorder. Poor access to grossly inadequate mental health services only adds to the suffering of mentally disordered women facing different types of violence. An unmarried woman with depression vividly described her situation:

> I cannot forget, sir, cannot forget at all. I cannot forget anything, sir [crying];... my torture, that boy's [she has relation with] torture, my family's torture. I am sick; I cannot sleep on bed, cannot eat, [and] cannot sleep. Where will my life go? ...I only want to live. I cannot take any more, my body cannot cope anymore.

The relationship between violence and mental disorders

We identified several patterns of relationship between violence against women and mental disorders. We found violence as a predisposing factor in some while in many a precipitator or maintenance factor. Sometimes, it was a mere coexistence and not perceived as unusually troublesome by the women with mental disorders. However, in many, it came as a consequence and often contributed to its maintenance. The type of violence and its severity perceived by women facing it sometimes played an important role in the development of a particular mental disorder. In the absence of adequate mental health facilities, women with severe and chronic mental disorders almost always faced some form of violence. It occurred when force was applied to restrain them from causing harm either towards self or others, it also happened when long exhausting caregiving took a huge toll on the care givers. Even the near ones themselves were either involved in perpetrating violence or kept silent when others were doing it. As shown in the Fig. 1, we found most of the time more than one category of violence was involved and played more than one role, which varied across different types of mental disorders.

We found physical violence, verbal abuse, or social humiliation played a role in predisposing a woman in developing mental disorder; emotional or psychological trauma played the most [Fig. 1]. We found emotional trauma resulting from negative remarks by their husband such as "you are black, you are not liked [by me], the girls outside are beautiful", extramarital affair or sex with other woman, and second marriages were likely to lead to mental disorders. A woman who tried to harm herself deliberately several times because of her husband's extramarital affairs alleged: "I have been hurt [emotionally] for the last year and a half. I have been tortured [emotionally], I have been dishonored".

We found violence predisposed an individual for mental disorder even in later life. A psychiatrist narrated his experience of treating a sexual dysfunctional patient which he believed to be the result of her childhood sexual abuse. The patient took around 2 years to see a psychiatrist because no physician had ever explored her past traumatized life:

This girl was sexually abused at an early age. This girl is now married, got married. After marriage, her sexual life, she does not like it. [I] mean she becomes afraid when she sees a man; terror strikes her. When her husband comes to her or touches [her], she develops seizure like feature, right. She becomes tense, develop seizure like feature and try her best to avoid her husband.

We understood, as illustrated in Fig. 1, physical, verbal, and emotional violence worked as precipitators in many, while social in some cases of mental disorder. They played at least some role in precipitating acute stress disorder, depressive disorder, conversion disorders, schizophrenia, bipolar mood disorders, and obsessive compulsive disorder. A respondent with depression recalled her physical and verbal abuse and social suffering when she declined to marry a person 20 years older than her when she was 14 years old:

After breaking the marriage, meanwhile when I decline, then [I endured] beating with shoes, beating with broom, keeping without food, not allowed to sleep at home. My aunty came and said, "she is a prostitute, where [she] has become prostitute from". Grand mother came and said, "pour some chili solution on her", mother said, "kill her", father came and beat me with stick, uncle came and say [the same], pulled my hair, [and] grandfather pushed me down.

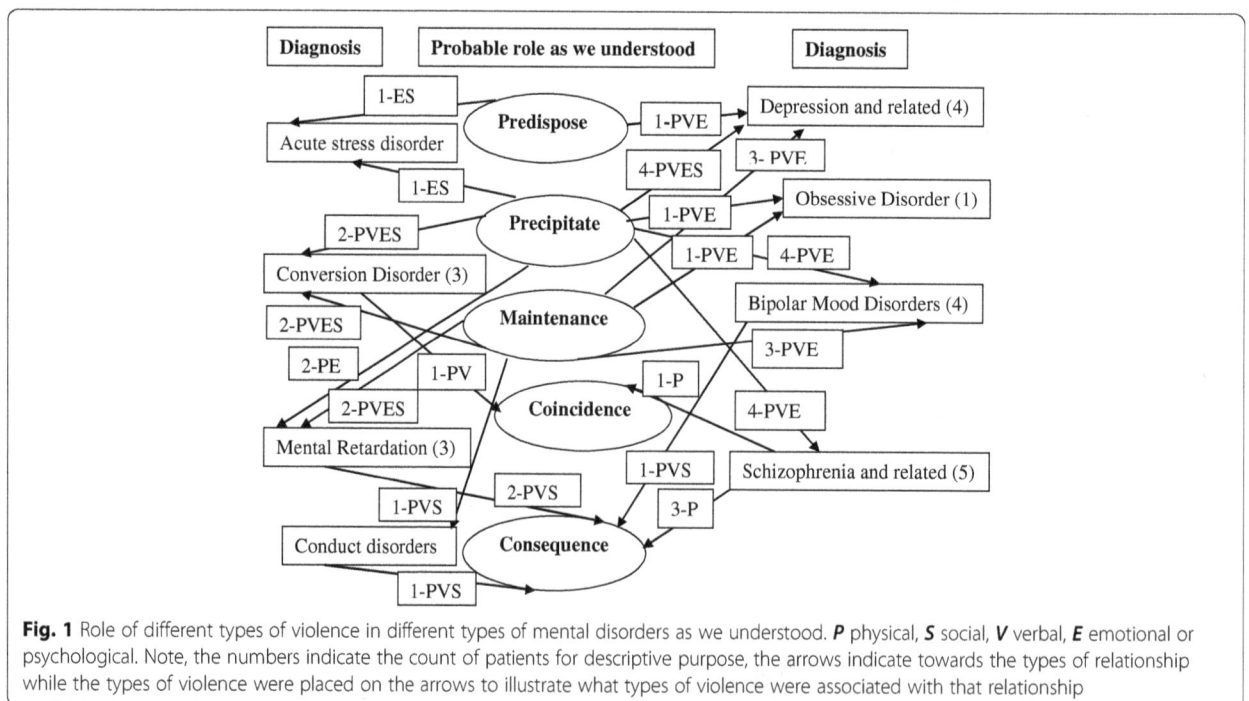

Fig. 1 Role of different types of violence in different types of mental disorders as we understood. *P* physical, *S* social, *V* verbal, *E* emotional or psychological. Note, the numbers indicate the count of patients for descriptive purpose, the arrows indicate towards the types of relationship while the types of violence were placed on the arrows to illustrate what types of violence were associated with that relationship

We found psychological trauma resulted from refusal of marriage by a boyfriend as precipitator of mental disorders. A woman developed brief psychotic disorder when her boyfriend refused to marry her after a physical relationship. Premarital sex was not acceptable in this culture and was stigmatized. Consequent teasing by others worsened her suffering as her mother said:

People are not good; have said *habijabi* [demeaning words], "you have married off alone, gone out alone" and the men [who the girl was in relation and had sex] said, "I will be married off [by my parents]. I do not love you; do not have any relationship [with you]". And father has forcibly brought her at night [because she went to her boyfriend house and living without marriage is not socially acceptable]. Various issues affected [her]. My daughter was healthy, that healthy daughter became crazy.

We found social violence or social humiliation stemmed from social politics and injustice as a precipitator in mental illness. A female school teacher was forced to ask for forgiveness from a lady who was in an extramarital affair with her husband. The unfair decision came from an arbitration meeting convened to resolve the issue where she could not establish her point, rather she was accused of defaming the lady engaged in the extramarital affair. This type of traditional dispute resolution is prevailing in Bangladesh which is often manipulated by local influential persons and delivers an unfair verdict [31]. Consequently, she developed acute stress disorder. She exclaimed: "The one who has broken my family she has not got any punishment. I have to seek forgiveness from her. [Interviewer: Is it more humiliating [then extramarital relationship]?] Yes."

We found violence often worked as a maintenance factor; physical, verbal, emotional, and even social abuse or negligence played some role in maintaining conversion disorder, mental retardation with conduct disorders, bipolar mood disorders, obsession, and depression. Often parents, in laws, and very near ones hurled abusive language or physically hurt patients without understanding the impact. The ongoing abuse contributed to the maintenance of mental illness. A woman patient said how her recent episode recurred after being verbally abused by in laws:

In spite of talking in a sympathetic way, they said, "why you do not recover? You have destroyed my brother's life. We have married our brother to such a women that my brother [has to suffer] throughout his whole life".

A mismatched marital relationship where the wife had an outgoing personality often brought on physical

violence by her husband and emotional suffering and contributed to the maintenance of mental disorders. A depressed lady English teacher who was often battered by her husband shared her feelings:

I do not have any thing in my life, sister [addressing the interviewer as her sister]. I have spent eight years of life like a prisoner, have not gone anywhere. Going out is a pastime, he does not have that. [Interviewer: Has your husband barred you to go out?]. [He] did not bar but who would I go with? He does not go anywhere, [he is] different.

We found mentally disordered people were considered as eccentric and down torn. People around them more often than not avoided them which were emotionally traumatic for the patient. This contributed to the deterioration of the existing mental disorder. A mother of a mentally retarded girl explained how her daughter felt when some visitors came to her house and did not talk to her:

That happens. When someone comes to my house and does not talk to her, then she feels bad in her heart. Again, when we go to somewhere to visit, when they talk to me but not to her, when a girl of her age comes but does not talk to her, she feels bad in her.

We found violence as a very common consequence of mental disorders; either by the patients towards themselves or by very close ones such as parents, brothers or sisters or even daughter or in laws and often by traditional healers. Patients with chronic mental disorders such as schizophrenia, bipolar mood disorders, mental retardation, and conduct disorders might face physical, verbal and social or sexual violence as a consequence of their condition [Fig. 1]. When the eccentric activities of a mentally disordered person went beyond tolerable limits; the caregivers might be burnt out and violence against the patient became a consequence irrespective of class and creed or understanding. Even the neighbors or people around often resorted to violence and parents used to endure that. A mother's opinions on the beating of her bipolar mood disorder daughter by her neighbor was:

I do not blame them. [They] wanted to keep my daughter good taking into consideration my deplorable situation. [The neighbor might have thought] Alas! [The lady] did not get peace with her husband [husband is sick]; the daughter is now doing this. Let see if we can make her good by beating [because they did not consider her as ill rather with ill behaviors]

"All beat me" was the response of a girl suffering from schizophrenia while an educated daughter of a schizophrenic confessed how the close ones behaved with her mother:

My father has raised hand [to beat her], then when she was very crazy, making trouble, my younger sister has beaten her. Then my brother also raised hand on [her] body. When we kept her in our maternal uncles' house, when she used to give trouble to them, maternal uncles have also beaten. We have our uncles where we are, they have beaten, beaten a lot.

When asked if the brothers and very close others understood that the patient was not mentally healthy, the daughter said: "[They] have understood, even then [they] have beaten [her]. Because, they understand that [she] is giving so much trouble, what would we do, let's kill, give beating; if cured after being beaten, it's a problem.". The other reason of violence might be social stigma as the KI said:

I think they do this, two reasons behind this; one, they think if we can calm them this way before going to hospital we can save our prestige [face]. The second reason is that going to the doctor will make the issue public, that is why many guardians [come] at last after doing this [corporal punishment]. They try themselves.

We found that violence came with traditional treatment as a consequence. The treatment included beating with a broom and shoe, inflicting pain, holding burned chili or grass or flame or smoke in front of the nose and forcing inhalation to drive out the *bhoot* (spirit). A mother influenced by a relative consulted a *kabiraj* (a type of traditional healer) and described her experience of the treatment which caused a burn injury on the face of the patient:

A new cloth was soaked with mustard oil [and set on fire], then the arms [of the patient] were held [firmly so that she could not move away] and [the *kabiraj*] kept [the burning cloth in front of the nose and mouth of the patient] and said "if there is *alga* [possession] it will leave." [Interviewer: [Had he] held the fire in front [of her face]?]. Yes. All these were burnt [pointing the burnt areas].

We found violence in the form of chaining used to restrain a mentally disordered person. Even at hospital it was in place. When asked why she fastened the chain around her daughter's leg, a mother said:

[I] cannot keep her at home by any means. [We] got her admitted here [the NIMH hospital] for 8 days including today. One day [she] ran away [from here]. [Interviewer: where did she go?] Outside,[she] will go away [outside of the hospital], this is the disease she is with, will go into hiding, [and] cannot be caught. [Interviewer: Did you chain her at home as well?] Yes, [I] keep her chained and a grill [an iron made structure used to secure the window or veranda] weighing 10 kg attached with it; she cannot go away with it.

We found psychological trauma as a consequence from avoidance, neglect, or negative attitude demonstrated to patients. Adults as well as children avoided or teased a person if s/he was known to have a mental disorder. It appeared that many times that violence, as mentioned above, did not fall under the category of gender violence because they were not related to gender identity but came as consequence of the mental disorder. It is never the less difficult to comment on this since we were only assessing the experience of women in the study.

Sometimes emotional trauma could come in a very different way as a consequence. One discussant said:

Violence can happen taking the opportunity of mental disorders such as some patients suffer from delusional disorders and under treatment, probably suspect husband. Now husbands take the opportunity. Because the wife already suspects him, everybody in society knows about it; the in laws know; all of the - girl's father's family know. The husband often indulges in extramarital relationships with two-three [women]. It is then seen that whatever the wife is saying, he is doing it, the wife also can sense it. The disease of the wife does not get better. He is doing the job but when told to all, nobody believes [it].

Apart from being victimized by others, some mental disorder patients often resort to violence against themselves, their family members or others because of the nature of the disease. When asked about a scar mark on a psychotic patient, her mother said:

Has bitten; bitten her, crazy [she] is. [Interviewer: has bitten herself?] Yes, has bitten herself. Has bitten all; her father, me, her brother, her sister and even her brother-in-law as well, did not spare from biting. Go this way, that way, if restrained, [she] bites.

Some patients developed mental disorders after their spouses with mental disorder indulged in violence against them. A gambler husband who has been beating his wife since their marriage, inflicted bruises over several areas and a head injury with bleeding inside as revealed by CT scan. He used to resort to violence when he needed money, when his wife protested about his gambling borrowing money from others or coming home late. Her sister described one incident: "After pushing her on *pacca* [concrete floor of the house] he kicked her. After that, [he] punched [her] head with both hands."

Some violence did not appear to be related to mental disorders. Occasional slapping or smacking was usual in some family environments in Bangladesh and are not considered to be problematic. The following dialog was with a woman diagnosed as conversion disorder because of her mental agony related to financial issues:

Interviewer (I): How is the relationship with your husband?

Respondent (R): Relationship [with husband] is good overall; occasionally [he] slaps-smacks, that are problems [smiling].

I: Do you feel bad with these slaps or smacks? Is [it] painful for you?

R: No

I: Do you feel good with these slaps or smacks?

R: Yes, [I] feel good.

I: You feel good if slapped or smacked?

R: Yes

I: Why do you say feel well? Why do you feel good?

R: Feel well, that is it.

I: No, I mean why do you feel good if slapped or smacked?

R: Because *Mohabbat* [feeling of affection] increases.

A lady trainee psychiatrist supported this in the discussion:

They largely, to a great extent take it normally. There is less salt in curry, will be beaten [by husband], this is normal. They do not take it very seriously [that] I have become victim of violence

and get upset, this is not the case. But, now, recently, there has been some change.

We came across a single type of violence which played multiple roles across different categories of mental disorders [Fig. 1] while more than one type were playing a single role in the same category of disorders. Some violence or conflict precipitated some category of mental disorder and then if continued contributed to its maintenance. Such type of disorders includes somatoform, dissociative or conversion disorders. A woman discussant said:

In conversion disorder, we see if there is some maintaining factors or continuous problem remaining, usually what happens in the case of tender aged young woman with conversion disorder, the main problem we get is some conflict with in laws, which [she] cannot overcome or cannot leave the in laws' house. In the case, [in] case of conversion disorder, [violence] works as a maintaining factor.

A leading psychiatrist explains how the impact of violence varies across different disorders and their course.

For example, in depression, anxiety it can precipitate. This type of behavior can precipitate every disease. In the case of mental retardation, what happens, they become the big victims; many a times they are sexually abused,[and] physically abused. It is a sorrow that they cannot do anything and cannot protest or protect nothing happened [to the perpetrators]; we perhaps cannot do anything for them. They are the most neglected and suffered. In other instances can precipitate or perpetuate. Perhaps we can consider it as etiological factor, but gender violence is contributing as precipitating or perpetuating factors. [Interviewer: Can it be a co-incidence? Because it is quite common in our culture, can it be that there is no relationship but a co-incidence?]. That can be.

We found a patient who was diagnosed with bipolar disorder endured enormous physical abuse, psychological (husband's spending money on having sex with other women] and verbal abuse by her husband and in laws. When asked by her mother, the patient narrated one of many incidence of her physical torture which in turn with psychological distress might result in her present mental disorder:

Mother, [he] watches TV all the night. I told him, can you please turn off the TV or switch off the light. I am going to sleep. He does not allow me to sleep. Then, because I have turned off the TV, he with rolling pin, used to prepare handmade bread hit me;

the rolling pin was broken. Then, [my] head was swollen and the place [pointing a place in the head] became black, the present condition resulted from this; I cannot rememberanythingnow. I do not understand myself what I say to whom, do not understand.

Discussion

We believe our qualitative study is the first one of its kind in understanding the experience of women suffering from mental disorders who came across some form of violence and exploring the relationship between violence and specific mental disorders in Bangladesh. The strength of the study is its findings extend beyond domestic or intimate partner violence and included a wide range of mental disorders. The context violence against women in Bangladesh is a male dominated society where violence against women often starts with marrying off when they are children. This is in line with the findings of others in similar cultural settings including Bangladesh [5, 32]. The negative influence of technology on the context of violence is also mentioned by others [33]. Corporal punishment and its cultural acceptability is common in other cultures as well [34]. Our findings of different types of violence with under reporting of sexual violence which often committed by close acquaintances were also reported elsewhere [35]. Our finding of mother in laws or sister in laws as instigators are consistent with other qualitative study in India and a mixed method study in Bangladesh [14, 36]. However, the findings of sons, brothers, sisters, or mothers as perpetrators were not mentioned previously in the literature as far as we know.

We found violence to be both predisposing and precipitating factors as well as a consequence or maintenance factors for mental disorders. The relationship is not straightforward as some quantitative or mixed method studies across different countries including Bangladesh have found [12, 19, 37]. In fact, the causes of mental disorders are multi factorial with complex interactions between factors [17]. Violence plays some role as other quantitative studies documented [9, 10, 38]. However, the effect varies across different disorders; sometimes it may predispose, many a time it may precipitate, it often results as a consequence and sometimes it is just a coincidence.

The strength of our study is that we looked in depth into how violence against women associated with specific mental disorders. Our study included all types of violence against women and all major categories of psychiatric disorders. The findings are supported by those of Naveed and Person on the triggers, risk factors and protective factors of violence in Bangladesh where violence would be a major modifiable risk factor [9, 39].

To reduce both the violence and mental disorders, we need to promote protecting factors and reduce facilitators through programmatic, healthcare resource strengthening, and regulatory measures. These views have the support of others [8, 9]. A qualitative exploration in a mixed method study found that social and spiritual support worked as a protective factor against mental disorders in women facing domestic violence [40, 41].

We found violence to be a common consequence of mental disorder, either committed by the patients on others or by others towards them. Other authors in quantitative and qualitative articles mentioned the issues [10, 42]. A qualitative study in India also found physical, social, and emotional violence facing patients with mental disorders [43]. However, all consequent violence women with mental disorder were facing was not because they were women as defined by others [8]; rather, they were victimized because of mental disorders as mentioned in other quantitative study [10]. They often faced violence because of "poor mental health literacy" among the general population and the caregivers [44]. The family and society usually take the role of sole care givers in Bangladesh, as mental services are grossly inadequate and poorly accessible [45]. Carers are often burnt out preventing harm caused by mentally disordered patients and may resort to violence as a mean of releasing their anger or of restraint and treatment because of supernatural beliefs [46, 47].

The main strength of our study in exploring the experience and understanding the role of violence against women with mental disorder was that all interviewers or analyst were qualified psychiatrists having a long familiarity with both the culture and the disease they were exploring. This allowed us to gather rich and valid information [24].

Limitation of the study

We, the clinician researchers, conducted all the interviews and which may have hindered "frank discussion". The long interviews taken place under a doctor patient relationship helped us to understand their experience without "fear, subconscious repression, and concealment" [28].

We did not interview other stakeholders such as general physicians or traditional healers. We did not visit the place where the incidence took place. We did not do it for various reasons; one was resource constraint and the other was our presence might raise undue attention which might be harmful to the respondent. However, we collected information from various sources and compared the emerging themes, finding our conclusions to be consistent across information sources. This we believe is the main essence of any qualitative research [48].

Conclusions

We identified four key theoretical understandings. Many women in Bangladesh with mental disorders have been and continue to be exposed to violence. Gender violence played some role in many mental disorders but not in all. The roles of violence varied; sometimes it predisposed the disorder, while other times it precipitated or maintained the disorder. Sometimes it was just a coexistence or a consequence. The relationships were complex and sometimes depended on the type of mental disorders, nature, and intensity of the violence. Interestingly, not all violence faced by mentally disordered women was because they were women. Rather, they were facing violence because of the disease they were suffering from. The findings can be used in structuring culturally appropriate, but valid programs aimed at reducing both violence and the mental disorders they are associated with. Further mixed method research is recommended to enrich and quantify our understanding.

Abbreviations
FGD: Focus group discussion; HARK: Humiliation, Afraid, Rape, and Kick; IDI: In-depth interview; KI: Key informant interview; NIMH: National Institute of Mental Health; WHO: World Health Organization

Acknowledgements
We acknowledge the kind contribution of Dr. Zinat De Laila, Dr. AKM Khaleequzzaman, Professor Md. Waziul Alam Chowdhury, and Professor Md. Faruq Alam in data collection and administrative support. We are grateful to Adrian Cameron and Nicola Nikolaou for their review of the manuscript. All respondents and the relevant staff of NIMH deserve special mention for their time and effort for the study.

Funding
Not applicable.

Authors' contributions
MMI designed, collected data, analyzed all data and wrote the draft of manuscript. NJ collected data, contributed to analysis and reviewed the draft manuscript. MDH contributed to designing, collected data and reviewed the draft manuscript. All authors read and approved the final manuscript.

Competing interests
The authors declare that they have no competing interests.

Author details
[1]Training Unit, icddr,b, 68, Shaheed Tajuddin Ahmed Sarani, Mohakhali, Dhaka 1212, Bangladesh. [2]Department of Psychiatry, BIRDEM General Hospital and IMC, Dhaka, Bangladesh. [3]National Institute of Mental Health, Sher-e-bangla Nagar, Dhaka 1207, Bangladesh.

References
1. Assembly, U.N.G. Declaration on the elimination of violence against women. 1993; Available from: http://www.un.org/documents/ga/res/48/a48r104.htm.
2. Ellsberg M, Heise L, editors. Researching violence against women: a practical guide for researchers and activists. Washington DC: World Health Organization, PATH; 2005.
3. Garg S, Singh R. Gender-violence and health care: how health system can step in. Indian J Public Health. 2013;57(1):4.
4. Kumar R. Domestic violence and. Mental Health. 2012;
5. García-Moreno C, Jansen HAFM, Ellsberg M. WHO multi-country study on women's health and domestic violence against women. Geneva: World Health Organization; 2005.
6. Åsling-Monemi K, Naved RT, Persson LÅ. Violence against women and the risk of fetal and early childhood growth impairment: a cohort study in rural Bangladesh. Arch Dis Child. 2009;94(10):775–9.
7. Afifi M. Gender differences in mental health. Singap Med J. 2007;48(5):385.
8. Heise L, Ellsberg M, Gottmoeller M. A global overview of gender-based violence. Int J Gynecol Obstet. 2002;78:S5–S14.
9. Devries K, et al. Violence against women is strongly associated with suicide attempts: evidence from the WHO multi-country study on women's health and domestic violence against women. Soc Sci Med. 2011;73(1):79–86.
10. Choe, J.Y., L.A. Teplin, and K.M. Abram, Perpetration of violence, violent victimization, and severe mental illness: balancing public health concerns. 2008.
11. Vachher AS, Sharma AK. Domestic violence against women and their mental health status in a Colony in Delhi. Indian Journal of Community Medicine : Official Publication of Indian Association of Preventive & Social Medicine. 2010;35(3):403–5.
12. Kumar S, Jeyaseelan L, Suresh S. Domestic violence and its mental health correlates in Indian women, vol. 187; 2005. p. 62–7.
13. Ayub M, et al. Psychiatric morbidity and domestic violence: a survey of married women in Lahore. Soc Psychiatry Psychiatr Epidemiol. 2009;44(11):953–60.
14. Naved RT, Akhtar N. Spousal violence against women and suicidal ideation in Bangladesh. Womens Health Issues. 2008;18(6):442–52.
15. Fischbach RL, Herbert B. Domestic violence and mental health: correlates and conundrums within and across cultures. Soc Sci Med. 1997;45(8):1161–76.
16. Islam MM, et al. Prevalence of psychiatric disorders in an urban community in Bangladesh. Gen Hosp Psychiatry. 2003;25(5):353–7.
17. Cooper B. Nature, nurture and mental disorder: old concepts in the new millennium, vol. 178; 2001. p. s91–s101.
18. Gelder M, Mayou R, Cowen P. Shorter Oxford textbook of psychiatry. 4th ed. Newdelhi: Oxford University Press; 2001.
19. Coid J. et al, Abusive experiences and psychiatric morbidity in women primary care attenders. Br J Psychiatry. 2003;183(4):332–9.
20. Davidson L, et al. Using qualitative research to inform mental health policy. The Canadian Journal of Psychiatry. 2008;53(3):137–44.
21. Tong A, Sainsbury P, Craig J. Consolidated criteria for reporting qualitative research (COREQ): a 32-item checklist for interviews and focus groups. Int J Qual Health Care. 2007;19(6):349–57.
22. Sohal H, Eldridge S, Feder G. The sensitivity and specificity of four questions (HARK) to identify intimate partner violence: a diagnostic accuracy study in general practice. BMC Fam Pract. 2007;8(1):49.
23. Groenewald, T., A phenomenological research design illustrated. 2004.
24. Patton MQ. Enhancing the quality and credibility of qualitative analysis. Health Serv Res. 1999;34(5 Pt 2):1189.
25. Baker C, Wuest J, Stern PN. Method slurring: the grounded theory/ phenomenology example. J Adv Nurs. 1992;17(11):1355–60.
26. Islam M, et al. A qualitative exploration of drug abuse relapse following treatment. Journal of Ethnographic & Qualitative Research. 2012;7(1).
27. Bailey J. First steps in qualitative data analysis: transcribing. Fam Pract. 2008; 25(2):127–31.
28. Havens L. Taking a history from the difficult patient. Lancet. 1978; 311(8056):138–40.
29. Davidsen AS. Phenomenological approaches in psychology and health sciences. Qual Res Psychol. 2013;10(3):318–39.
30. Anderson S. Why dowry payments declined with modernization in Europe but are rising in India. J Polit Econ. 2003;111(2):269–310.
31. Khondker HH. Modern Law, Traditional 'Shalish' and Civil Society Activism in Bangladesh, in The Sociology of Shari'a: Case Studies from around the World, A. Possamai, J.T. Richardson, and B.S. Turner, Editors. 2015, Springer International Publishing: Cham. p. 31–49. Available from: https://link. springer.com/chapter/10.1007%2F978-3-319-09605-6_3.

32. Ali, T.S., Living with violence in the home: exposure and experiences among married women, residing in urban Karachi, Pakistan. 2011.

33. Sen R. Not all that is solid melts into air? Care-experienced young people, friendship and relationships in the 'digital age'. Br J Soc Work. 2015;46(4): 1059–75. https://academic.oup.com/bjsw/article/46/4/1059/2472229.

34. Lansford JE, et al. Physical discipline and Children's adjustment: cultural Normativeness as a moderator. Child Dev. 2005;76(6):1234–46.

35. Watts C, Zimmerman C. Violence against women: global scope and magnitude. Lancet. 2002;359(9313):1232–7.

36. Kaur R, Garg S. Domestic violence against women: a qualitative study in a rural community. Asia Pac J Public Health. 2010;22(2):242–51.

37. Fulu E, et al. Prevalence of and factors associated with male perpetration of intimate partner violence: findings from the UN multi-country cross-sectional study on men and violence in Asia and the Pacific. Lancet Glob Health. 2013;1(4):e187–207.

38. Dillon G, et al. Mental and physical health and intimate partner violence against women: a review of the literature. International Journal of Family Medicine. 2013;2013:313909.

39. Naved RT, Persson LÅ. Factors associated with spousal physical violence against women in Bangladesh. Stud Fam Plan. 2005;36(4):289–300.

40. Anderson KM, Renner LM, Danis FS. Recovery: resilience and growth in the aftermath of domestic violence. Violence Against Women. 2012;18(11):1279–99.

41. Friedman SH, et al. Intimate partner violence victimization and perpetration by Puerto Rican women with severe mental illnesses. Community Ment Health J. 2011;47(2):156–63.

42. Hsu M-C, Tu C-H. Adult patients with schizophrenia using violence towards their parents: a phenomenological study of views and experiences of violence in parent–child dyads. J Adv Nurs. 2014;70(2):336–49.

43. Mathias K, et al. Under the banyan tree - exclusion and inclusion of people with mental disorders in rural North India. BMC Public Health. 2015;15:446.

44. Jorm AF. Mental health literacy: public knowledge and beliefs about mental disorders. Br J Psychiatry. 2000;177(5):396–401.

45. Hossain MD, et al. Mental disorders in Bangladesh: a systematic review. BMC psychiatry. 2014;14(1):216.

46. Mullick MS, et al. Beliefs about jinn, black magic and evil eye in Bangladesh: the effects of gender and level of education. Mental Health, Religion & Culture. 2013;16(7):719–29.

47. Fazel S, et al. Schizophrenia and violence: systematic review and meta-analysis. PLoS Med. 2009;6(8):e1000120.

48. Merriam SB. Introduction to qualitative research. Qualitative research in practice: Examples for discussion and analysis. 2002;1:1–17.

3

Risk perceptions, attitudes, and knowledge of chikungunya among the public and health professionals: a systematic review

Tricia Corrin[1,2*] (iD), Lisa Waddell[1], Judy Greig[1], Ian Young[3], Catherine Hierlihy[1,2] and Mariola Mascarenhas[1]

Abstract

Background: Recently, attention to chikungunya has increased due to its spread into previously non-endemic areas. Since there is no available treatment or vaccine, most intervention strategies focus on mosquito bite prevention and mosquito control, which require community involvement to be successful. Thus, our objective was to systematically review the global primary literature on the risk perceptions, attitudes, and knowledge of chikungunya among the public and health professionals to inform future research and improve our understanding on which intervention strategies are likely to be successful.

Methods: Potentially relevant articles were identified through a standardized systematic review (SR) process consisting of the following steps: comprehensive search strategy in seven databases (Scopus, PubMed, CINAHL, CAB, LILACS, Agricola, and Cochrane) and a grey literature search of public health organizations, relevance screening, risk of bias assessment, and data extraction. Two independent reviewers performed each step. Reporting of this SR follows PRISMA reporting guidelines.

Results: Thirty-seven relevant articles were identified. The majority of the articles were published since 2011 (83.8%) and reported on studies conducted in Asia (48.7%) and the Indian Ocean Islands (24.3%). The results were separated into four categories: general knowledge and perceptions on chikungunya; perceptions on the risk and severity of chikungunya; knowledge of chikungunya-harboring vectors and transmission; and knowledge, perceptions, and attitudes on mitigation practices. Overall, the systematic review found that risk perceptions, attitudes, and knowledge of chikungunya among the public and health professionals vary across populations and countries and knowledge is higher in areas that have experienced an outbreak.

Conclusion: The results suggest that most of the affected populations in this study do not understand mosquito borne diseases or chikungunya and are therefore less likely to protect themselves from mosquito bites. While more research is required to improve the generalizability of this dataset, it appears that a lack of knowledge is an important barrier for motivating community level interventions and personal protection against mosquitoes.

Keywords: Chikungunya, Systematic review, Attitudes, Knowledge, Perceptions

* Correspondence: triciacorrin@gmail.com
[1]Public Health Risk Sciences Division, National Microbiology Laboratory, Public Health Agency of Canada, Guelph, ON, Canada
[2]Department of Population Medicine, University of Guelph, Guelph, ON, Canada
Full list of author information is available at the end of the article

Background

Chikungunya is an alphavirus that is transmitted to humans through mosquito bites. It causes a non-specific illness including high fever, severe joint pain, muscle pain, headache, nausea, fatigue, and rash in infected individuals [1, 2]. While most people recover from the acute illness in 1–2 weeks, there are a proportion of individuals that continue to suffer from chronic joint pain which can persist for weeks to years following infection [1, 2].

Historically, chikungunya virus (CHIKV) has circulated in Africa, Asia, and the Indian and Pacific Ocean Islands [2]. In 2013, the virus spread to the Americas and caused outbreaks in countries that harbor the vectors, *Aedes aegypti* and *Aedes albopictus* [2–4]. Cases of infected travelers in Europe and North America returning from CHIKV-affected countries have been documented as well as several small outbreaks in Europe due to importation of the virus into an area with suitable vectors [3, 5].

Chikungunya is an important public health concern as the virus continues to emerge into previously non-endemic areas such as the Americas, which have reported more than 1.7 million suspected or confirmed cases since 2013 [6]. In the USA, chikungunya has been a notifiable disease since 2015, and in the same year, the Centers for Disease Control and Prevention reported 679 travel-related cases of chikungunya from 44 states [3]. Canada has reported several hundred travel-related cases of chikungunya since it spread to the Americas [7].

Most intervention strategies have focused on mosquito control and mosquito bite prevention as there is currently no treatment or vaccine for CHIKV infection in humans [8]. The success of these intervention strategies relies on social factors such as knowledge, attitudes, and perceptions of the disease. It is important to understand how affected populations understand and perceive chikungunya, its transmission cycle, and the importance of control measures to determine what prevention strategies are likely to be successful. In addition, how and why the target population chooses to take preventative action against mosquito borne diseases like CHIKV is necessary to inform future education and control strategies. Thus, a systematic review was conducted to identify, assess, and analyze the global evidence on the knowledge, attitudes, and perceptions of CHIKV and its transmission in affected populations.

Methods

Research question, team, and protocol

This systematic review was conducted following internationally recognized procedures and is reported in accordance with the PRISMA guidelines [9–11].

The systematic review question is "what are risk perceptions, attitudes and/or knowledge of chikungunya among the public and health professionals?" A multidisciplinary team with expertise in knowledge synthesis, epidemiology, risk assessment, public health, and information science conducted the review.

Prior to the systematic review, a pre-specified systematic review protocol was developed which included the research question, definitions, inclusion criteria for relevance screening, risk of bias tool, and data extraction forms. The systematic review protocol and citation list of relevant articles is available in supplementary material (Additional files 1 and 2), and the dataset resulting from this review is available upon request.

Search strategy and eligibility criteria

A scoping review of the global literature on chikungunya, conducted at the Public Health Agency of Canada (personal communication M. Mascarenhas 2017), served as the starting point for this systematic review. Briefly, the scoping review aimed to identify all relevant research on chikungunya; a search was conducted to capture all primary research in English, French, Spanish, or Portuguese. Seven electronic sources were selected based on their relevance to the scoping review. These were accessed through the Public Health Agency of Canada Library and included Scopus, PubMed, The Cumulative Index to Nursing and Allied Health Literature (CINAHL), CAB, LILACS (South America), Agricola, and the Cochrane Library for any relevant trials in the trial registry. The initial search was conducted on May 27, 2015, using a pre-tested search algorithm (Chikungunya OR CHIK OR CHIKV) OR (alphavirus AND mosquito* AND control). An updated search using the same electronic sources and algorithms was completed on January 6, 2017. A grey literature search of pre-specified public health organization ($n = 19$, list available upon request) websites was undertaken to identify any non-peer-reviewed studies or surveillance data that was not captured in the electronic search. All studies on any aspect of chikungunya or CHIKV were included and characterized. One of the scoping review categories was on studies describing "Public and health professionals/physicians' knowledge, attitudes and/or risk perceptions towards chikungunya and potential prevention and control strategies." The 45 studies from this category were considered for inclusion in this systematic review. Further details on the scoping review protocol and methods are available upon request.

Relevance confirmation, risk of bias assessment, and data extraction

To ensure that the studies from the scoping review were applicable to the research question, a single relevance question appeared at the beginning of the risk of bias assessment and data extraction form to allow the reviewer to eliminate any irrelevant studies.

All studies were evaluated for their risk of bias using a pre-designed risk of bias assessment form (Additional file 1). The form was created to address both qualitative (8 criteria) and quantitative (11 criteria) studies. Previously designed critical appraisal tools for qualitative and quantitative studies were used to create this risk of bias form [12–14]. Each study received an overall risk of bias score where studies conducted to minimize bias in the results were assigned a low risk of bias ranking. If one or more criteria could not be assessed due to lack of reporting, an unclear risk of bias was appointed. Studies received a high risk of bias if one or more criteria were not met. A data extraction form was used to extract relevant information and results from each quantitative study. The extraction form included 9 questions designed to extract information on study design, demographics, and the results of the studies that fell into the following categories: perceptions about the severity of chikungunya disease; knowledge, perceptions, and attitudes on mitigation practices; knowledge on chikungunya; and knowledge on CHIKV harboring vectors and how CHIKV is transmitted. Outcomes more generally related knowledge, perceptions, and attitudes on mosquito borne diseases (MBDs), and mosquito control reported in relevant papers on chikungunya and chikungunya-affected populations were also captured to examine if general attitudes, perceptions, and knowledge were more closely correlated to knowledge, attitudes, and perceptions on the use of personal protective measures than knowledge on chikungunya or CHIKV specifically.

Both forms were pre-tested by all team members to ensure clarity of the questions, extraction of the right information to address our research question, and to ensure process consistency. Once pre-testing was completed, two reviewers extracted the data and evaluated the risk of bias for each paper independently. During both stages, conflicts between reviewers were resolved by consensus.

Review management and data analysis

The scoping review steps, data extraction, and risk of bias assessment were conducted using the web-based systematic review software DistillerSR (Evidence Partners, Ottawa, Canada). The data was then exported to Microsoft Excel (Microsoft Corporation 2010) for descriptive analysis. Results with reference to "n" refer to the total number of samples, subjects, or participants for the presented outcome.

Meta-analysis models were developed using the statistical software STATA13 (StatCorp 2015). The metaprop package was used to obtain weighted average prevalence estimates for two outcomes: the proportion of the general public sample population that were aware of chikungunya in outbreak and non-outbreak populations and the proportion of the sample population that had

knowledge on mosquito transmission of CHIKV by country. Based on the assumption that the prevalence estimates would have some heterogeneity between study populations, a random effects meta-analysis was conducted using the DerSimonian and Laird method [15]. In some cases, more than one observation per study was included in the meta-analysis. We did not account for the potential similarity of these results as they were all independent observations on different sampling frames. We evaluated how much heterogeneity between studies was not explained by random error using the value I^2 [16]. High heterogeneity, $I^2 > 60\%$, was expected, and our goal was to investigate whether there were study level variables that explained the heterogeneity and to provide a graphic of the studies for the reader. We caution readers not to use the summary estimates as an estimate of the average outcome across studies given that estimates were obtained from very different populations and no study level variables explained all the heterogeneity between studies. In the forest plots, $p = 0.00$ is actually $p < 0.01$. This is an output of STATA13 (StatCorp 2015) and is not open for the user to alter or redefine.

Qualitative research studies were synthesized using a narrative review approach [17]. This included two reviewers independently reviewing the results of each study and descriptively summarizing the key results as reported by the study authors. Summaries from both reviewers were discussed and consolidated to arrive at the final narrative description. Only two relevant qualitative studies were identified in this review; therefore, we decided not to use a formal coding procedure in the analysis or develop interpretive across-study themes.

Results
Systematic review descriptive statistics

There were 6820 citations screened for relevance in the scoping review project, of which 1921 studies were considered to be relevant primary research on chikungunya (Additional file 3). Only 45 of these were categorized to address knowledge, perceptions, and attitudes toward chikungunya and potential prevention and control strategies. Eight of these studies were deemed irrelevant during relevance confirmation, resulting in 37 total articles included in this systematic review. The flow of information through the systematic review process is depicted in Fig. 1.

All studies were published between 2007 and 2016, with 83.8% ($n = 37$) published since 2011. The majority of the articles (73.0%) reported on studies conducted in Asia (48.7%) and the Indian Ocean Islands (24.3%). Specifically, most of the research originated from India (41.0%) and La Réunion (18.0%), as shown in Table 1. The most widely used study design was cross-sectional (75.7%), followed by quasi-experiment (13.5%), qualitative (5.4%), case-control (2.7%), and longitudinal (2.7%). The main population

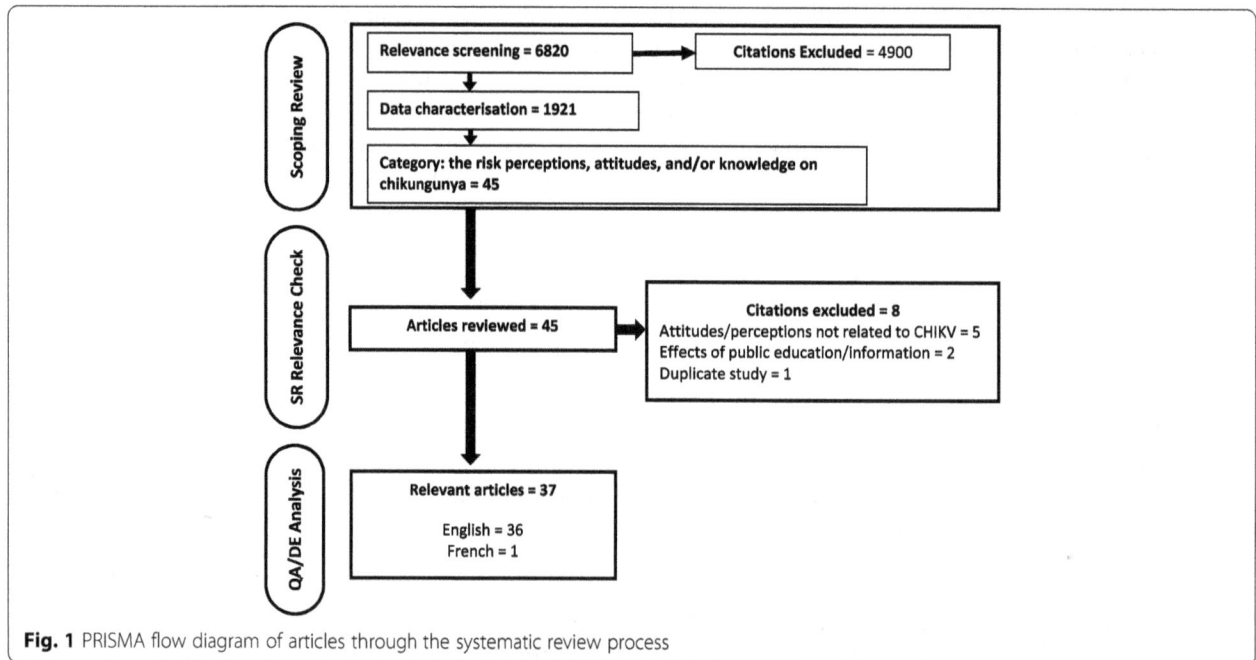

Fig. 1 PRISMA flow diagram of articles through the systematic review process

studied was the general public (86.5%), and only a few studies had data collection processes that were informed by established theories of behavior change (24.3%).

The 35 quantitative studies were ranked as having a low (45.7%), unclear (45.7%), or high (8.6%) overall risk of bias. The most common reason for an unclear risk of bias score was due to a lack of reporting on potential confounders (56.3%, $n = 16$) and a lack of clarity on whether tools to measure outcomes (e.g., questionnaires) were reliably tested and validated (81.3%, $n = 16$). For the two qualitative studies, the main quality assessment deficiencies were that the method of analysis, research design, and data collection were not clearly described in either study.

General knowledge and perceptions on chikungunya

Awareness of chikungunya was evaluated in nine studies. Eight studies conducted in Asia ($n = 7$) and the Caribbean ($n = 1$) dichotomized results and reported awareness of chikungunya among the general public, which varied from 7–96% as shown in Fig. 2 [18–25]. The meta-analysis in Fig. 2 shows that awareness of chikungunya was highest in the four studies where an outbreak was on-going [19, 22, 23] and among urban link workers who are responsible for implementing anti-larval measures through door-to-door visits in their community [21]. In contrast, a study conducted in Sri Lanka where an outbreak was occurring only reported an awareness rate of 7% [24]. However, it is unclear from the study if chikungunya was an emerging disease and whether any previous public education had occurred.

Before traveling from the USA to the Dominican Republic, 19% of community service volunteers ($n = 102$) reported they had knowledge of chikungunya [26]. Of these volunteers, 87% ($n = 102$) had visited a health-care provider for a pre-travel consultation [26]. In Nicaragua, 93.5% of individuals ($n = 848$) from a general population sample considered themselves informed about chikungunya, but actual knowledge was not evaluated [27]. Whereas in a study in India, only 8.9% of the surveyed population ($n = 740$) had correct knowledge about the virus etiology [28]. When students in French Guiana were asked about the duration of chikungunya, 51% ($n = 1462$) answered correctly 3 weeks to several months [29].

Three studies evaluated general knowledge of mosquito borne diseases [30–32]. One of the studies attempted to gauge the level of understanding about mosquito borne diseases in the population by sampling 1506 individuals and having them rank their knowledge on a scale of 0–10, with 0 being "do not understand at all" and 10 being "understand completely" [30]. The mean score was 5.6 (SD 2.85), indicating some knowledge, but a lack of in-depth understanding [30]. General knowledge on mosquito borne diseases in India among a group of health-care workers was 83% ($n = 100$) [31] whereas in a different study 88.1% ($n = 119$) [32] of the general population sample was considered to have general knowledge.

Gender was shown to be a significant predictor of knowledge of chikungunya as a mosquito borne disease in two studies from India [20, 33]. In both studies, females were shown to have more knowledge about

Table 1 General characteristics of 37 included primary research publications

Category		Count (percentage)
Continent/country[a,b]		
Asia	India	16 (41.0%)
	Singapore	1 (2.6%)
	Sri Lanka	1 (2.6%)
Europe	France	2 (5.1%)
	Italy	1 (2.6%)
	Spain	1 (2.6%)
Indian Ocean Islands	La Réunion	7 (18.0%)
	Mauritius	2 (5.1%)
	Mayotte	2 (5.1%)
Americas	USA	2 (5.1%)
	Colombia	1 (2.6%)
	French Guiana	1 (2.6%)
	Nicaragua	1 (2.6%)
	US Virgin Islands	1 (2.6%)
Language		
	English	36 (97.3%)
	French	1 (2.7%)
Date of publication		
	2007–2010	6 (16.2%)
	2011–2016	31 (83.8%)
Risk of bias assessment[c]		
	Low risk of bias	16 (45.7%)
	Unclear risk of bias	16 (45.7%)
	High risk of bias	3 (8.6%)
Study design		
	Cross-sectional	28 (75.7%)
	Quasi-experiment	5 (13.5%)
	Qualitative	2 (5.4%)
	Case-control	1 (2.7%)
	Longitudinal	1 (2.7%)
Population		
	General public	32 (86.5%)
	Health professionals	5 (13.5%)
Theory of behavior change used		
	None	28 (75.7%)
	Health belief model	3 (8.1%)
	Stages of change theory	2 (5.4%)
	Theory of planned behavior	4 (10.8%)

[a]Total number sums to >37 as studies can fall into more than one category
[b]Total percentages do not equal 100 due to rounding
[c]Total number sums to 35 as qualitative studies were not given an overall risk of bias score

mosquito borne disease (13.8%, $n = 350$) compared to males (4.8%, $n = 350$), p value 0.01 [20] and chikungunya (OR 1.37; 95% CI 1.11–1.71; $p = 0.003$; $n = 1674$) [33]. Other significant socio-economic factors included less knowledge among illiterate participants (OR 0.65; 95% CI: 0.51–0.82); $p < 0.001$) and participants over the age of 30 (OR 0.67; 95% CI: 0.54–0.83; $p < 0.01$) compared to those that were literate or between the age of 18–30 [33].

Eight studies measured knowledge of chikungunya [22, 30, 31, 34, 35] and mosquito borne disease [29, 36, 37] symptoms among populations affected by the disease. Knowledge of the signs and symptoms of chikungunya varied across different study populations; however, joint pain, fever, and swelling were commonly identified [22, 30, 35]. In a group of health-care workers in India, 22% ($n = 100$) had knowledge on chikungunya symptoms [31]. The results of a case-control study where the cases were diagnosed with chikungunya showed that those with first-hand experience of the disease were more aware of the symptoms of the disease in comparison with the non-cases [35]. In a study of health-care workers and medical students in two Colombian cities, participants correctly identified polyarthralgia and fever as the most frequent symptoms of chikungunya: 91.9% in Pereira ($n = 99$) and 86.9% in Cartagena ($n = 107$) [34]. For mosquito borne diseases, the most frequently reported symptoms included limb swelling, fever, headache, myalgia, arthralgia, and skin rashes [29, 36]. In one study, knowledge about the symptoms of mosquito borne disease varied depending on whether larval breeding sites were identified around the home [37]. In the absence of larval breeding sites on an individual's property, 37.5% surveyed ($n = 160$) had no knowledge of the symptoms of mosquito borne diseases compared to 62.5% of individuals where larval breeding sites were identified on their property [37]. Larval breeding sites around homes was used as a surrogate measure for risk of exposure, and knowledge of symptoms is presumably due to personal experience with someone in the home being ill from CHIKV.

Perceptions on the treatment of chikungunya were addressed in four studies, two of which sampled populations of health professionals [26, 30, 38, 39]. A group of final year medical students ($n = 314$) from Singapore were surveyed and 20.1% believed that it is necessary to isolate patients who have chikungunya [38]. Five doctors (100%) surveyed in India believed that the traditional system of medicine called Ayurveda was more effective than other systems of medicine to treat chikungunya [39]. In addition, these same doctors all believed that homeopathic medicine can cure chikungunya completely, but only 60% were aware of the efficacy and adverse effects of the treatment used [39]. In France, 1506 participants from the general public gave a mean score of 7.01

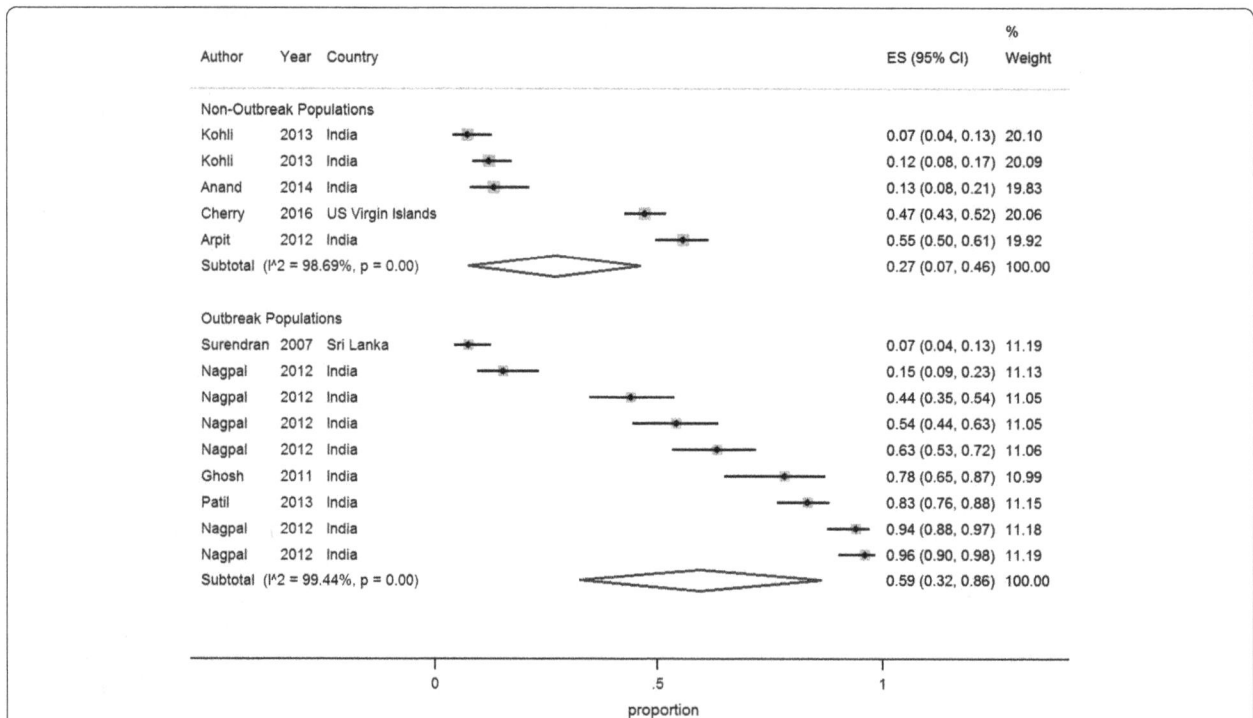

Fig. 2 Meta-analysis of the proportion (ES, 95% CI) of the general public sample population that were aware of chikungunya in outbreak and non-outbreak populations

(SD 2.24) out of 10 that treatment can help with mosquito borne diseases including chikungunya, where 0 indicates no effect of treatment and 10 indicates treatment is highly effective [30]. From a group of community service volunteers in the USA with knowledge on chikungunya, 68% (n = 19) believed there was no available treatment for the disease [26].

Perceptions on the risk and severity of chikungunya

Six studies looked at perceptions of the risk and severity of chikungunya among populations of the general public that were recently affected by an outbreak (Table 2) [26, 29, 40–43]. The perceived severity of the disease was deemed to be high or moderate by 20.5–93.4% of the participants across three studies (n = 1021, n = 880) conducted on the Indian Ocean Islands [41, 43] and 94.5% (n = 18) in a group of USA community volunteers traveling to the Dominican Republic [26]. Following a small CHIKV outbreak in Italy, 49.8% (n = 293) of the population in the affected region perceived a high risk associated with chikungunya, and 83.2% (n = 291) were worried about the disease in the near future [40]. Whereas a study conducted in France (n = 1506) reported that the perceived severity of mosquito borne diseases was moderate, mean score of 7.07 (SD 1.94), and they were less concerned about the risk of contracting a mosquito borne disease, mean score 4.89 (SD 3.15), which may be because many mosquito borne diseases are not endemic in France

[30]. Another study conducted in the USA reported that 63% of the surveyed population (n = 87) were a little or very worried about contracting a mosquito borne disease such as chikungunya or dengue, but only 15% (n = 88) believed it was likely that someone they knew would contract a mosquito borne disease [44].

Knowledge of chikungunya-harboring vectors and transmission

Twenty-four studies assessed what proportion of a study population knew that CHIKV is transmitted to humans through mosquito bites [19, 22–30, 32–36, 40–42, 45–50]. All of these studies looked at the general population with the exception of one study that looked at a group of health professionals in Colombia. The results of the meta-analysis in Fig. 3 indicate that knowledge levels on transmission of CHIKV by mosquitoes range widely between 2 and 97% across studies.

A few studies of the general public conducted on the Indian Ocean Islands found that there are misconceptions on how and why CHIKV is transmitted. One study (n = 1035) reported 73.3% (n = 989) of participants were aware that mosquitoes transmit CHIKV; however, participants also believed that CHIKV could be transmitted through the air (36.5%, n = 996) and/or direct human contact (33.9%, n = 999) [41]. When asked how CHIKV was introduced to the island, responses varied from the bodies of tsunami victims that reached the island (33.1%,

Table 2 Perceived risk and severity of chikungunya and mosquito borne diseases (MBDs) among the general public

REF	Author (year)	Location	Sample size	Proportion or mean score	Description of outcome
Chikungunya					
[29]	Fritzell (2016)	French Guiana	1462	Mean score = 5.37 95% CI: 5.12–5.63	Perceived risk of exposure to chikungunya
[40]	Moro (2010)	Italy	293	49.8%	Perceived a high risk associated with chikungunya
[40]	Moro (2010)	Italy	291	83.2%	Worried about chikungunya in the near future
[41]	Setbon (2008)	La Réunion	1021	2.7% (score: 0–3) 20.5% (score: 4–6) 76.8% (score: 7–10)	Perceived severity of chikungunya on a scale of 0–10 (0 - low, 10 - high)
[42]	Thuilliez (2014)	La Réunion	1024	47.7%	Perceived risk of a new chikungunya outbreak was reasonable or high
[43]	Raude (2009)	Mayotte	880	93.4% (high or moderate) 6.6% (low or none)	Perceived severity of chikungunya
[26]	Millman (2016)	USA	18	94.5%	Perceived possible risk of exposure in Dominican Republic
Mosquito borne diseases (MBD)					
[30]	Raude (2012)	France	1506	Mean score = 7.07 SD = 1.94	Perception on how serious MBDs are on a scale of 0–10 (0 – not serious, 10 – serious)
[30]	Raude (2012)	France	1506	Mean score = 4.89 SD = 3.15	Worried about the risk of contracting MBDs on a scale of 0–10 (0 – not worried at all, 10 – extremely worried)
[33]	Boratne (2010)	India	1674	54.9%	Perceived MBDs as a serious problem in the area (54.9%)
[24]	Surendran (2007)	Sri Lanka	162	29% (severe) 71% (moderate)	Perception of the mosquito problem
[61]	Boyer (2014)	La Réunion	Not reported	78.9%	Good knowledge of vectorial risk
[25]	Cherry (2016)	US Virgin Islands	443	43% (not concerned) 49.5% (mildly concerned) 7.5% (very concerned)	Concerned about getting a MBD during their trip
[44]	Adalja (2016)	USA	87	37% (had not thought about it or were not worried at all) 63% (a little worried or very worried)	Level of worry about MBDs like dengue or chikungunya
[44]	Adalja (2016)	USA	88	85% (very unlikely, unlikely, or uncertain) 15% (likely or very likely)	Perceived likelihood that someone they know could contract dengue or chikungunya while living in their community

MBD mosquito borne disease, SD Standard deviation, 95% CI = 95% confidence interval

n = 983), crews of quarantined ships (61.7%, n = 981) to intentional introduction by secret agents (26.8%, n = 965) [41]. A large proportion of a population in Mayotte (n = 888) believed that the proximate cause of CHIKV is mosquitoes (77%, n = 835), but the ultimate cause is God's punishment (55.4%, n = 802), migrants (36.8%, n = 742), and witchcraft/sorcery (12.5%, n = 807) [43]. This same group of participants (n = 888) also believed the virus can be transmitted by blood transfusion (64%), sexual intercourse (40%), animals (30%), and by shaking the hand of an infected person (21%) [48].

Knowledge of the general public on mosquito breeding sites was assessed in ten studies [18, 20, 23, 31–33, 35, 36, 45, 51]. With the exception of one study from Spain, all were conducted in India. Between 2008 and 2010, 84.9% of a studied population in Spain (n = 820) knew about the larval habitats of tiger mosquitoes [51]. In

India, 89% of a surveyed group of health-care workers (n = 100) had knowledge of mosquito breeding sites [31]. Across all studies (Table 3), stagnant water (29–85%) [18, 20, 23, 33, 36] and coconut shells (4.2–73%) [20, 33, 35, 45] were most commonly identified as places where mosquitoes breed. Other breeding places such as cement baths [35], vehicle tires [20, 33], water storage jars [35], broken utensils [45], cracks in the wall, drain and polluted water [32], and desert coolers [20] were cited with lower frequency. Those with first-hand experience of the disease in a case-control study conducted in India were found to have less knowledge on mosquito breeding sites than those who were selected as non-cases [35]. For example, 73% of individuals who did not have the disease (n = 450) knew that mosquitoes breed in coconut shells as opposed to 35% of those who had contracted chikungunya (n = 150) [35].

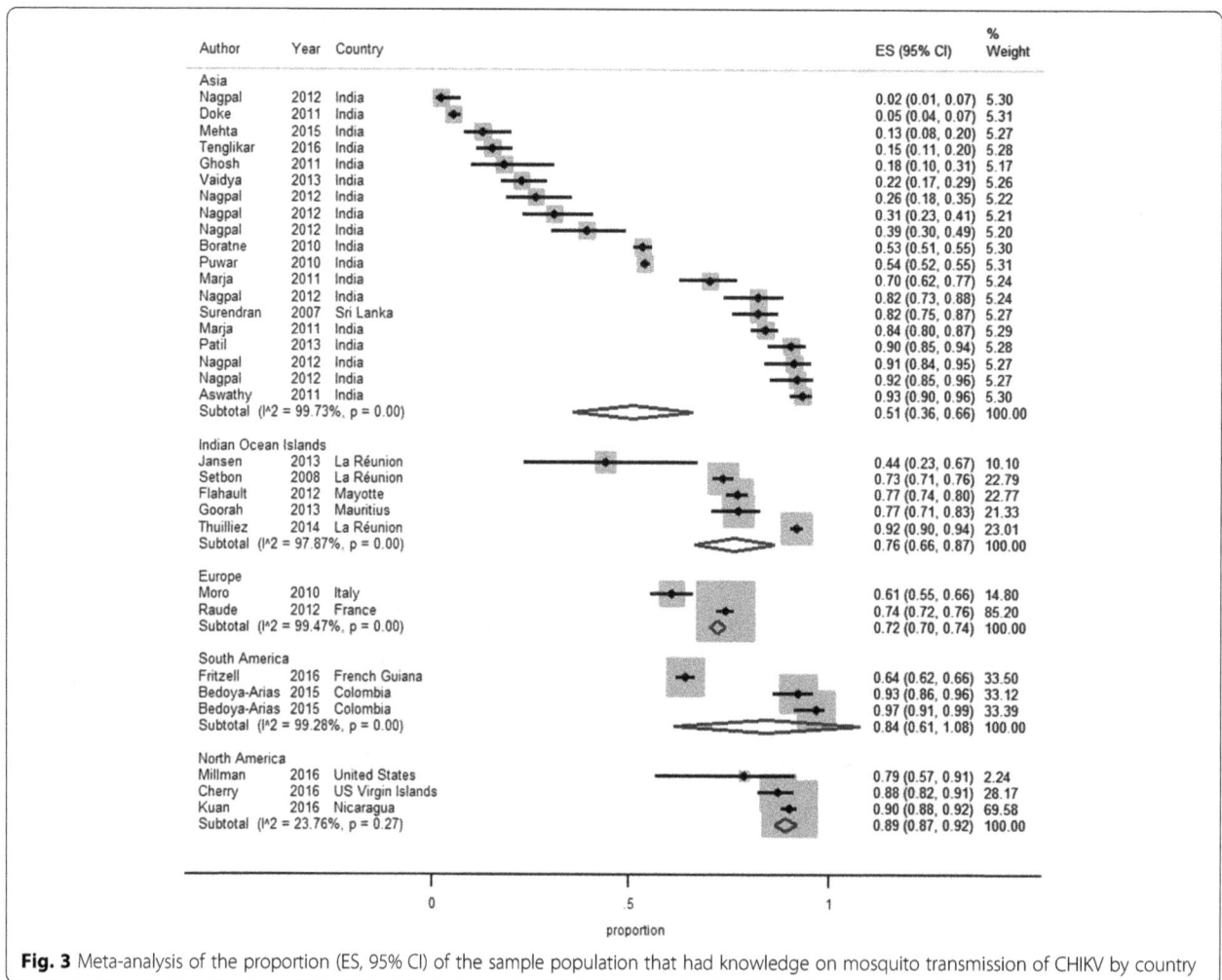

Fig. 3 Meta-analysis of the proportion (ES, 95% CI) of the sample population that had knowledge on mosquito transmission of CHIKV by country

Knowledge, perceptions, and attitudes on mitigation practices

The perception of personal control or "self-responsibility" for mitigation of CHIKV varied among four studies of the general public. In a study conducted in India, 42.7% of participants (n = 178) believed that they were personally responsible for the mitigation of CHIKV [46]. On the Indian Ocean Islands where a large chikungunya outbreak was occurring for the first time, 54% (n = 1021) [41] did not believe they had any control over the disease whereas another study on the island reported that 83.9% (n = 888) [43] believed that chikungunya is controllable. In France, participants indicated they have a moderate level of control over their risk of contracting mosquito borne diseases, mean 7.12 (SD 2.39) on a scale of 0–10, with 0 having absolutely no control and 10 having an extreme amount of control [30].

Knowledge on government measures for the prevention and control of mosquito borne diseases varied across three studies conducted in India, 21.1% (n = 1674), 84% (n = 100), and 88.9% (n = 135) [18, 32, 33]. Following an

outbreak in La Réunion, 55% (n = 999) of the study participants from the general public believed that public authorities had done everything in their power to stop the spread of chikungunya [41]. However, during the same outbreak, the management directives from health authorities in La Réunion were perceived as ineffective by 60.4% (n = 91) of health professionals [52]. Variation on the perceived effectiveness of mitigation measures was also seen between studies of the general public. The perceived effectiveness of CHIKV protective measures was positive in Mayotte (79.7%, n = 888) and La Réunion (64.8%, n = 1024) [42, 43], but in India, only 14% (n = 84) and 28.3% (n = 120) of participants from two studies believed the protective measures to be adequate [18, 32]. The participants from one of the studies in India cited corruption, a late reactive approach, and a lack of accountability in the system as reasons for the inadequacy and ineffective mitigation [18].

Thirteen studies [18–23, 31–33, 35, 43, 45, 46] captured knowledge of the general public on vector control and personal protective measures. The majority (92.3%,

Risk perceptions, attitudes, and knowledge of chikungunya among the public and health...

31

Table 3 General public's knowledge on mosquito breeding sites

REF	Author (year)	Location	Sample size	Results
Stagnant water				
[18]	Anand (2014)	India	100	Stagnant polluted water (29%), stagnant clean water (68%)
[33]	Boratne (2010)	India	1674	Stagnant water (60.7%), ditches (35%), ponds (24%)
[20]	Kohli (2013)	India	350	Stagnant water (60.9%), blocked drains (40%)
[23]	Ghosh (2011)	India	50	Stagnant water (66%)
[36]	Tenglikar (2016)	India	247	Dirty stagnant water (85%)
[32]	Mehta (2015)	India	119	Drain and polluted water (58.8%)
Water - storage and other				
[35]	Majra (2011)	India	150 cases, 450 non-cases	Water storage jars—cases (48%), non-cases (66%)
[32]	Mehta (2015)	India	119	Clean water collection (27.7%)
[36]	Tenglikar (2016)	India	247	Artificial collection of water/water storage (14.6%)
Small containers				
[18]	Anand (2014)	India	100	Desert coolers (20%)
[45]	Aswathy (2011)	India	300	Coconut shells and broken utensils (69%)
[33]	Boratne (2010)	India	1674	Vehicle tires (2.6%); coconut shells (4.2%)
[20]	Kohli (2013)	India	350	Old tires, broken pots and coconut shells (41.4%), desert coolers (26.3%)
[35]	Majra (2011)	India	150 cases, 450 non-cases	Coconut shells—cases (35%), non-cases (73%), tires—cases (13%), non-cases (54%)
Other				
[23]	Ghosh (2011)	India	50	Cracks in walls (2%), earth and air (2%)
[35]	Majra (2011)	India	150 cases, 450 non-cases	Cement baths—cases (28%), non-cases (66%)

$n = 13$) of these studies were conducted in India. Table 4 shows many differences between knowledge of various protective measures across studies. Knowledge on the vector control measures using larvicides (0.8–79.2%) [19, 31, 35] and biological measures (2.9–54.7%) [21, 23, 33] were the least known control measures. Whereas knowledge on using insecticides (5–83.2%) [19, 21, 22, 31, 32, 35] and "chemicals" (34–79.2%) [21, 32, 33], which is likely synonymous with insecticides were widely understood mosquito control measures.

Studies reported a large range in knowledge of personal protective measures (PPMs) (Table 5). Knowledge of the general public and health-care workers on the use of mosquito repellents and bed nets ranged from 0 to 92% in five studies from India [19, 21, 22, 32, 35], while knowledge of wearing protective clothing ranged (1–30%) across two studies from India [22, 45].

When a group of 1462 students in Nicaragua were surveyed about the effectiveness of several preventative measures against mosquito bites, the most commonly reported measures were bed nets (60.6%), sprays (60.5%), window nets (58.6%), and the removal of stagnant water from containers (58.5%) [29]. Wearing protective clothing (35%) and closing windows (33%) were perceived by this group to be less effective at reducing mosquito bites [29].

Knowledge on the availability of a vaccine for chikungunya was assessed in two studies [26, 29]. In a group of students from French Guiana ($n = 1462$), 16% believed there was a vaccine for chikungunya [29]. Of the community service volunteers from the USA traveling to the Dominican Republic who had self-reported pre-travel knowledge on chikungunya, 67% ($n = 19$) correctly answered there is no vaccine available for chikungunya [26]. A community opinion survey on the use of genetically modified mosquitoes as a method of mosquito management was conducted in the USA [44]. This novel approach to mosquito control was opposed by 58% of the respondents ($n = 86$) and the remaining 42% were either neutral or supported the method [44]. When multiple vector control measures were ranked on a scale of 1–5 (1 being the method they support the most and 5 the least), this group was most supportive of draining water on private property to reduce mosquito breeding (mean = 1.98) and least supportive of genetically modified mosquitoes to reduce the mosquito population (mean = 4.14) [44].

Qualitative studies

Two qualitative research articles were identified from the same author [50, 53], both focusing on local experiences and responses to the 2005–2007 chikungunya epidemic in

Table 4 Knowledge of the general public on vector control

	Author (year)	Location	Sample size	Proportion	Preventative measure	Description of outcome
Source reduction of mosquito breeding areas						
[18]	Anand (2014)	India	100	47%	Source reduction	Knowledge on prevention of MBDs
[19]	Patil (2013)	India	154	12.5%	Source reduction	Knowledge on preventing chikungunya
[22]	Nagpal (2012)	India	1000	4–69% across study states	Source reduction	Knowledge on how to eliminate mosquito breeding
[45]	Aswathy (2011)	India	300	39%	Environmental sanitation	Knowledge of the means to prevent mosquito breeding
[33]	Boratne (2010)	India	1674	20.8%	Environmental	Knowledge on vector control measures
[21]	Arpit (2012)	India	274	34.7%	Environmental	Knowledge on mosquito control measures
[20]	Kohli (2013)	India	350	49.7%	Prevent stagnation of water	Knowledge on prevention of MBDs
[31]	Thakor (2015)	India	100	34.7%	Environmental	Knowledge on vector control measures
[32]	Mehta (2015)	India	120	31.6%	Regular cleaning of drainage	Knowledge of government measures to prevent MBDs
[32]	Mehta (2015)	India	103	66%	Keeping surroundings clean and proper drainage	Knowledge on prevention of MBDs
Source reduction from drinking water containers						
[18]	Anand (2014)	India	100	20%	Draining water and cleaning coolers	Knowledge on prevention of MBDs
[45]	Aswathy (2011)	India	300	20.7%	Overturning plastic cups, containers, and other receptacles	Knowledge of measures to prevent mosquito breeding
[20]	Kohli (2013)	India	350	41.1%	Cover water containers	Knowledge on prevention of MBDs
[20]	Kohli (2013)	India	350	21.1%	Cleaning of coolers	Knowledge on prevention of MBDs
[35]	Majra (2011)	India	150 cases, 450 non-cases	36% cases 64% non-cases	Changing stored water frequently	Knowledge on preventative measures
[35]	Majra (2011)	India	150 cases, 450 non-cases	40% cases 68% non-cases	Turning containers upside down	Knowledge on preventative measures
Biological						
[33]	Boratne (2010)	India	1674	2.9%	Biological	Knowledge on vector control measures
[23]	Ghosh (2011)	India	50	8%	Fish	Knowledge on mosquito control
[21]	Arpit (2012)	India	274	54.7%	Biological	Knowledge on mosquito control measures
[31]	Thakor (2015)	India	100	54.7%	Biological	Knowledge on vector control measures
Larvicides						
[19]	Patil (2013)	India	154	0.8%	Larvicides	Knowledge on preventing chikungunya
[35]	Majra (2011)	India	150 cases, 450 non-cases	4% cases 10% non-cases	Using abate	Knowledge on preventative measures
[31]	Thakor (2015)	India	100	79.2%	Anti-larval method	Knowledge on vector control measures
Insecticides						
[19]	Patil (2013)	India	154	33.1%	Insecticide spraying	Knowledge on preventing chikungunya
[22]	Nagpal (2012)	India	1000	5–48% across study States	Treatment with insecticides	Knowledge on how to eliminate mosquito breeding

Table 4 Knowledge of the general public on vector control *(Continued)*

[35]	Majra (2011)	India	150 cases, 450 non-cases	64% cases 68% non-cases	Spraying insecticides	Knowledge on preventative measures
[21]	Arpit (2012)	India	274	83.2%	Space spray	Knowledge on mosquito control measures
[31]	Thakor (2015)	India	100	83.2%	Space spray	Knowledge on vector control measures
[32]	Mehta (2015)	India	120	34.2%	Spraying and fogging	Knowledge of government measures to prevent MBDs
Unspecified Chemical						
[33]	Boratne (2010)	India	1674	61.1%	Chemical	Knowledge on vector control measures
[21]	Arpit (2012)	India	274	79.2%	Chemical	Knowledge on mosquito control measures
[32]	Mehta (2015)	India	103	34%	Spraying chemicals on water and keeping the surrounding clean	Knowledge on prevention of MBDs
[32]	Mehta (2015)	India	120	34.2%	Chemical spraying and cleaning of garbage	Knowledge of government measures to prevent MBDs
Other						
[43]	Raude (2009)	Mayotte	888	59.2%	Vector control	Knowledge of vector control
[33]	Boratne (2010)	India	1674	0.6%	Integrated	Knowledge on vector control measures
[20]	Kohli (2013)	India	350	38.6% 12%	Cleaning up garbage Putting kerosene oil in coolers	Knowledge on prevention of MBDs
[21]	Arpit (2012)	India	274	4%	Genetic method	Knowledge on mosquito control measures

MBD mosquito borne disease

La Réunion. The first article reported on an anthropological study consisting of interviews with 16 residents who believed they had been ill with the disease [53]. Participants had differing beliefs regarding the etiology of chikungunya, with seven participants leaning toward biomedical explanations of CHIKV as vector-borne, while others thought that the infection was air-borne or due to poor sanitary conditions [53].

"Although *bann la* [they, all of them] said that chikungunya is a mosquito, I don't think so because mosquitoes have always existed here in Réunion" (quote from participant, reported in Jansen, 2012).

The second study reported on a discourse analysis of 111 local newspaper articles published in La Réunion during the chikungunya epidemic [50]. These newspapers functioned as a secondary source to communicate local perceptions and experiences with the epidemic [50]. The analysis revealed that coverage of the epidemic began as informational, but became increasingly political at the height of the epidemic, with criticisms of the government's response [50]. For instance, many Réunionese did not believe that chikungunya was transmitted by mosquitoes, but rather that the state was keeping important information from them [50].

Discussion

Risk perceptions, attitudes, and knowledge of chikungunya among the public and health professionals vary across populations and countries as shown in this systematic review. The results suggest that the majority of the populations in the captured studies are uncertain, unaware, or do not understand chikungunya and/or mosquito borne diseases. This is a potential barrier to community and personal protective actions.

Based on the studies captured in this review, there has been limited research on this subject. By employing the scoping and systematic review methodologies and including studies in multiple languages (English, French, Spanish, and Portuguese), we attempted to identify and include all the relevant research on this topic. However, it is possible that some non-indexed studies or studies in other languages were missed. Many of the identified studies investigated participants' knowledge, perceptions, and attitudes of general mosquito borne diseases rather than chikungunya specifically. Also, in many of the countries where people are at risk of contracting chikungunya, they are also at risk of contracting malaria or dengue, which tend to be more well-known diseases among the general public [18]. This may explain why

Table 5 Knowledge of the general public on personal protective measures (PPMs)

	Author (year)	Location	Sample size	Proportion	Preventative measure	Description of outcome
Mosquito repellents						
[21]	Arpit (2012)	India	274	53.3%	Repellents	Knowledge on personal control measures
[22]	Nagpal (2012)	India	1000	12–52% across study states	Repellents	Knowledge on how to protect yourself from mosquitoes
[35]	Majra (2011)	India	150 cases, 450 non-cases	72% cases 30% non-cases	Repellents	Knowledge on preventative measures
[31]	Thakor (2015)	India	100	53.3%	Repellents	Knowledge on personal protection
Mosquito nets						
[21]	Arpit (2012)	India	274	71.9%	Mosquito nets	Knowledge on personal control measures
[22]	Nagpal (2012)	India	1000	0–85% across study states	Bed nets	Knowledge on how to protect yourself from mosquitoes
[35]	Majra (2011)	India	150 cases, 450 non-cases	60% cases 92% non-cases	Mosquito nets	Knowledge on preventative measures
[31]	Thakor (2015)	India	100	71.9%	Mosquito nets	Knowledge on personal protection
Mosquito nets and repellents						
[19]	Patil (2013)	India	154	23.2%	Mosquito nets and repellents	Knowledge on preventing chikungunya
Protective clothing						
[22]	Nagpal (2012)	India	1000	1–30% across study states	Wear body covering clothing	Knowledge on how to protect yourself from mosquitoes
[35]	Majra (2011)	India	150 cases, 450 non-cases	7% cases 24% non-cases	Wearing full dresses	Knowledge on preventative measures
Mosquito proofing home						
[22]	Nagpal (2012)	India	1000	0–6% across study states	Make house mosquito proof	Knowledge on how to protect yourself from mosquitoes
[35]	Majra (2011)	India	150 cases, 450 non-cases	30% cases 70% non-cases	Screening of houses	Knowledge on preventative measures
Other						
[20]	Kohli (2013)	India	350	5.7%	Using PPMs	Knowledge on prevention of MBDs
[43]	Raude (2009)	Mayotte	888	60.5%	Self-protective behavior	Knowledge of self-protective behavior
[18]	Anand (2014)	India	100	93%	PPMs	Knowledge on prevention of MBDs
[46]	Vaidya (2013)	India	178	74.2%	Cleaning	Knowledge on protective measures

MBD mosquito borne disease

some populations were knowledgeable on vector control and personal protective measures but have low levels of awareness on chikungunya. Although the disease is endemic in many areas of Africa, Asia, and the Pacific and Indian Ocean Islands, the majority of the studies to date (43%, $n = 37$) were conducted in India which has recorded outbreaks of chikungunya for several decades, or La Réunion Island, which experienced a large outbreak in 2005–2006. Based on the geographic distribution of chikungunya, the current studies do not represent all chikungunya-affected populations or even a representative sample. Thus, the knowledge, attitudes, and perceptions

of chikungunya-affected populations that are not represented may be different and their absence is a knowledge gap in this review.

The risk of bias assessment and data extraction revealed that the studies captured in this review were not well reported and were missing some critical details. This decreases our confidence in the findings of the studies identified and prevents a reliable interpretation of their results. Across studies, the outcomes reported were not comparable to each other thus preventing synthesis of results or comparisons across populations. Future standardization of outcomes would improve the comparability of results across studies making them easier to synthesize and draw more generalizable conclusions about the consistency, direction, and magnitude of the results.

There was a lack of qualitative research on the topic, and it was suggested that there is a need for greater understanding and consideration of varying cultural explanations and for conceptualizations of CHIKV etiology to more effectively address and respond to outbreaks in affected communities [53]. This is supported by some of the beliefs and misunderstandings of respondents in several surveys from this systematic review. The importance of cultural practices and community perception can be critical to the success of epidemic control measures as was the case during the 2014 Ebola outbreak in West Africa [54]. Social stigmatization and deeply ingrained cultural practices such as ritual washing of the deceased and the consumption of bush meat threatened the success of mitigation efforts [55, 56]. Investigating underlying social factors associated with chikungunya and barriers and facilitators to potential mitigation options through qualitative research would be useful for designing future education and control strategies.

Risk perceptions, attitudes, beliefs, and knowledge are important predictors of an individuals' behavior toward mosquito borne disease [57, 58]. The relationship between these variables and an individuals' behavior can be explained and predicted by different theories of behavior change, such as the Health Belief Model, Theory of Planned Behavior, and the Stages of Change Model [59]. These theories provide formal and structured frameworks for investigating predictors of health behaviors and for designing health behavior change inventions; however, only nine studies in this review used a formal theory of behavior change to guide their data collection [22, 25, 29, 34, 36, 40, 45, 46, 60]. Future studies should use theories of behavior change to investigate the psychosocial risk factors for chikungunya prevention and to design future education and control strategies for CHIKV.

Studies that looked at the general knowledge and perceptions on chikungunya varied across populations and countries. As expected, higher awareness of chikungunya was found in areas affected by an outbreak. This is most likely due to public education, media, and personal experience with the disease. There may also be a difference between recognizing a disease with no depth in knowledge, which is perceived as being informed, compared to factual knowledge about the disease. One study identified literacy, a socio-economic factor that can be considered a surrogate for education and knowledge, as a significant confounder [33]. Other studies found that gender and age were predictors of higher knowledge levels; however, these findings were less consistent and should be investigated further.

Limited studies were conducted on the perceptions of the risk and severity of chikungunya. Two studies that found a high perceived severity of the disease were both conducted on the Indian Ocean Islands [41, 43]. This is to be expected as the studies occurred shortly after the large outbreak in 2005–2006. In contrast, the study in France, where many mosquito borne diseases are not endemic, showed that although the participants recognized the severity of mosquito borne diseases, they were not worried about contracting them [30].

There was a lot of heterogeneity in the level of knowledge on transmission of CHIKV by mosquitoes between studies, likely due to the outbreak status of the area and the amount of public education that had occurred. Knowledge on general mosquito breeding sites was generally higher, which could be attributed in part to the fact that malaria and dengue are endemic in many of these countries and are well-known diseases among the general public. Higher knowledge about vector control and personal protective measures in endemic countries such as India are also likely the result of the presence of many endemic mosquito borne diseases.

The perception of personal control or "self-responsibility" for mitigation was only investigated in a few studies. Since self-efficacy is one of the most important variables in most of the theories of behavior change [59], it would be useful to study perception of control over protection from CHIKV or mosquito borne diseases as a determinant of personal protective behaviors and what education strategies are most likely to empower the individual to participate in proposed mitigation strategies.

This review encompassed knowledge, attitudes, and perceptions of both the general public and health professionals. However, the majority (86.5%, $n = 37$) of studies were conducted on the general public. There were no direct comparisons done between the general public and health professionals. Only one outcome, knowledge of CHIKV transmission by mosquitoes, looked at both populations. As expected, health professionals had higher levels of knowledge that mosquitoes transmit CHIKV than the general public. Most of the studies with health professionals measured knowledge of symptoms and perceptions on various treatments. Information from different populations is needed to inform the design of future education and control strategies.

Almost all populations in the studies included in this review were from developing countries with a large proportion of poorly educated individuals that have little to no disposable income. Thus, the affordability of mitigation measures needs to be considered when developing control strategies. For example, although it was shown that insecticides were the most commonly known mitigation strategy, that might not be the best strategy for a community with no disposable income for the insecticides.

Conclusion

Overall, this review identified, assessed, and analyzed the global literature on the knowledge, attitudes, and perceptions of CHIKV and its transmission in affected populations. The results indicated that there is variability across populations and countries, but most of the captured populations are uncertain, unaware, or do not understand chikungunya and/or mosquito borne diseases. As the disease continues to spread into previously non-endemic areas, it is recommended that research efforts be increased to close some of the knowledge gaps or better understand the uncertainty identified in this SR with respect to the impact knowledge, attitudes, and perceptions of chikungunya and personal protective measures can have on affected and non-affected populations. Investigations into what motivates individuals to adopt personal protective and vector control measures at home and within their communities will aid in the design and implementation of effective education and control strategies. Researchers in this area are encouraged to follow guidelines on conduct and reporting based on study design to minimize bias in their research and enhance the clarity of their article for use by other researchers and decision makers.

Abbreviations

CHIKV: Chikungunya virus; CINAHL: The Cumulative Index to Nursing and Allied Health Literature; LILACS: Latin American and Caribbean Health Sciences Literature; MBD: Mosquito borne disease; PPM: Personal protective measure; PRISMA: Preferred Reporting Items for Systematic Reviews and Meta-Analyses; SR: Systematic review

Acknowledgements

Not applicable.

Funding

This research did not receive any specific grant from funding agencies in the public, commercial, or not-for-profit sectors.

Authors' contributions

TC analyzed and interpreted the data. The data was extracted from all studies, and risk of bias was assessed by TC and CH. LW and MM provided extensive feedback and mentorship throughout the project. All authors read, provided feedback, and approved the final manuscript.

Competing interests

The authors declare that they have no competing interests.

Author details

[1]Public Health Risk Sciences Division, National Microbiology Laboratory, Public Health Agency of Canada, Guelph, ON, Canada. [2]Department of Population Medicine, University of Guelph, Guelph, ON, Canada. [3]School of Occupational and Public Health, Ryerson University, Toronto, ON, Canada.

References

1. Staples EJ, Breiman RF, Powers AM. Chikungunya fever: an epidemiological review of a re-emerging infectious disease. Clin Infect Dis. 2009. doi:10.1086/605496.
2. Thiberville SD, Moyen N, Dupuis-Maguiraga L, Nougairede A, Gould EA, Rogues P, et al. Chikungunya fever: epidemiology, clinical syndrome, pathogenesis and therapy. Antivir Res. 2013. doi:10.1016/j.antiviral.2013.06.009.
3. Centers for Disease Control and Prevention. Chikungunya virus. 2015. https://www.cdc.gov/chikungunya/geo/united-states-2015.html. Accessed 22 July 2016.
4. Weaver SC, Forrester NL. Chikungunya: evolutionary history and recent epidemic spread. Antivir Res. 2015. doi:10.1016/j.antiviral.2015.04.016.
5. European Centre for Disease Control and Prevention. Chikungunya. 2016. https://ecdc.europa.eu/en/chikungunya. Accessed 19 July 2016.
6. Pan American Health Organization. Chikungunya. 2016. http://www.paho.org/hq/index.php?option=com_topics&view=article&id=343&Itemid=40931. Accessed 19 July 2016.
7. Drebot MA, Holloway K, Zheng H, Ogden NH. Travel-related chikungunya cases in Canada, 2014. Canada communicable disease report CCDR. 2015. http://www.phac-aspc.gc.ca/publicat/ccdr-rmtc/15vol41/dr-rm41-01/rapid-eng.php. Accessed 22 July 2016.
8. World Health Organization. Neglected tropical diseases. 2016. http://www.who.int/neglected_diseases/vector_ecology/VCAG/en/. Accessed 22 July 2016.
9. Henderson LK, Craig JC, Willis NS, Tovey D, Webster AC. How to write a Cochrane systematic review. Nephrology. 2010. doi:10.1111/j.1440-1797.2010.01380.x.
10. Moher D, Liberati A, Tezlaff J, Altman DG, PRISMA Group. Preferred reporting items for systematic reviews and meta-analyses: the PRISMA statement. Ann Intern Med. 2009;151:264–9.
11. Tranfield D, Denyer D, Smart P. Towards a methodology for developing evidence-informed management knowledge by means of systematic review. Brit J Manage. 2003;14:207–22.
12. Critical Appraisal Skills Programme. 2013. http://www.casp-uk.net/. Accessed 3 Aug 2016.
13. GRADE. 2016. http://www.gradeworkinggroup.org/. Accessed 3 Aug 2016.
14. Lundh A, Gøtzsche PC. Recommendations by Cochrane review groups for assessment of the risk of bias in studies. BMC Med Res Methodol. 2008. doi:10.1186/1471-2288-8-22.
15. DerSimonian R, Laird N. Meta-analysis in clinical trials. Control Clin Trials. 1986;7:177–88.
16. Higgins JP, Thomson SG, Deeks JJ, Altman DG. Measuring inconsistency in meta-analyses. BMJ. 2003. doi:10.1136/bmj.327.7414.557.
17. Mays N, Pope C, Popay J. Systematically reviewing qualitative and quantitative evidence to inform management and policy-making in the health field. J Health Serv Res Policy. 2005;10(Suppl 1):6–20.
18. Anand T, Kumar R, Saini V, Meena G, Ingle G. Knowledge and use of personal protective measures against mosquito borne diseases in a resettlement Colony of Delhi. Ann Med Health Sci Res. 2014. doi:10.4103/2141-9248.129048.
19. Patil SS, Patil SR, Durgawale PM, Patil AG. A study of the outbreak of Chikungunya fever. J Clin Diagn Res. 2013. doi:10.7860/JCDR/2013/5330.3061.
20. Kohli C, Kumar R, Meena GS, Singh MM, Ingle GK. Awareness about mosquito borne diseases in rural and urban areas of Delhi. J Commun Disord. 2013;45:201–7.
21. Arpit P, Sonal P, Manish F, DV B. Impact of educational intervention regarding mosquito borne diseases and their control measures among the link Workers of Urban Health Centers (UHCs) of Ahmedabad City. Natl J Community Med. 2012;3:178–82.
22. Nagpal BN, Saxena R, Srivastava A, Singh N, Ghosh SK, Sharma SK, et al. Retrospective study of chikungunya outbreak in urban areas of India. Indian J Med Res. 2012;135:351–8.
23. Ghosh SK, Chakaravarthy P, Panch SR, Krishnappa P, Tiwari S, Ojha VP, et al. Comparative efficacy of two poeciliid fish in indoor cement tanks against chikungunya vector Aedes Aegypti in villages in Karnataka. India BMC Public Health. 2011. doi:10.1186/1471-2458-11-599.
24. Surendran SN, Kannathasan S, Kajatheepan A, Jude PJ. Chikungunya-type fever outbreak: some aspects related to this new epidemic in Jaffna district, northern Sri Lanka. Trop Med Health. 2007;35:249–52.
25. Cherry CC, Beer KD, Fulton C, Wong D, Buttke D, Staples JE, et al. Knowledge and use of prevention measures for chikungunya virus among visitors––Virgin Islands National Park, 2015. Travel Med Infect Dis. 2016. doi:10.1016/j.tmaid.2016.08.011.

26. Millman AJ, Esposito DH, Biggs HM, Decenteceo M, Klevos A, Hunsperger E, et al. Chikungunya and dengue virus infections among United States community service volunteers returning from the Dominican Republic, 2014. Am J Trop Med Hyg. 2016. doi:10.4269/ajtmh.15-0815.

27. Kuan G, Ramirez S, Gresh L, Ojeda S, Melendez M, Sanchez N, et al. Seroprevalence of anti-Chikungunya virus antibodies in children and adults in Managua, Nicaragua, after the first Chikungunya epidemic, 2014–2015. PLoS Negl Trop Dis. 2016. doi:10.1371/journal.pntd.0004773.

28. Doke PP, Dakhure DS, Patil AV. A clinico-epidemiological study of chikungunya outbreak in Maharashtra state. India Indian J Public Health. 2011. doi:10.4103/0019-557X.92413.

29. Fritzell C, Raude J, Adde A, Dusfour I, Quenel P, Flamand C. Knowledge, attitude and practices of vector-borne disease prevention during the emergence of a new Arbovirus: implications for the control of Chikungunya virus in French Guiana. PLoS Negl Trop Dis. 2016. doi:10.1371/journal.pntd.0005081.

30. Raude J, Chinfatt K, Huang P, Betansedi CO, Katumba K, Vernazza N, et al. Public perceptions and behaviours related to the risk of infection with Aedes mosquito-borne diseases: a cross-sectional study in southeastern France. BMJ Open. 2012. doi:10.1136/bmjopen-2012-002094.

31. Thakor NC, Vikani SK, Nagar AA. Impact of educational intervention regarding mosquito-borne diseases and their control measures among multipurpose health workers (MPHWs) of Patan district, Gujarat, India. Int J Med Sci Public Health. 2015;4:1620–3.

32. Mehta D, Solanki H, Patel P, Umat P, Chauhan R, Shukla S, et al. A study on knowledge, attitude & practice regarding mosquito borne diseases in an urban area of Bhavnagar. Health. 2015;6:29–32.

33. Boratne AV, Jayanthi V, Datta SS, Singh Z, Senthilvel V, Joice YS. Predictors of knowledge of selected mosquito-borne diseases among adults of selected peri-urban areas of Puducherry. J Vector Borne Dis. 2010;47:249–56.

34. Bedoya-Arias JE, Murillo-García DR, Bolaños-Muñoz E, Hurtado-Hurtado N, Ramírez-Jaramillo V, Granados-Álvarez S, et al. Healthcare students and workers' knowledge about epidemiology and symptoms of chikungunya fever in two cities in Colombia. J Infect Dev Ctries. 2015. doi:10.3855/jidc.6445.

35. Majra JP, Acharya D. Impact of knowledge and practices on prevention of chikungunya in an epidemic area in India. Ann Trop Med PH. 2011;4:3–6.

36. Tenglikar PV, Hussain M, Nigudgi SR, Ghooli S. Knowledge and practices regarding mosquito borne disease among people of an urban area in Kalaburgi, Karnataka. Natl J Community Med. 2016;7:223–5.

37. Claeys C, Robles C, Bertaudiere-Montes V, Deschamps-Cottin M, Megnifo HT, Pelagie-Moutenda R, et al. Socio-ecological factors contributing to the exposure of human populations to mosquito bites that transmit dengue fever, chikungunya and zika viruses: a comparison between mainland France and the French Antilles. Environ Risque Sante. 2016;15:318–25.

38. Hsu LY, Jin J, Ang BS, Kurup A, Tambyah PA. Hand hygiene and infection control survey pre- and peri-H1N1-2009 pandemic: knowledge and perceptions of final year medical students in Singapore. Signapore Med J. 2011;52:486–90.

39. Dilip C, Saraswathi R, Krishnan PN, Azeem AK, Raseena A, Ramya JJ. Comparative evaluation of different systems of medicines and the present scenario of chikungunya in Kerala. Asian Pac J Trop Med. 2010. doi:10.1016/S1995-7645(10)60106-X.

40. Moro ML, Gagliotti C, Silvi G, Angelini R, Sambri V, Rezza G. Knowledge, attitudes and practices survey after an outbreak of chikungunya infections. Int Health. 2010. doi:10.1016/j.inhe.2010.07.003.

41. Setbon M, Raude J. Chikungunya on Réunion Island: social, environmental and Behavioural factors in an epidemic context. Population. 2008. doi:10.3917/popu.803.0555.

42. Thuilliez J, Bellia C, Dehecq JS, Reilhes O. Household-level expenditure on protective measures against mosquitoes on the island of La Reunion. France PLoS Negl Trop Dis. 2014. doi:10.1371/journal.pntd.0002609.

43. Raude J, Setbon M. The role of environmental and individual factors in the social epidemiology of chikungunya disease on Mayotte Island. Health Place. 2009. doi:10.1016/j.healthplace.2008.10.009.

44. Adalja A, Sell TK, McGinty M, Boddie C. Genetically modified (GM) mosquito use to reduce mosquito-transmitted disease in the US: a community opinion survey. PLoS Curr. 2016. doi:10.1371/currents.outbreaks.

45. Aswathy S, Dinesh S, Kurien B, Johnson AJ, Leelamoni K. A post-epidemic study on awareness of vector habits of Chikungunya and vector indices in a rural area of Kerala. J Commun Disord. 2011;43:209–15.

46. Vaidya V, Sawant S. A KAP study in Pune City involving school children as a strategy for effective vector control in Chikungunya. Indian J Public Health. 2013. doi:10.5958/j.0976-5506.4.4.181.

47. Puwar T, Sheth JK, Kohli V, Yadav R. Prevalence of chikungunya in the city of Ahmedabad, India, during the 2006 outbreak. WHO Dengue Bulletin. 2010. http://apps.who.int/iris/bitstream/10665/170980/1/db2010v34p40.pdf. Accessed 7 June 2016.

48. Flahault A, Aumont G, Boisson V, de Lamballerie X, Favier F, Fontenille D, et al. An interdisciplinary approach to controlling chikungunya outbreaks on french islands in the south-west indian ocean. Med Trop (Mars). 2012;72:66–71.

49. Goorah S, Dewkurun MK, Ramchurn SK. Assessing the sustainability of individual behavior change against mosquitos after the outbreak of a vector-borne disease in Mauritius: a case study. IJMU. 2013;8:9–16.

50. Jansen KA. The 2005-2007 Chikungunya epidemic in Reunion: ambiguous etiologies, memories, and meaning-making. Med Anthropol. 2013; doi:10.1080/01459740.2012.679981.

51. Abramides GC, Roiz D, Guitart R, Quintana S, Giménez N. Control of the Asian tiger mosquito (Aedes Albopictus) in a firmly established area in Spain: risk factors and people's involvement. Trans R Soc Trop Med Hyg. 2013; doi:10.1093/trstmh/trt093.

52. Fenétrier E, Sissoko D, Vernazza-Licht N, Bley D, Gaüzère BA, Malvy D. Feedback from primary care practitioners two years after the chikungunya epidemic on Reunion. Bull Soc Pathol Exot. 2013; doi:10.1007/s13149-013-0295-8.

53. Jansen KA. The printed press's representations of the 2005–2007 chikungunya epidemic Réunion: political polemics and (post)colonial disease. J Afr Media Stud. 2012;4:227–42.

54. Scott V, Crawford-Browne S, Sanders D. Critiquing the response to the Ebola epidemic through a Primary Health Care Approach. BMC Public Health. doi:10.1186/s12889-016-3071-4.

55. Alexander KA, Sanderson CE, Marathe M, Lewis BL, Rivers CM, Shaman J, et al. What factors might have led to the emergence of Ebola in West Africa? PLoS Negl Trop Dis. 2015; doi:10.1371/journal.pntd.0003652.

56. Phua KL. Meeting the challenge of Ebola virus disease in a holistic manner by taking into account socioeconomic and cultural factors: the experience of West Africa. Infect Dis (Auckl). 2015; doi:10.4137/IDRT.S31568.

57. Beaujean DJMA, Bults M, van Steenbergen JE, Voeten HACM. Study on public perceptions and protective behaviors regarding Lyme disease among the general public in the Netherlands: implications for prevention programs. BMC Public Health. 2013; doi:10.1186/1471-2458-13-225.

58. Trumbo CW, Harper R. Perceptual influences on self-protective behavior for West Nile virus, a survey in Colorado. USA BMC Public Health. 2015; doi:10.1186/s12889-015-1918-8.

59. Edberg MC. Essentials of health behaviour. Burlington: Social and Behavioural Theory in Public Health. Jones and Bartlett Publishers, Inc; 2007.

60. Vilain P, Larrieu S, Renault P, Baville M, Filleul L. How to explain the re-emergence of chikungunya infection in Reunion Island in 2010? Acta Trop. 2012. doi:10.1016/j.actatropica.2012.03.009.

61. Boyer S, Foray C, Dehecq JS. Spatial and temporal heterogeneities of Aedes albopictus density in La Reunion Island: rise and weakness of entomological indices. PLoS One. 2014. doi:10.1371/journal.pone.0091170.

4

Efficacy and safety of praziquantel against *Schistosoma haematobium* in the Ikata-Likoko area of southwest Cameroon

Calvin Bisong Ebai[1*], Helen Kuokuo Kimbi[1,2], Irene Ule Ngole Sumbele[1], Jude Ebah Yunga[1] and Leopold Gustave Lehman[3]

Abstract

Background: Schistosomiasis remains a parasitic infection of public health importance especially in Africa south of the Sahara including Cameroon. Chemotherapy using praziquantel has been the most effective and widespread control measure used. However, there are reports of reduced efficacy of the drug. The aim of this study was to assess the efficacy and safety of praziquantel against *Schistosoma haematobium* among infected individuals in the Ikata-Likoko area of southwest Cameroon. Following a baseline study, *S. haematobium* egg load was determined using the urine filtration technique and microscopy. Participants were treated with a unique dose of praziquantel of 40 mg/Kg body weight. A control test was carried out on the 42nd day post-treatment to determine the proportion of positive participants with viable eggs (cure rate) and the egg loads. The egg loads obtained during the control and at baseline were used to calculate the egg reduction rate (ERR) used as the main indicator of praziquantel efficacy according to the WHO, 2013 protocol.

Results: At baseline, the prevalence of *S. haematobium* was 34.3% (177/516). Out of these a total of 174 participants aged between 4 and 76 years were recruited into the study. A total of 130 participants came for follow up on day 42. Among them, 22.3% (29) were positive for eggs of *S. haematobium* but none of the eggs were viable giving a cure rate of 100%. The overall mean egg load per 10 mL (MEL/10 mL) of urine reduced from 31 (1–400) at baseline to 6.0 (1–35) on day 42. The overall ERR was reduced (80.3%). However, the efficacy was satisfactory (ERR ≥ 90%) in females, children < 5 years, and some localities and for individuals with heavy infection intensity. Fifteen (8.6%) of the participants presented minor adverse events including abdominal disorders, headache and vomiting but did not last for more than 24 h.

Conclusions: Treatment with praziquantel was efficacious and safe showing reduction in prevalence as well as mean egg load in some individuals with few adverse events recorded. The distribution of praziquantel in the area should be extended to other age groups and not just school-age children. A study with multiple drug doses and longer period of evaluation could reveal more information on praziquantel efficacy in the area.

Keywords: Cameroon, Efficacy, Egg reduction rate, Praziquantel, Safety, *Schistosoma haematobium*

* Correspondence: ebaipi2000@yahoo.com
[1]Department of Zoology and Animal Physiology, Faculty of Science, University of Buea, P.O. Box 63, Buea, SWR, Cameroon
Full list of author information is available at the end of the article

Background

Schistosomiasis remains a parasitic infection of public health importance in many tropical and subtropical countries especially in Africa south of the Sahara. The World Health Organization (WHO) estimates that up to 218.8 million people in the world with a majority of them in sub-Saharan Africa required treatment for schistosomiasis in 2015 [1]. Effectively, more than 66 million received preventive chemotherapy with praziquantel (PZQ). In addition to chemotherapy, other measures to fight against the disease include snail (intermediate host) control, basic sanitation, supply of safe water and health education either separately or in combination [2]. Globally, chemotherapy has been the most widespread antischistosomal measure used. Although, several drugs have been found to be efficacious against all five species of *Schistosoma* [3], praziquantel has been the most widely used. It is a pyrazinoquinoline derivative whose safety and efficacy have ensured its widespread usage. Although it is found to be associated with minor adverse events such as abdominal disorder, nausea and vomiting [4, 5], PZQ remains active against adult schistosomes [6]. It has also been reported to improve on the morbidity of the disease, with some clinical signs and symptoms such as haematuria, abdominal pain and dysuria subsiding shortly following treatment [7–9]. Considering that the disease has a focal distribution, the WHO recommends that distribution of praziquantel should be done following the prevalence in the communities. In this regard, in high-risk communities where parasitological prevalence is ≥ 50% and visible haematuria is ≥ 30%, children of school age and adults considered to be at risk should be treated once a year. Meanwhile, in moderate-risk communities where parasite prevalence is ≥ 10% but < 50%, all school-age children and adults considered to be at risk should receive treatment once every 2 years. In the same light, in low-risk communities where parasite prevalence is < 10%, all school-age children should be treated twice during primary school age while praziquantel is made available in health care institutions for treatment of suspected cases. Unfortunately, reports have indicated the availability of suboptimal brands of the drug in the market thus adding to the already existing pressure on the drug and to the reported resistance developed by the parasites [10, 11].

Urinary schistosomiasis caused by *Schistosoma haematobium* is reportedly prevalent in Cameroon [12–16], and its main control measure has been mass distribution of PZQ to school children since 2004. Unfortunately, there have been reports about the increasing problem of reduced efficacy of the drug in some countries [17] such as Zimbabwe [18], Egypt [19] and Cameroon [10, 15]. However, there has been no assessment of its efficacy in many foci in the Southwest Region of Cameroon including the Ikata-Likoko area in the Mount Cameroon Region where the disease is prevalent [14, 16]. Against this background, this study was carried out to assess the efficacy and safety of PZQ in the Ikata-Likoko area of southwest Cameroon.

Methods
Study area

This study was carried out in the Ikata-Likoko area comprised of four rural localities, Ikata, Bafia, Mile 14 and Likoko in the southwest of Cameroon. Ikata is located between longitudes 9.363 E and 9.352 E and latitudes 4.329 N and 4.328 N and between 87 and 132 m above sea level. Bafia is between longitudes 9.324 E and 9.311 E and latitudes 4.350 N and 4.363 N and is 229 to 256 m above sea level. Mile 14 is located between longitudes 9.302 E and 9.292 E and latitudes 4.396 N and 4.401 N and between 157 and 168 m above sea level. Likoko is located between longitudes 9.319 E and 9.320 E and latitudes 4.399 N and 4.393 N and is between 108 and 116 m above sea level. Access to these villages from the main town is through an earth road which is usually muddy in the rainy season. The topography of the area is characterized by hills and valleys. Rainfall averages 3126.7 mm annually while temperature varies between 23 and 33 °C with an annual average of about 26.2 °C. There are two major seasons in the area, the rainy (March to October) and the dry (November to February) seasons. The vegetation is mainly the tropical forest type. More details on the study area were already published with baseline data of this study by Ebai et al. [20]. Earlier studies by Ntonifor et al. [14] and Kimbi et al. [16] carried out in localities near this study area have shown that only *S. haematobium* is present in the area. Mass distribution of praziquantel by the Ministry of Health in Cameroon is done in schools. Personal communication with village authorities and participants indicate that the last distribution of praziquantel in the schools dated more than 2 years before this study was started.

Study population

Participants in this study were individuals who had spent at least 2 months in the study area, were aged 1 year and above, were positive for *S. haematobium* in the baseline study and who gave their informed consent. Assent for minors was obtained from parents or legal guardians.

Participants with signs of chronic or severe illness, such as cardiac, renal or hepatic disease, HIV/AIDS, severe diarrhoea, and dehydration, and those with history of treatment with PZQ in the past 2 months, with hypersensitive reaction to PZQ, and pregnant or breast feeding mothers were excluded from the study [3]. Also, participants with residence out of the study area and those who violated the study protocol, used other antischistosomal drug, and withdrew their assent or consent or could not be attended to during follow up were excluded from the study.

Study design

This was a prospective study carried out between June and September, 2014. After obtaining administrative and ethical clearances, visits to the village authorities were scheduled during which the procedures and the benefits of the study as well as the dates and collection venues for the study were presented. A structured questionnaire was used to collect data on the socio-demography of the participants. Urine samples were collected and transported to the Malaria Research Laboratory of the University of Buea for parasitological analyses. Individuals who were positive for *S. haematobium* were treated with praziquantel and enrolled into the study. The follow up was done on the 42nd day post-treatment, during which parasitological analyses were repeated to detect the presence, density and viability of *S. haematobium* eggs.

Administration of questionnaire

Socio-demographic data collected through the use of questionnaire included age, sex, level of educational attainment, religion and occupation. The body weight was measured using a floor scale (Seca GmbH & Co. Germany). Concerning general health, participants were asked if they were suffering from any chronic disease, were on any treatment or had taken PZQ within the last 6 months. Questionnaires were administered in English and exceptionally in Pidgin English where necessary.

Urine sample collection and laboratory analyses

Labelled 50-mL containers were given to participants for the collection of urine samples. Collection was done between 10 a.m. and 2 p.m. which is the period corresponding with the peak excretion of schistosome eggs [21]. Immediately after collection, the samples were tested biochemically for the presence of blood (haematuria) using urine test strips (Medi test Combi 9, Germany). The urine containers were corked and transported in cool boxes to the Malaria Research Laboratory of the University of Buea for parasitological analyses.

Ten milliliter of each urine sample was analysed for schistosome eggs using the syringe filtration method as described by Cheesbrough [21]. Filtration was done by passing 10 mL of urine through a filter (STERLITECH Corporation, USA) which retains the schistosome eggs. The filter was placed on a microscope slide and examined under × 10 objective of a light microscope (Olympus, USA). The number of eggs counted was reported per 10 mL of urine. Eggs detected were tested for viability by adding a drop of methylene blue on every positive slide. Viable eggs remained colourless while non-viable eggs were stained blue [21]. Participants who had ≤ 50 eggs/10 mL of urine were classified as light infections while those with > 50 eggs/10 mL of urine were heavy infections.

Treatment and follow up of *S. haematobium* infection

Participants who were positive for eggs of *S. haematobium* were treated with praziquantel oral tablets (Cesol™ 600, Germany, batch number M25343) at 40 mg/Kg body weight in a unique dose alongside snacks as recommended by WHO [3]. Those who received the tablets were under observation for at least 4 h, and any adverse events were recorded. Adverse events were defined as any manifestation that was absent at baseline but present after swallowing the praziquantel tablets. On day 42 post-treatment, urine samples were collected from the participants and analysed for *S. haematobium* eggs. When found, the eggs were counted and tested for viability. Participants who did not show up for the control were contacted on telephone and attended to in their homes. Those who were not attended to on this day were excluded from the study. This was to avoid reinfection cases.

Endpoints for follow up of praziquantel efficacy

The primary endpoint of this study was the efficacy of PZQ which was classified into three levels by comparing the observed egg reduction rate (ERR) with the 90% reference value [3]. Hence, the drug efficacy was either of the following: satisfactory if the ERR ≥ 90%, reduced if the ERR ≥ 80% but < 90% or doubtful if the ERR < 80%. The secondary endpoints were the prevalence at follow up and the cure rate. A cured participant in this study was defined as one who was positive for urinary schistosomiasis (US) with viable eggs on day 0, received PZQ treatment and was negative for US on day 42, or was positive for US but the eggs detected were non-viable [3].

Statistical analysis

Data was entered into Excel version 2013 and analysed using IBM Statistical Package for Social Sciences (IBM SPSS) version 20 (IBM Inc. 2012). Results were summarized into proportions and means. Proportions were compared using the Cramer's (V) and chi-square (χ^2) tests, and the Mann-Whitney test (U) was used to compare mean egg loads for two groups while the Kruskall-Wallis test (H) was used to compare mean egg loads for more than two groups. The Wilcoxon signed-rank test (Z) was used to compare mean egg loads at day 0 and day 42. The ERR was calculated from the formula: ERR (%) = 100 × 1 – [arithmetic mean egg counts on day 42/ arithmetic mean egg counts at baseline] [3]. The level of significance was set at $P < 0.05$.

Results

Characteristics of the study population

At baseline, the prevalence of *S. haematobium* was 34.3% (177/516). Out of the 177 participants who were positive for *S. haematobium*, a total of 174, 84 males and 90 females, with an age range of 4–76 years and mean age ± SD of 23.8 ± 17.5 years were enrolled into the study (Table 1). They had a MEL/10 mL of urine of 30 (1–400). All the eggs detected were viable. None of the participants had taken anti-schistosomal treatment during the past 6 months before the commencement of the study. Out of the 174 participants enrolled, 130 (74.7%) came for follow up on day 42 out of which 29 (22.3%) were positive for US with all the eggs being non-viable, giving a cure rate of 100%. On day 42 post-treatment, the overall MEL/10 mL of urine was 6.0 (range, 1–35). The overall efficacy was reduced with an egg reduction rate (ERR) of 80.3%.

Efficacy of praziquantel with respect to gender and age

With respect to gender, the prevalence of US reduced significantly in both sexes following treatment, from 100% on day 0 to 10.0% on day 42 for the male participants and from 100 to 12.3% for the females. Comparing the prevalence and mean egg load after treatment for

males and females did not show any statistically significant difference (Table 2). On the contrary, there were significant reductions in MEL/10 mL of urine from 32 to 12 for the males (Z = 3.854, P < 0.001) and from 29 to 3 for the females (Z = 4.231, P < 0.001). The ERR was satisfactory in females (90%) but doubtful in males (62.5%).

There were significant reductions in the prevalence of US in all age groups (P = 0.0004) following treatment as well as the MEL/10 mL (P = 0.02). The ERR was highest in children less than 5 years (100%) when compared with other age groups.

Efficacy of praziquantel with respect to socio-demographic factors

In terms of occupation, a statistically significant reduction in prevalence (V = 0.2, P = 0.0007) was observed with the highest reduction recorded among farmers, from 100% (66) on day 0 to 7.0% (9) on day 42 while, the least reduction was among semi-skilled workers, from a prevalence of 100% (7) to 1.5% (2). Although there was a reduction in the mean egg loads/10 mL of urine among the different occupations, the difference was not statistically significant (H = 3.5, P = 0.32) (Table 3).

A significant reduction in prevalence post-treatment was observed in all the localities, with the highest reduction occurring in Mile 14 from 100% (73) to 10% (13), whereas the least prevalence was recorded in Likoko, from 100% (48) to 2.3% (3). MEL/10 mL of urine reduced significantly in three of the localities (P < 0.05) except in Bafia (Z = − 1.572, P = 0.116). Satisfactory ERR were observed in Bafia (90.6%) and Ikata (93.8%), whereas those of Likoko (65%) and Mile 14 (74.3%) were doubtful.

The prevalence of US reduced significantly (χ^2 = 4.25, P = 0.04) by day 42 in both groups of levels of educational attainment. Among participants with no formal or primary education, the prevalence reduced from 100% (130) to 16.1% (21) after treatment while that for participants who had attained secondary or tertiary education reduced from 100% (44) to 6.0% (8). No significant differences in MEL/10 mL of urine were observed on day 0 and day 42, with respect to level of education (U = 1730, P = 0.61). On the other hand, the ERR was higher in participants with no formal or primary education (83.8%) than their counterparts with secondary or tertiary education (73.3%).

Efficacy of praziquantel with respect to initial infection intensity

With respect to infection intensity, the difference in US prevalence between day 0 and day 42 was statistically significant between participants with initial heavy infections (1.6%) and those with light infections (20.8%) down from 100% on day 0 (V = 0.3, P < 0.0001). A statistically significant difference was observed in MEL/10 mL of

Table 1 Characteristics of participants in the monitoring of praziquantel efficacy on *S. haematobium* in the Ikata-Likoko area of southwest Cameroon (n = 174)

Characteristics	Category	Frequency/value	Percentage (%)
Sex	Male	84	48.3
	Female	90	51.7
Age group (years)	< 5	23	13.2
	5–15	54	31
	> 15	97	55.8
Mean age ± SD (years)		23.8 ± 17.5	
Prevalence of *S. haematobium*	Day 0	177/516	34.3
Number admitted into the study	Day 0	174	
Overall mean egg load/10 mL of urine	Day 0	30 (range, 1–400)	
Highest level of school attainment	No formal education and primary	130	74.7
	Secondary and tertiary	44	25.3
Occupation	Semi-skilled workers	7	4.0
	Farmers	66	38.0
	Housewife	6	3.4
	Pupils and students	95	54.6

Table 2 Efficacy of praziquantel against *S. haematobium* with respect to gender and age in the Ikata-Likoko area of southwest Cameroon

Characteristic	Category	Prevalence on day 0 (*n*) (*N* = 174)	Prevalence on day 42 (*n*) (*N* = 130)	Mean egg load on day 0 (range)	Mean egg load on day 42 (range)	*Z* test *P* value	ERR (%)
Sex	Male	100 (84)	10.0 (13)	32 (1–400)	12 (2–35)	3.854 < 0.001	62.5
	Female	100 (90)	12.3 (16)	29 (1–300)	3 (1–10)	4.231 < 0.001	90.0
Level of significance		$\chi^2 = 0.06, P = 0.80$		$U = 1854.5, P = 0.109$			
Age	< 5	100 (23)	0.0 (0)	38 (1–300)	0.0	2.805 0.005	100
	5–15	100 (54)	9.2 (12)	36 (1–200)	6 (1–35)	3.626 < 0.001	83.3
	> 15	100 (97)	13.1 (17)	24 (1–400)	6 (1–35)	3.847 < 0.001	75.0
Level of significance		$\chi^2 = 15.55, P = 0.0004$		$H = 2.03, P = 0.02$			

urine in both categories (Table 4). For the light infections, the MEL/10 mL of urine reduced from 15.53 to 6.15 ($Z = 5.33, P < 0.001$) while for the heavy infections, it reduced from 153.58 to 6.0 ($X = 2.03, P = 0.04$). The ERR was satisfactory and higher in individuals with heavy infections (96.1%) than those with light infections (60.4%).

Also, it was observed that before treatment, 60 (34.5%) participants who were positive for US presented with haematuria, but after treatment, all of them were negative for haematuria.

With respect to mean egg loads in the different categories, it was also observed that a majority of participants with higher mean egg load at admission had

Table 3 Efficacy of praziquantel against *S. haematobium* with respect to socio-demographic factors and locality

Characteristic	Category	Prevalence at day 0 (*n*) (*N* = 174)	Prevalence at day 42 (*n*) (*N* = 130)	Mean egg load on day 0 (range)	Mean egg load on day 42 (range)	*Z* test *P* value	ERR (%)
Occupation	Semi-skilled worker	100 (7)	1.5 (2)	15 (4–50)	3 (1–5)	1.604 0.109	80.0
	Farmers	100 (66)	7.0 (9)	25 (1–400)	7 (1–35)	1.605 0.108	72.0
	Housewife	100 (6)	1.5 (2)	30 (5–50)	5 (1–10)	2.821 0.005	83.3
	Pupil/student	100 (95)	12.3 (16)	34 (1–300)	6 (1–35)	1.342 0.180	82.4
Level of significance		$V = 0.20, P = 0.0007$		$H = 3.5$ $P = 0.32$			
Locality	Bafia	100 (20)	4.6 (6)	53 (1–400)	5 (1–10)	1.572 0.116	90.6
	Ikata	100 (33)	5.4 (7)	48 (2–300)	3 (1–6)	2.154 0.012	93.8
	Likoko	100 (48)	2.3 (3)	20 (1–200)	7 (2–35)	3.117 0.002	65.0
	Mile 14	100 (73)	10.0 (13)	23 (1–50)	9 (1–35)	3.923 < 0.001	74.3
Level of significance		$V = 0.163, P = 0.242$		$H = 6.1, P = 0.12$			
Highest level of school attainment	No formal or primary	100 (130)	16.1 (21)	31 (1–400)	5 (1–35)	4.919 < 0.001	83.8
	Secondary/ tertiary	100 (44)	6.0 (8)	30 (1–200)	8 (1–35)	1.965 0.049	73.3
Level of significance		$\chi^2 = 4.25, P = 0.04$		$U = 1730, P = 0.61$			

Table 4 Efficacy of praziquantel against *S. haematobium* on day 42 post-treatment with respect to initial infection intensity in the Ikata-Likoko area of southwest Cameroon

Characteristic	Category	Prevalence day 0 (*n*) (*N* = 174)	Prevalence day 42 (*n*) (*N* = 130)	Mean egg load on day 0 (range)	Mean egg load on day 42 (range)	*Z* test *P* value	ERR (%)
Infection intensity	Light ≤ 50 eggs/ 10 mL	100 (155)	20.8 (27)	15.53 (1–50)	6.15(1–35)	5.33 < 0.001	60.4
	Heavy > 50 eggs/10 mL	100 (19)	1.6 (2)	153.58 (56–400)	6.00(4–8)	2.03 0.04	96.1
	Level of significance	*V* = 0.3, *P* < 0.0001		*U* = 4.32, *P* = 0.13			
Overall		100 (174)	22.3(29)	31 (1–400)	6 (1–35)	5.73 < 0.001	80.3

higher ERRs. In the age category, children below 5 years who presented with the highest initial egg load had the highest ERR of 100%. Similarly, in terms of occupation, housewives and pupils/students who had relatively lower initial MEL/10 mL of urine of 30 and 34, respectively, had ERR of 83.3 and 82.5%. These were higher than the values observed in farmers and semi-skilled participants with lower initial egg loads. In like manner, participants of Bafia and Ikata with higher initial MEL/10 mL of urine of 53 and 48, respectively, had higher ERR of 90.6 and 93.8% than those of Mile 14 and Likoko with lesser initial MEL/10 mL of urine as shown on Fig. 1.

Adverse events post-treatment with praziquantel

Some participants (15, 8.6%) amongst the 174 recruited manifested adverse events such as abdominal pain (6, 3.4%), nausea (7, 4.0%) and headache (6, 3.4%) hours after treatment with praziquantel. The prevalence of adverse events amongst participants was comparable. Two (1.1%) participants had all three adverse events. Nonetheless, these events did not last for more than a day in all the participants.

Discussion

Treatment with praziquantel is the mainstay for the control of schistosomiasis in endemic areas. However, with reports on decreased cure rates in some endemic areas including Cameroon [15, 17, 18], there is a need for continuous monitoring of its efficacy while continuing to seek a possible replacement when the need arises.

The results obtained from this study indicate that a single dose of PZQ (40 mg/kg body weight) had a reduced efficacy (ERR, 80.3%) 42 days post-treatment with respect to the 90% efficacy recommended by WHO protocol [3]. The efficacy observed in this study is less than that recorded by Tchuem-Tchuente et al. in the Littoral Region of Cameroon [10]. It is however similar to that recorded by Tchuem-Tchuente et al. in the Northern and Central Regions of Cameroon [15] and Ojurongbe et al. in Nigeria [8]. This observed efficacy could be due to reasons including the fact that follow up was done once, for a shorter period, and that only a unique dose of the drug was administered. Similar studies with multiple doses of treatment and longer periods of follow up [8, 10] have reported higher efficacies. Longer periods of follow up may depict constant reduction

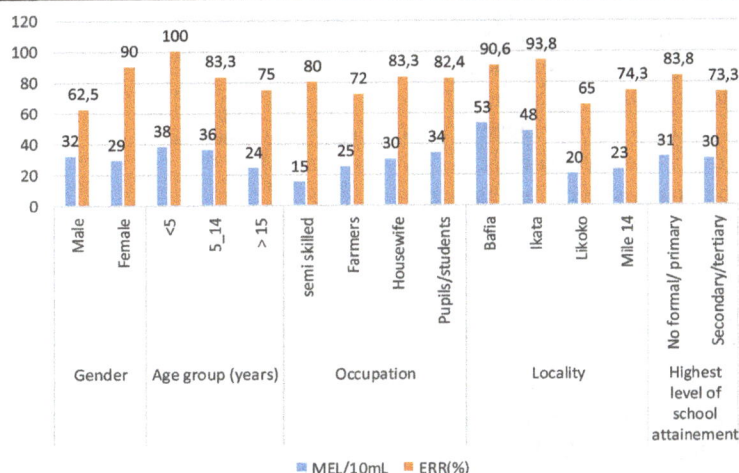

Fig. 1 Variation in ERR on day 42 post praziquantel treatment with mean egg loads per category on day 0

in egg loads with time. Given that schistosomiasis is generally chronic, egg release in most cases starts way before treatment is sought especially in areas where praziquantel is not readily available. Some eggs may be trapped in tissues and some probably excreted after treatment. Egg excretion in a majority of cases continues months after the death of the worms [22]. The late excretion of eggs results in a reduction in the observed efficacy of the drug given that the mean egg load on the follow-up day is increased.

Variation in efficacy was noted with some factors such as sex, age and locality, where the females, children < 5 years and those from Bafia as well as Ikata showed satisfactory efficacies. This variation could be due to factors associated with individuals, such as general health condition, cognisant of the fact that not all health conditions were excluded in this study. Also, it could be due to parasite loads which varied in the different categories of participants or prevailing environmental factors. These findings are similar to those obtained by Senghor et al. in Senegal [23]. However, the higher efficacy observed in females could be buttressed by the fact that female hormones increase antibody response to specific parasites resulting in a higher female resistance against several parasitic infections [24, 25]. Also, females may have better complied to advice given them during the study knowing that they are more exposed to infection as their daily domestic activities bring them in regular contact with infested water bodies. Similarly, following treatment, the prevalence and egg loads of S. haematobium reduced in the study population, an indication that the adult schistosomes were effectively killed by the drug. The reduction in prevalence and egg load varied within some of the categories including age, occupation, level of education and initial infection intensity. Further studies on the influence of these factors on the bioavailability and pharmacokinetics of the praziquantel may provide more information on the efficacy of the medication.

With respect to infection intensity, the higher ERRs observed in participants with higher initial infection intensity probably suggests a higher efficacy of praziquantel on heavy intensity infections than light ones. These results are contrary to the findings of Ojurongbe et al. in Abeokuta, Nigeria [8] and Tchuem-Tchuente et al. [15] in Cameroon. In addition, factors such as high pretreatment egg intensities, poor drug absorption and a high rate of PZQ catabolism, rather than parasite resistance, have been attributed to reduced PZQ cure rate in some endemic areas [18].

The decrease in prevalence of haematuria among participants after treatment is a confirmation of the efficacy of praziquantel in the reduction of morbidity associated with US as reported by earlier studies [8, 26]. The elimination of the worms by the drug would lead to a corresponding decrease in the number of eggs laid.

Eventually, the egg numbers that traverse blood vessels in the bladder reduce and so the amount of blood lost as haematuria is reduced.

Conclusion

Based on ERR rate, the efficacy of praziquantel in the Ikata-Likoko area was reduced although it varied from doubtful to satisfactory with respect to sociodemographic factors. On the other hand, the efficacy in terms of cure rate was 100% since no viable eggs were detected among all positive individuals during control on day 42. Treatment with PZQ showed variation in the reduction of prevalence between age groups, occupations, level of education, initial infection intensity and variation in the mean egg load of the different age groups. Praziquantel can be described as safe due to the few minor adverse events observed. Efficacy is also confirmed since a significant decrease in haematuria was observed after treatment. The distribution of PZQ in the area should be extended to other age groups and not just to school children. Another study with a prolonged period of assessment could improve the evaluation of efficacy of PZQ on urinary schistosomiasis in the study area.

Abbreviations

ERR: Egg reduction rate; H: Kruskall-Wallis test; IBM SPSS: IBM Statistical Package for Social Sciences; MEL/10 mL: Mean egg load per 10 mL; PZQ: Praziquantel; U: Mann-Whitney test; US: Urinary schistosomiasis; WHO: World Health Organization; χ^2: Chi-square test; Z: Wilcoxon signed-rank test

Acknowledgements

The authors appreciate all the participants and authorities of the four localities for their collaboration during this study. We also thank the authorities of the Department of Zoology and Animal Physiology of the University of Buea for material and logistic assistance. Our appreciation goes to the National Program for the Control of Schistosomiasis in Cameroon for providing praziquantel tablets.

Authors' contributions

CBE, HKK, IUNS and LGL conceived the study. CBE, HKK, IUNS and JEY performed the field and laboratory work. CBE analyzed the data. All authors contributed materials for the study. CBE wrote the manuscript. HKK, IUNS and LGL supervised and revised the manuscript. All authors read and approved the final manuscript.

Funding

No funding was received for this study. Financing came from the authors.

Author details

[1]Department of Zoology and Animal Physiology, Faculty of Science, University of Buea, P.O. Box 63, Buea, SWR, Cameroon. [2]Department of Medical Laboratory Sciences, Faculty of Health Sciences, University of Bamenda, P O Box 39, Bambili, NWR, Cameroon. [3]Department of Animal Biology, Faculty of Science, University of Douala, P.O. Box 24157, Douala, Cameroon.

References

1. World Health Organization: Schistosomiasis. http://www.who.int/mediacentre/factsheets/fs115/en/ (2017). Accessed 1 June 2017.
2. World Health Organization: Schistosomiasis Control and Preventive Chemotherapy. http://www.who.int/schistosomiasis/strategy/en (2014). Accessed 5 Jan 2015.
3. World Health Organization: Assessing the Efficacy of Antihelminthic Drugs Against Schistosomiasis and Soil Transmitted Helminthiasis. http://www.who.int/iris/bitstream/10665/79019/1/9789241564557_eng.pdf. (2013); Accessed 5 Feb 2014.
4. Erko B, Degarege A, Tadesse K, Mathiwos A, Legesse M. Efficacy and side effects of praziquantel in the treatment of *Schistosomiasis mansoni* in schoolchildren in Shesha Kekele Elementary School, Wondo Genet, Southern Ethiopia. Asian Pac J Trop Biomed. 2012;2(3):235–9. https://doi.org/10.1016/S2221-1691(12)60049-5 PMCID: PMC360928.
5. Garba A, Lamine MS, Barkiré N, Djibo A, Sofo B, Gouvras AN, Labbo R, Sebangou H, Webster JP, Fenwick A, Utzinger J. Efficacy and safety of two closely spaced doses of praziquantel against Schistosoma haematobium and *S. mansoni* and re-infection patterns in school-aged children in Niger. Acta Trop. 2013;128(2):334–44.
6. Doenhoff MJ, Cioli D, Utzinger J. Praziquantel: mechanisms of action, resistance and new derivatives for schistosomiasis. Curr Opin Infect Dis. 2008;21(6):659–67.
7. Mekonnen A, Legesse M, Belay M, Tadesse K, Torben W, Teklemariam Z, Erko B. Efficacy of praziquantel against *Schistosoma haematobium* in Dulshatalo village, western Ethiopia. BMC Res Notes. 2013; https://doi.org/10.1186/1756-6-392.
8. Ojurongbe O, Sina-Agbaje OR, Busari A, Nkem PO, Ojurongbe TA, Akindele AA. Efficacy of praziquantel in the treatment of *Schistosoma haematobium* infection among school-age children in rural communities of Abeokuta, Nigeria. Infect Dis Poverty. 2014;3:30.
9. WHO. Schistosomiasis and soil transmitted helminth infections—preliminary estimates of the number of children treated with albendazole or mebendazole. http://www.who.int/schistosomiasis/resources/who_wer8116/en/ (2006). Accessed 8 Feb 2014.
10. Tchuem-Tchuenté LA, Shaw DJ, Polla L, Cioli D, Vercruysse J. Efficacy of praziquantel against *Schistosoma haematobium* infection in children. Am J Trop Med Hyg. 2004;71:778–82.
11. Herwig J F, De Cnodder Tinne. Schistosomiasis: artenimol-based combination therapy for the curative treatment of schistosomiasis. 2012. https://www.researchgate.net/publication/221922170_Artenimol-Based_Combination_Therapy_for_the_Curative_Treatment_of_Schistosomiasis. Accessed 6 Feb 2014.
12. Ndamukong KJN, Ayuk MA, Dinga JS, Akenji TN, Ndiforchu VA, Titanji VPK. Prevalence and intensity of urinary schistosomiasis in primary school children of the Kotto Barombi health area, Cameroon. East Afri Med J. 2001;78:6.
13. Nkengazong L, Njiokou F, Tenkeng F, Enyong P, Wanji S. Reassessment of endemicity level of urinary schistosomiasis in the Kotto Barombi focus (South West Cameroon) and impact of mass drug administration (MDA) on the parasitic indices. J Cell Ani Biol. 2009;3(9):159–64.
14. Ntonifor HN, Mbunkur GN, Ndaleh NW. Epidemiological survey of urinary schistosomiasis in some primary schools in a new focus behind Mount Cameroon, South West Region. Cameroon East Afri Med J. 2012;89(3):82–8.
15. Tchuem-Tchuenté LA, Momo SC, Stothard JR, Rollinson D. Efficacy of praziquantel and reinfection patterns in single and mixed infection foci for intestinal and urogenital schistosomiasis in Cameroon. Acta Trop. 2013; 128(2):275–83.
16. Kimbi HK, Wepnje GB, Anchang-Kimbi J, Tonga C, Ayukenchengamba B, Njabi C, Nono LK, Nyabeyeu HN, Lehman LG. Active case detection and prevalence of urinary schistosomiasis and malaria in pupils of Kotto Barombi, southwest Cameroon using the CyScope® fluorescence microscope. IJTDH. 2015;8(1):1–12. ISSN: 2278–1005
17. Barakat R, Morshedy HE. Efficacy of two praziquantel treatments among primary school children in an area of high *Schistosoma mansoni* endemicity, Nile Delta. Egypt Parasitol. 2011;138:440–6.
18. Midzi N, Sangweme D, Zinyowera S, Mapingure MP, Brouwer KC, Kumar N, Mutapi F, Woelk G, Mduluza T. Efficacy and side effects of praziquantel treatment against *Schistosoma haematobium* infection among primary school children in Zimbabwe. Trans R Soc Trop Med Hyg. 2008;102:759–66.
19. Chai JY. Praziquantel treatment in trematode and cestode infections: an update. Infect Chemother. 2013;45:32–43.
20. Ebai CB, Kimbi HK, Sumbele IUN, Yunga JE, Lehman LG. Prevalence and risk factors of urinary schistosomiasis in the Ikata-Likoko area of southwest Cameroon. IJTDH. 2016;17(2):1–10.
21. Cheesbrough, M. District Laboratory Practice in Tropical Countries, Parts 1 & 2 Cambridge University Press. United Kingdom; 2014.
22. Webster BL, Diaw OT, Seye MM, Faye DS, Stothard JR, Sousa Figueiredo JC, Rollinson D. Praziquantel treatment of school children from single and mixed infection foci of intestinal and urogenital schistosomiasis along the Senegal River Basin: monitoring treatment success and reinfection patterns. Acta Trop. 2012;28:292–302.
23. Senghor S, Diallo A, Sylla SN, Doucouré S, Ndiath MO, Gaayeb L, et al. Prevalence and intensity of urinary schistosomiasis among school children in the district of Niakhar, region of Fatick, Senegal. Parasit Vectors. 2014;5 https://doi.org/10.1186/1756-3305-7-5.
24. Schuurs AHWM, Verheul HAM. Effects of gender and sex steroids on the immune response. J Steroid Biochem. 1990;35:157–72.
25. Roberts CW, Satoskar A, Alexander J. Sex steroids, pregnancy associated hormones and immunity to parasitic infections. Parasitol Today. 1996;12:382–8.
26. Koukounari A, Gabrielli AF, Toure S, Elisa BO, Zhang Y, Sellin B, Donnelly CA, Fenwick A, Webster JP. *Schistosoma haematobium* infection and morbidity before and after large-scale administration of praziquantel in Burkina Faso. JID. 2007;196:659–69.

5

Individual and household factors associated with incidences of village malaria in Xepon district, Savannakhet province, Lao PDR

Nouhak Inthavong[1,2,3], Daisuke Nonaka[1,2*], Sengchanh Kounnavong[3], Moritoshi Iwagami[2,4,5], Souraxay Phommala[3], Jun Kobayashi[1,2], Bouasy Hongvanthong[2,6], Tiengkham Pongvongsa[2,7], Paul T. Brey[2,5] and Shigeyuki Kano[2,4]

Abstract

Background: In the Lao PDR, the incidence of malaria greatly differs among villages even within a subdistrict, and the reasons for this difference are poorly understood. The objective of this study was to identify differences in villagers' behavior and the household environment between villages with high incidences and those with low incidences of malaria in a rural district of the Lao PDR.

Methods: A case-control study was conducted in Xepon district, Savannakhet province. Case villages were defined as those with a high incidence (> 10 cases per 1000 population per year), and control villages were those with a low incidence (0–10 cases per 1000 population per year). Data were collected from 178 households in the six case villages and six control villages between December 2016 and January 2017. The data collection consisted of an interview survey with the heads of households and an observational survey in and around the house. Logistic regression was used to assess the association between the case-control status and individual-level behavioral factors and household-level environmental factors adjusted for socio-demographic and economic factors.

Results: Compared to the household members in the control villages, household members in the case villages were significantly more likely to work at night in the forest (adjusted odds ratio 1.95; 95% confidence interval 1.28 to 2.98) and more likely to sleep overnight in the forest (adjusted odds ratio 1.94; 95% confidence interval 1.13 to 3.33). Additionally, compared to the households in the control villages, households in the case villages were significantly more likely to have an open space on the house surface (adjusted odds ratio 3.64; 95% confidence interval 1.68 to 7.84).

Conclusions: There were significant differences in nighttime working and sleeping behaviors in the forest and the presence of an open space on the house surface in the case versus control villages. These differences can partly explain the difference in the incidences of malaria among the villages. The Lao National Malaria Control Program should recommend that villagers use personal protection when working and sleeping in the forest and to reduce any open space on the house surfaces.

Keywords: Malaria, Incidence, Risk factor, Behavior and Laos

* Correspondence: laodaisuke@hotmail.co.jp
[1]Department of Global Health, Graduate School of Health Sciences, University of the Ryukyus, Uehara 207, Nishihara-cho, Okinawa 903-0215, Japan
[2]SATREPS Project for Parasitic Diseases, Vientiane, Lao People's Democratic Republic
Full list of author information is available at the end of the article

Background

The Lao People's Democratic Republic (Lao PDR) is a lower-middle-income country in Southeast Asia, bordering with China on its north border, Vietnam in the east and northeast, Cambodia in the south, Thailand in the west, and Myanmar in the northwest (Fig. 1). The country comprises 18 provinces with 148 districts and 8500 villages. The total land area is 23.68 million hectares, 79% of which is mountainous. The population of the Lao PDR was 7.0 million in 2016 [1], of which 80% live in rural areas and 85–90% are dependent upon subsistence farming [2].

Since 1992, the Lao PDR has implemented a nationwide malaria control program. The current malaria control strategies emphasize the promotion of long-lasting insecticide-treated bed nets (LLINs), early diagnosis by microscopic examination and rapid diagnostic tests, and prompt treatment with an artemisinin-based combination therapy (ACT). Since 2008, the use of the ACT has gradually been scaled-up to cover the entire public health sector, including village health volunteers (community health workers), some businesses in the private sector, and registered private pharmacies [3].

Since 2010, the Lao National Malaria Control Program has adopted stratification-based planning and implementation of control activities; villages are stratified into three strata according to village-level incidences of malaria, and different control strategies are applied to different strata. In stratum I villages, which are defined by an annual incidence of less than 0.1 cases per 1000 population, control activities focus on the maintenance of existing bed nets. In stratum II villages, which are defined by an annual incidence of 0.1 to 10 cases per 1000 population, control activities include the distribution of LLINs and the implementation of village-level diagnosis and treatment with rapid diagnostic tests and ACTs, respectively, and the maintenance of existing bed nets. In stratum III villages, which are defined by an annual incidence of more than 10 cases per 1000 population, additional control activities are the distribution of single LLINs to mobile members of the population and the provision of insect repellent [3].

During the period between 2000 and 2010, the Lao PDR significantly reduced its malaria burden by reducing the number of annual malaria deaths from 350 to 24. The number of confirmed cases had also declined from around 75,000 cases in 2000 to 30,000 cases in 2010. However, the national annual parasite incidence rose from 2.66/1000 population in 2011 to 7.3/1000 population in 2014 [4]. Currently, the malaria burden is concentrated in the southern provinces; approximately 90% of the malaria cases were reported in the five southernmost provinces, i.e., Savannakhet, Saravan, Sekong, Attapeu, and Champasak [3, 5].

In a total of 15 districts in Savannakhet province, malaria was endemic in four districts including Xepon district, which is located on the Vietnamese border, approximately 600 km to the southeast of the Vientiane capital. Xepon has a total area of 21,774 km^2 and 45,000 people. According to the Xepon District Health Office, most of them are ethnic minorities, specifically the Tri and Mangkong people, comprising 75% of the total district population. They have their own distinctive languages, have limited formal education, and live in mountainous and forested areas that are far from health care facilities. The majority of the population is farmers

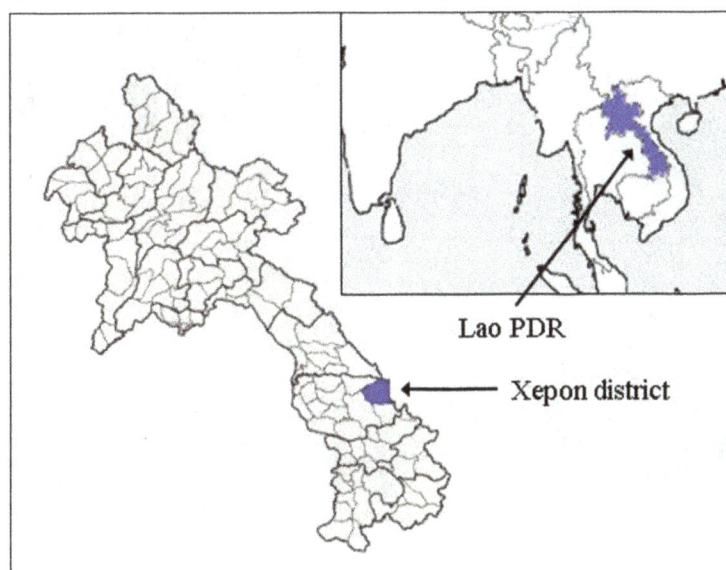

Fig. 1 The location of the Lao PDR and Xepon district

engaged in rice farming. Their houses are surrounded by vegetation and puddles, and cattle are often kept in fenced enclosures near the houses. According to the surveillance data obtained from the Center of Malariology, Parasitology and Entomology, the Xepon District Hospital recorded 225 cases of malaria including 208 *Plasmodium falciparum* mono-infections, 16 *Plasmodium vivax* mono-infections, and 6 co-infections of *P. falciparum* and *P. vivax* in 2015.

A number of studies conducted in the Lao PDR or neighboring countries have emphasized the importance of behavioral and environmental factors on the risk of malaria infection. In the Lao PDR, inappropriate use of bed nets [6] and sleeping away from home (e.g., sleeping in a farming hut) have been reported as risk factors [7, 8]. In Thailand, the relative risk of malaria infection was three times higher among people who slept in farm huts than in people staying in residential villages [9]. In Sri Lanka, the incidence of malaria among residents of poor-quality housing was higher compared with a population living in improved housing [10]. A study conducted in the Lao PDR also showed that house construction material, veranda style, kitchen location, and cow ownership were significantly associated with the house entry of *Anopheles* mosquitoes [11]. In addition, a study in Vietnam mentioned that living in a wooden/bamboo house was significantly related to malaria infection [12]. Hence, the present study hypothesized that individual behavioral factors and household environmental factors would be significantly different between villages with high incidences and villages with low incidences of malaria in Xepon district, Savannakhet province, Lao PDR.

Methods
Study site and population
This was a case-control study that was conducted in the 12 villages in the catchment area of the Dongsavanh Health Center, Xepon district (Fig. 2). A case village was defined as a stratum III village, and the control villages were defined as stratum I or II villages. Of the 43 villages in the catchment area, 13 stratum I and II villages were excluded, either because the number of households was less than the required number for a survey or because these villages were located near the health center and were thus not comparable to stratum III villages that were located far from the health center. Then, 6 case villages were randomly selected from 19 stratum III villages. Similarly, 6 control villages were randomly selected from 11 stratum I and II villages, 3 from the 7 stratum I villages and 3 from the 4 stratum II villages. The number of villages and households to be selected was mainly determined by the availability of human and time resources.

In each of the selected villages, 15 households were randomly selected, using a household list obtained from the heads of the villages; however, the survey failed to include 15 households in one village. All members of the selected households were included. Overall, this study collected data on 1070 individuals from 178 households.

The names (and number of eligible households) of the selected case villages were Lakheum-Tai (26), Palai (52), Alang-Noy (22), Satheum (53), Ahor (39), and Kaengkhai (43), and those of the selected control villages were Haengluoang (17), Kaengpae-Yai (18), Sky-Yai (60), Vangsalor (20), Tanang (33), and Alai-Noy (34).

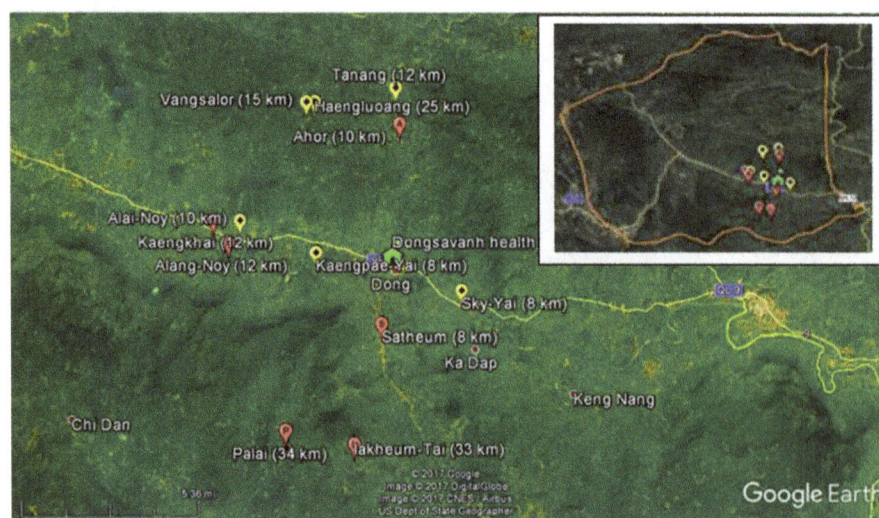

Fig. 2 Map of the study villages. The maps show the villages in which the present study was conducted. The red points indicate the locations of case villages, and the yellow points indicate the locations of control villages along with the distance of each from Xepon district hospital according to the hospital's data

Data collection

Data were collected between December 2016 and January 2017 through an interview survey and an observational survey. The trained surveyors, who were health workers at the Xepon District Health Office, visited the selected households and conducted interviews with the heads of households. Information on every member of each household was collected via the heads of households. When the head of a household was absent during the survey, another adult member of the household (e.g., spouse of the head) was recruited. When the respondent was unable to communicate with surveyors in the Lao language, the head of the village or other villagers who were able to speak both the local language and the Lao language were asked to assist the surveyors. For the observational survey, surveyors observed the household characteristics in and around the houses using a checklist.

Factors and measurements

Selection of the factors that were measured in this study was based on the conceptual framework depicted in Fig. 3. The conceptual model was developed principally on the basis of the findings of malaria studies that were conducted in the Lao PDR or neighboring countries [6–14]. The interview survey measured socio-demographic and economic factors and individual behavioral factors, whereas the observational survey measured household environmental factors.

Individual behavioral factors included preventive behavior (i.e., frequency of sleeping under a bed net in the past month), occupational behavior (i.e., experience of working in the forest at night or early morning in the past 1 year, sleeping in the forest in the past 1 year), and seeking behavior for malaria treatment in the past 1 year.

Household environmental factors included housing structure (i.e., wall and floor materials); presence of an open space that was larger than the size of an A4 sheet of paper on the surface of the house (i.e., lack of a door or no window coverings, no ceiling, and open eaves); kitchen location; type of water resources for bathing, washing clothes, and other daily use; keeping cattle near the house; presence of weeds within 10 m of the house in the household compound; and household bed net density (i.e., person per net ratio defined as the number of household members divided by the number of available bed nets in the household [15]). When measuring the presence of an open space, surveyors paid attention to and included only an open space that was larger than approximately the size of an A4 sheet of paper, ignoring an open space that was smaller than approximately the size of an A4 sheet of paper.

Socio-demographic factors included age, gender, and number of members in each household. Socio-economic factors included educational attainment, occupation of each member of the households, and household relative wealth determined by the household possession of assets including a motorbike, mobile phone, television, DVD/CD, car/tractor, and refrigerator. Principal component analysis was used to assess the weight of household assets by scoring factors for wealth index variables (Table 1) and to build a household wealth index [16]. Households were ranked by the household wealth index and divided into quartiles. As a result of the analysis, six components were extracted and the first component, which explained 41.3% of the total variance with the eigenvalue of 2.48, was used for the wealth index. For each asset variable, a scoring factor was derived from the weight of a variable divided by the eigenvalue. The wealth index of a household was expressed as the sum of the product between the scoring factor of an

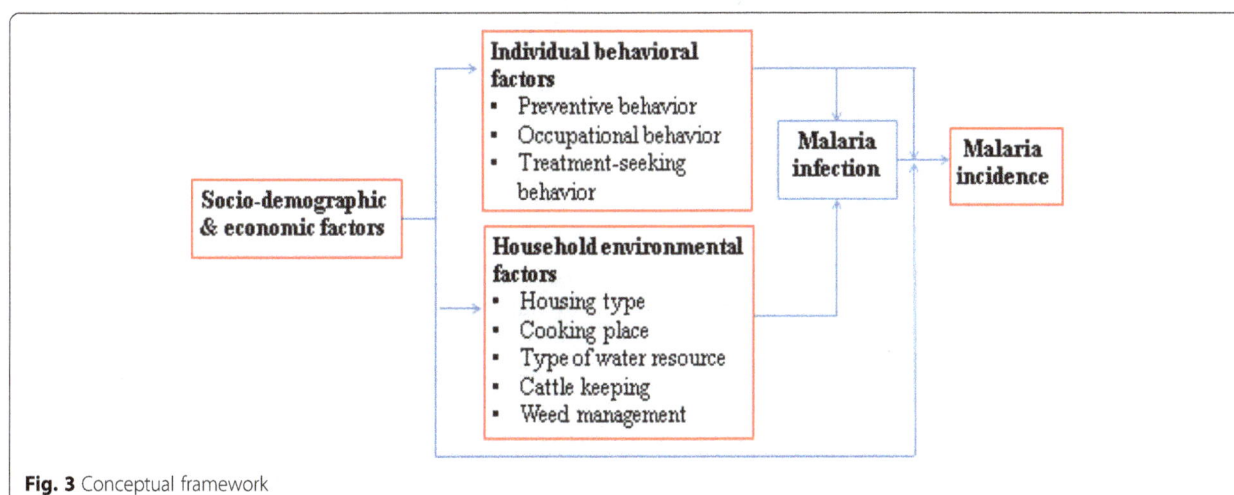

Fig. 3 Conceptual framework

Table 1 Scoring factors for wealth index variables

Variables	Scoring factor
Car/tractor	0.216
Motorbike	0.232
Mobile phone	0.262
Television	0.323
DVD/CD	0.301
Refrigerator	0.198

asset variable and the household's standardized score of the variable.

Data analysis

Frequencies, percentages, and medians with interquartile ranges were computed to summarize the data. Bivariate analyses were conducted to assess an association between a predictive factor and the case-control status, using Fisher's exact test. Multivariate analyses that adjusted for the effect of other predictive factors were conducted to assess an association between a predictive factor and the case-control status using logistic regression. According to Katz [17], regardless of a p value obtained from the bivariate analyses, variables that are theoretically important or those that have been reported as risk factors were included in the multivariate model. Two multivariate models were built: one included individual-level predictive variables and the other included only household-level predictive variables. The amount of multicollinearity (i.e., two or more predictive variables are correlated each other) in the multivariate model was estimated by the variance inflation factor (VIF). A VIF ≥ 4 was considered as the sign of multicollinearity. A p value < 0.05 was considered statistically significant. Statistical analyses were performed using SPSS version 24.

Results

Associations between individual-level characteristics and case-control status

The proportion of household members who worked in the forest at night was significantly higher in the case villages than in the control villages (21.8 vs. 15.6%, $p = 0.010$) (Table 2). In contrast, the proportion of household members who worked in the forest in the early morning was significantly lower in the case villages than in the control villages (19.1 vs. 24.4%, $p = 0.038$). Additionally, the proportion of household members who slept overnight in the forest (12.4 vs. 8.1%, $p = 0.026$), who had a malaria episode in past 1 year (13.8 vs. 6.3%, $p = <0.001$), and who sought a place for malaria treatment (48.7 vs. 0.0%, $p = <0.001$) was significantly higher in the case villages versus the control villages. No significant differences were observed in gender, age,

Table 2 Bivariate analysis of differences in individual-level characteristics

Characteristics	Respondents in cases ($n = 550$)		Respondents in controls ($n = 520$)		p value[a]
	n	%	n	%	
Gender					
Male	272	49.5	261	50.2	0.854
Female	278	50.5	259	49.8	
Age					
< 15 years	271	50.4	239	47.0	0.293
≥ 15 years	267	49.6	270	53.0	
Educational attainment					
No formal education	389	70.7	367	70.6	1.000
Primary school or higher	161	29.3	153	29.4	
Occupation					
Farmer	290	52.7	275	52.9	0.978
Child	159	28.9	152	29.2	
Student	101	18.4	93	17.9	
Frequency of using a bed net					
Everyday	455	82.7	428	82.3	0.872
Sometimes/never	95	17.3	92	17.7	
Working in the forest at nighttime in the past year					
No	430	78.2	439	84.4	0.010
Yes	120	21.8	81	15.6	
Working in the forest in the early morning in the past year					
No	445	80.9	393	75.6	0.038
Yes	105	19.1	127	24.4	
Sleeping overnight in the forest in the past year					
No	482	87.6	478	91.9	0.026
Yes	68	12.4	42	8.1	
Malaria episode in past 1 year					
No	474	86.2	487	93.7	< 0.001
Yes	76	13.8	33	6.3	
Place for the treatment of the episode					
Health center	36	47.4	30	90.9	< 0.001
Village health volunteer	37	48.7	0	0.0	
Other	3	3.9	3	9.1	

[a]Fisher's exact test

educational attainment, occupation, and frequency of using a bed net.

Among the household members who worked in the forest at night, the proportion of household members who slept overnight in the forest was not significantly different between the case and control villages (43.3 vs. 48.1%, $p = 0.564$) (data not shown in table).

After adjusting for the effects of other individual-level predictive variables in the multivariate analysis, the associations observed in the bivariate analysis remained significant (Table 3); working in the forest at night (adjusted odds ratio [AOR] 1.95; 95% confidence interval [CI] 1.28 to 2.98), working in the forest in the early morning (AOR 0.51; 95% CI 0.36 to 0.73), and sleeping overnight in the forest (AOR 1.94; 95% CI 1.13 to 3.33). Although the difference in age groups was not significant in the bivariate analysis, it became significant in the multivariate analysis (AOR 0.61; 95% CI 0.38 to 0.98). There was no sign of multicollinearity between the variables in the multivariate analysis.

Associations between household-level characteristics and case-control status

The proportion of households that used flooring materials other than wood was significantly lower in the case villages than in the control villages (21.1 vs. 36.4%,

Table 3 Multivariate analysis of differences in individual-level characteristics and case-control status

Predictive factors	Crude odds ratio (95% CI)	Adjusted odds ratio[a] (95% CI)
Gender		
Male	1.00	1.00
Female	0.97 (0.76–1.23)	1.22 (0.93–1.61)
Age		
< 15 years	1.00	1.00
≥ 15 years	0.87 (0.68–1.11)	0.61 (0.38–0.98)
Education attainment		
No formal education	1.00	1.00
Primary school and higher	0.99 (0.76–1.29)	0.88 (0.58–1.32)
Occupation		
Child	1.00	1.00
Student	1.03 (0.72–1.48)	1.33 (0.78–2.25)
Farmer	1.00 (0.76–1.33)	1.46 (0.87–2.45)
Frequency of using bed net		
Everyday	1.00	1.00
Sometimes/never	0.97 (0.70–1.33)	0.80 (0.57–1.14)
Working in the forest at nighttime in the past year		
No	1.00	1.00
Yes	1.51 (1.10–2.06)	1.95 (1.28–2.98)
Working in the forest in the early morning in the past year		
No	1.00	1.00
Yes	0.73 (0.54–0.97)	0.51 (0.36–0.73)
Sleeping overnight in the forest in the past year		
No	1.00	1.00
Yes	1.60 (1.07–2.40)	1.94 (1.13–3.33)

[a]Adjusted for age, gender, occupational attainment, education, frequency of using a bed net, working in the forest at nighttime in the past year, working in the forest in the early morning in the past year, and sleeping overnight in the forest in the past year

$p = 0.031$). The proportion of households with an open space was significantly higher in the case villages than in the control villages (77.8 vs. 50.0%, $p = <0.001$) (Table 4). No other significant differences were found in the bivariate analysis.

After adjusting for the effects of other household-level variables in the multivariate analysis, the association with flooring materials other than wood was significant (AOR 0.25; 95% CI 0.09–0.68) (Table 5). The presence of an open space also remained significant (AOR 3.64; 95% CI 1.68 to 7.84). Although the bivariate analysis did not show a significant difference in the proportion of household wealth quartiles, the multivariate analysis showed that compared to the proportion of the first-quartile households, the proportion of the fourth-quartile households was significantly higher in the case villages than in the control villages (AOR 6.16; 95% CI 1.92 to 19.72). There was no sign of multicollinearity between the variables in the multivariate analysis.

Risk behaviors in households

There was no tendency that risk behaviors concentrated in some particular households; 68.9% (62/90) of the households in the case villages and 67.0% (59/88) of the households in the control villages had at least one member who worked in the forest at night. Additionally, 51.1% (46/90) of the households in the case villages and 37.5% (33/88) of the households in the control villages had at least one member who slept in the forest at night (data not shown in table).

Discussion

This study found that a number of individual-level and household-level factors were associated with village-level incidences of malaria. The results showed that the household members in the case villages were significantly more likely to work at night and more likely to sleep overnight in the forest, as compared with those in the control villages. These differences of behaviors could be the reason why the incidences of malaria were higher in the case villages than in the control villages. A case-control study conducted in Attapeu province, Lao PDR reported that study participants who slept away from home in the past 2 weeks had significantly higher odds of malaria infection than those who did not [7, 8]. A cross-sectional study that was conducted in Savannakhet province, Lao PDR reported that staying overnight in the forest was associated with *P. viviax* mono-infections [18]. A cross-sectional study conducted in Vietnam reported that working and sleeping at night in the forest was a risk factor for malaria infection [13], and a similar finding was also reported from Thailand [14]. In the study district, *Anopheles dirus* is thought to be the main malaria vector [19]. The biting time of *A. dirus* is

Table 4 Bivariate analysis of the associations between household-level characteristics

Characteristics	Respondents in cases (n = 90)		Respondents in controls (n = 88)		p value[a]
	n	%	n	%	
Number of household members					
< 5	27	30.0	27	30.7	0.994
5–7	40	44.4	39	4.3	
≥ 8	23	25.6	22	25.0	
Median (interquartile range)	6	4–8	6	4–8	
Household that hung a bed net					
No	0	0.0	4	4.5	0.058
Yes	90	100	84	95.5	
Household that hung long-lasting insecticide-treated bed net					
No	3	3.3	9	10.2	0.079
Yes	87	96.7	79	89.8	
Person per net ratio					
≤ 2.5	49	54.4	44	52.4	0.879
> 2.5	41	45.6	40	47.6	
Type of water used for daily life					
Stream water	41	45.6	44	50.0	0.653
Water other than stream water	49	54.4	44	50.0	
Wealth index quartiles					
First (least poor)	19	21.1	30	34.1	0.121
Second	21	23.3	22	25.0	
Third	18	20.0	17	19.3	
Fourth (poorest)	32	35.6	19	21.6	
Wall materials					
Brick	48	53.3	45	51.1	0.881
Other	42	46.7	43	48.9	
Flooring materials					
Wood	71	78.8	56	63.6	0.031
Other	19	21.1	32	36.4	
Roofing materials					
Zinc	82	91.1	73	83.0	0.121
Other	8	8.9	15	17.0	
Open space in the house (size larger than A4 sheet)					
No	20	22.2	44	50.0	< 0.001
Yes	70	77.8	44	50.0	
Percent of open spaces in the house (%)					
≤ 10	23	32.9	13	29.5	0.837
> 10	47	67.1	31	70.5	
Median (interquartile range)	11.2	0.9–21.5	0.6	0.0–18.4	

Table 4 Bivariate analysis of the associations between household-level characteristics *(Continued)*

Characteristics	Respondents in cases (n = 90)		Respondents in controls (n = 88)		p value[a]
	n	%	n	%	
Kitchen location					
Inside the house	58	64.4	61	69.3	0.527
Outside the house	32	35.6	27	30.7	
Cattle keeping near the house					
No	53	58.9	58	65.9	0.357
Yes	37	41.1	30	34.1	
Weed management within 10 m around the house					
Poor	52	57.8	42	47.7	0.230
Good	38	42.2	46	52.3	

[a]Fisher's exact test

between 19:00 and 06:00 with the peak at midnight [8, 20]. This vector behavior can also support our causal inference that the statistical associations with working and sleeping at night in the forest represent a cause-effect relation.

In rural areas of the Lao PDR, people work in the forest during nighttime to sustain their lives. The purposes of nighttime working in the forest include seeking forest products, hunting, and protecting crops in a slash-and-burn field from animals. Therefore, it is difficult to stop their behavior. Considering the risk of malaria infection of the behavior, the Lao National Malaria Control Program has already promoted devices for protection. Mosquito repellent lotions and single LLINs for this mobile population have been made available in the stratum III villages where the incidences of malaria are high. However, little is known about whether the villagers are actually using these devices. In addition to these protective devices, wearing long-sleeved shirts should be recommended to villagers who work in the forest at nighttime. A cross-sectional study that was conducted with hill tribes in Thailand showed that when working outdoors, people who wore long-sleeved clothes were significantly less likely to have malaria infection, as compared with those who did not [21].

The present study also showed that the houses in the case villages were significantly more likely to have an unprotected open space on their surfaces, as compared to the houses in the control villages. The difference in the presence of an open space between the case and control houses could be one reason for the higher incidence of malaria in the case villages than in the control villages. Such open spaces can make it easier for vector mosquitoes to enter the house, thus increasing human-vector contacts. Although no study has been conducted in the Lao PDR and neighboring countries, a number of

Table 5 Multivariate analysis of the associations between household characteristics and case-control status

Predictive factors	Crude odds ratio (95% CI)	Adjusted odds[a] ratio (95% CI)
Number of household members		
≤ 6	1.00	1.00
> 6	1.16 (0.63–2.12)	1.48 (0.70–3.13)
Person per net ratio		
≤ 2.5	1.00	1.00
> 2.5	0.92 (0.50–1.67)	0.83 (0.40–1.71)
Type of water used for daily life		
Stream water	1.00	1.00
Water other than stream water	1.19 (0.66–2.15)	1.50 (0.70–3.21)
Wealth index quartiles		
First (least poor)	1.00	1.00
Second	1.50 (0.65–3.45)	1.67 (0.63–4.38)
Third	1.67 (0.69–4.02)	2.35 (0.77–7.14)
Fourth (poorest)	2.65 (1.18–5.96)	6.16 (1.92–19.72)
Wall materials		
Brick	1.00	1.00
Other	0.96 (0.50–1.64)	0.97 (0.40–2.35)
Flooring materials		
Wood	1.00	1.00
Other	0.46 (0.24–0.91)	0.25 (0.09–0.68)
Roofing materials		
Zinc	1.00	1.00
Other	0.47 (0.19–1.18)	0.61 (0.21–1.75)
Open space in the house		
No	1.00	1.00
Yes	3.50 (1.82–6.70)	3.64 (1.68–7.84)
Kitchen location		
Inside the house	1.00	1.00
Outside the house	1.24 (0.66–2.33)	0.94 (0.35–2.48)
Cattle keeping near the house		
No	1.00	1.00
Yes	1.35 (0.73–2.48)	1.78 (0.85–3.74)
Weed management within 10 m around the house		
Poor	1.00	1.00
Good	0.66 (0.36–1.20)	0.67 (0.32–1.39)

[a]Adjusted for number of household members, person per net ratio, type of water used for daily life, wealth index, wall materials, flooring materials, roofing materials, open space in the house, kitchen location, cattle keeping near the house, weed management within 10 m around the house

studies conducted in Sri Lanka or African countries have shown an association between the presence of an open space or non-screened space on the surface of a house and malaria infections among the residents of the house [10, 22–25]. An open space under the eaves is considered to be the most critical for house entry of malaria vectors [23, 25, 26]. A randomized controlled trial of house screening intervention showed that the number of mosquitoes inside the house and the incidences of childhood anemia were significantly lowered in the intervention group [23].

There are at least two concerns about promoting net screens in the study district. One is the increased temperature due to installing net screens. A study in Gambia showed that houses with net screens were a little hotter than houses without any screens; full screened houses were 0.26 °C hotter at night than houses with screened ceilings and 0.51 °C hotter than houses with no screening (28.43 °C). Nonetheless, only 9% of full screened house users complained about the heat [27]. Another concern is the cost for installing net screens. Because many households in malaria-prone villages of the study district may not afford to buy nets for screening by themselves, the Lao National Malaria Control Program should consider subsidizing a part of the cost. The Lao National Malaria Control Program has already experienced the distribution of bed nets and repellent spays to the target population at a subsidized price.

Although the difference in household bed net density measured by person per net ratio was not significant between the case and controls, it should be noted that 45.6% of the households in the case villages did not possess an adequate number of bed nets to protect all members of the household. This finding suggests the need for increasing the availability of LLINs in malaria-prone villages.

In the present study, the poorest households were significantly more abundant in the case villages than in the control villages. It has been frequently reported from many countries that poorer households are at higher risk of malaria [26, 28, 29]. In this study site, there are at least two possible explanations for why poor households are at risk of malaria. First, poor households would be more reluctant to seek treatment for malaria as compared to non-poor households. Although treatment for malaria is free of charge in the Lao PDR, treatment seeking requires opportunity costs including transportation costs. Second, as compared to better-off households, poor households would be more likely to be exposed to malaria infection because protective materials including long-sleeved clothes or insecticides are less likely available among these households.

The present study compared individual and household characteristics between the case villages and control villages. The result showed that there were significant differences in these characteristics. However, because the case villages and control villages were not necessarily comparable, caution is necessary when interpreting the results. If case and control individuals are recruited in the same village, then there might be no significant differences in individual and household characteristics. However, a previous case-control study that recruited cases and controls in the same village in Lao PDR also showed that there were significant differences in individual and household characteristics, i.e., not using a bed net, sleeping away from home, and houses closed to a vector breeding site [8].

A cross-sectional study that was conducted in Xepon district by Pongvongsa et al. showed that malaria infections were highly clustered at the household level. Pongvongsa et al. suggested two possible reasons for such household clustering. One is that household members share the same environmental risk factors including the proximity of housing location to breeding sites and housing type. Another is that household members share the same risk behaviors such as not using a bed net and working in the forest [30]. The results of the present study partly support their speculation. The present study found that houses with an open space were significantly more common in villages with high incidences than in those with low incidences of malaria, suggesting the importance of housing conditions. The present study also found that some households did not own any LLINs, suggesting that all members of the households are equally not protected by nets. The present study, however, did not find that risk behaviors were highly clustered at the household level; individuals who practiced risk behaviors did not concentrate on particular households.

There are four limitations in the present study. Firstly, the case villages were not matched with the control villages on the basis of village-level characteristics. Therefore, the risk of malaria infection could be different between the two. The stratum III case villages were more likely to be located far from the health center as compared with the stratum I and II control villages. Thus, the case villages were likely to be at higher risk of malaria infections, as compared to control villages. The ethnicity of the study population was, however, the same between the case and control villages, i.e., Tri and Mangkong. To minimize the impact of the absence of matching, the present study excluded the stratum I and II villages that were located within 7 km of the health center. Secondly, although people in the study site might have sought malaria treatment from the private sector, the village-level incidence of malaria used in the present study relied solely on records from the public health sector. Thus, the present study could underestimate the village-level incidence. However, the impact of the underestimation would be very low because access to the private health sector was available only in the center of Xepon district, which was located at least 8 km from

the study villages, and as shown in Table 2, more than 90% of the study households reported treatment seeking from the public sector for past malaria episodes. Thirdly, because in the present study the outcome measurement was not at the individual level but at the village level, the present study was unable to take the village and household clustering into account in the analyses. Therefore, the present study possibly overestimated the significance of the statistical associations. Finally, because small villages in which the total number of households was 14 or fewer were excluded, the results of the present study were not free from selection bias. However, the impact of the selection bias would be small as the total number of households was 15 or larger in the most of the villages of the study district.

Although in the present study the study site was confined to the catchment area of one health center in Xepon district, the findings of the present study can be generalized to a wider area in Savannakhet province. This is because the same ethnic groups such as Tri and Mangkong are predominant in the malaria-prone villages of the province including the study villages of the present study. Additionally, ecological characteristics are similar among the malaria-prone villages of the province.

Conclusion

There were significant differences in personal behaviors and household environment between the villages with high and those with low incidences of malaria. Villagers in the villages with high incidences of malaria were significantly more likely to work and sleep in the forest at night as compared with those in villages with low incidences. Houses in villages with high incidences were significantly more likely to have open spaces on their surfaces that could facilitate mosquito entry. These differences can partly explain the difference in the incidences of malaria between the villages. The Lao National Malaria Control Program should recommend that villagers use personal protection such as repellent lotions, single LLINs, and long-sleeved clothes when they work and sleep in the forest and to reduce open spaces on house surfaces by installing net screens.

Acknowledgements

The authors thank the study participants and heads of the study villages for their cooperation. The authors also thank Dongsavanh Health Center, Xepon District Health Office, and Savannakheth Provincial Health Department for their contributions.

Funding

This study was supported by a JICA/AMED SATREPS project for the "Development of innovative research technique in genetic epidemiology of malaria and other parasitic diseases in the Lao PDR for containing their expanding endemicity" and the Grant for National Center for Global Health and Medicine (28-4).

Authors' contributions

NI was the principal investigator and drafted the manuscript with the help of DN, MI, and SKA. SKO, SP, JK, BH, and PTB contributed to the conception of the study. TP contributed to data collection. DN contributed to the data analysis. All of the authors have read and approved the final manuscript.

Competing interests

The authors declare that they have no competing interests.

Author details

[1]Department of Global Health, Graduate School of Health Sciences, University of the Ryukyus, Uehara 207, Nishihara-cho, Okinawa 903-0215, Japan. [2]SATREPS Project for Parasitic Diseases, Vientiane, Lao People's Democratic Republic. [3]National Institute of Public Health, Ministry of Health, Ban Kaognot, Samsenthai Road, Sisattanak District, Vientiane, Lao People's Democratic Republic. [4]Department of Tropical Medicine and Malaria, Research Institute, National Center for Global Health and Medicine, 1-21-1 Toyama, Shinjuku-ku, Tokyo 162-8655, Japan. [5]Institut Pasteur du Laos, Ministry of Health, Sisattanak District, Vientiane, Lao People's Democratic Republic. [6]Center of Malariology, Parasitology and Entomology, Ministry of Health, Vientiane, Lao People's Democratic Republic. [7]Savannakhet Provincial Health Department, Thahea village, Kaysone-Phomvihan District, Savannakhet, Lao People's Democratic Republic.

References

1. Lao Statistics Bureau. Vientiane capital: Ministry of Planning and Investment, Lao PDR. 2016. http://www.lsb.gov.la/lsb/en/#.WfcXzVu0O00. Accessed 30 Oct 2017.
2. Midgley S, Bennett J, Samontry X, Stevens P, Mounlamai K, Midgley D, et al. Enhancing livelihoods in Lao PDR through environmental services and planted-timber products. Canberra: Australian Centre for International Agricultural Research; 2012. p. 14–5.
3. Ministry of Health: Lao People's Democratic Republic. National strategy for malaria control and pre-elimination 2011–2015. Lao People's Democratic Republic: Ministry of Health; 2010.
4. Ministry of Health: Lao People's Democratic Republic. National strategy for malaria control and elimination 2016–2030. Lao People's Democratic Republic: Ministry of Health; 2016.
5. Kounnavong S, Gopinath D, Hongvanthong B, Khamkong C, Sichanthongthip O. Malaria elimination in Lao PDR: the challenges associated with population mobility. Infect Dis Poverty. 2017;6:81.
6. Nonaka D, Laimanivong S, Kobayashi J, Chindavonsa K, Kano S, Vanisaveth V, et al. Is staying overnight in a farming hut a risk factor for malaria infection in a setting with insecticide-treated bed nets in rural Laos? Malar J. 2010;9:372.
7. Khaminsou N, Kritpetcharat O, Daduang J, Kritpetcharat P. A survey of malaria infection in endemic areas of Savannakhet province, Lao PDR and comparative diagnostic efficiencies of Giemsa staining, acridine orange staining, and semi-nested multiplex PCR. Parasitol Int. 2008;57:143–9.
8. Vythilinggam I, Sidavong B, Chan ST, Phonemixay T, Vanisaveth V, Sisoulad P, et al. Epidemiology of malaria in Attapeu province, Lao PDR in relation to entomological parameters. Trans R Soc Trop Med Hyg. 2005;99:833–9.
9. Somboon P, Aramrattana A, Lines J, Webber R. Entomological and epidemiological investigations of malaria transmission in relation to population movements in forest areas of north-west Thailand. Southeast Asian J Trop Med Public Health. 1998;29:3–9.
10. Gunawardena DM, Wickremasinghe AR, Muthuwatta L, Weerasingha S, Rajakaruna J, Senanayaka T, et al. Malaria risk factors in an endemic region of Sri Lanka, and the impact and cost implications of risk factor-based interventions. Am J Trop Med Hyg. 1998;58:533–42.
11. Hiscox A, Khammanithong P, Kaul S, Sananikhom P, Luthi R, Hill N, et al. Risk factors for mosquito house entry in the Lao PDR. PLoS One. 2013;8:5.
12. Abe T, Honda S, Nakazawa S, Tuong TD, Thieu NQ, Hungle X, et al. Risk factors for malaria infection among ethnic minorities in Binh Phuoc, Vietnam. Southeast Asian J Trop Med Public Health. 2009;40:18–29.
13. Erhart A, Thang ND, Ky PV, Tinh TT, Overmeir CV, Speybroeck N, et al. Epidemiology of forest malaria in central Vietnam: a large scale cross-sectional survey. Malar J. 2005;4:58.
14. Chaveepojnkamjorn W, Pichainarong N. Behavioral factors and malaria infection among the migrant population, Chiang Rai province. J Med Assoc Thail. 2005;88:1293–301.
15. Nonaka D, Pongvongsa T, Nishimoto F, Nansounthavong P, Sato Y, Jiang H, et al. Households with insufficient bednets in a village with sufficient bednets: evaluation of household bednet coverage using bednet distribution index in Xepon district. Lao PDR Trop Med Health. 2015;43:95–100.
16. Vyas S, Kumaranayake L. Constructing socio-economic status indices: how to use principal components analysis. Health Policy Plan. 2006;21:459–68.
17. Katz HM. Multivariable analysis: a practical guide for clinicians and public health researchers. 3rd ed. Cambridge: Cambridge University Press; 2011.
18. Phommasone K, Adhikari B, Henriques G, Pongvongsa T, Phongmany P, von Seidlein L, et al. Asymptomatic plasmodium infections in 18 villages of southern Savannakhet province, Lao PDR (Laos). Malar J. 2016;15:296.
19. Pongvongsa T, Ha H, Thanh L, Marchand RP, Nonaka D, Tojo B, et al. Joint malaria surveys lead towards improved cross-border cooperation between Savannakhet province, Laos and Quang Tri province. Vietnam Malar J. 2012;11:262.
20. Kobayashi J, Phompida S, Toma T, Looareensuwan S, Toma H, Miyagi I. The effectiveness of impregnated bed net in malaria control in Laos. Acta Trop. 2004;89:299–30.
21. Pichainarong N, Chaveepojnkamjorn W. Malaria infection and life-style factors among hilltribes along the Thai-Myanmar border area, northern Thailand. Southeast Asian J Trop Med Public Health. 2004;35:834–9.
22. Lindsay SW, Emerson PM, Charlwood JD. Reducing malaria by mosquito-proofing houses. Trends Parasitol. 2002;18:510–4.
23. Kirby MJ, Ameh D, Bottomley C, Green C, Jawara M, Milligan PJ, et al. Effect of two different house screening interventions on exposure to malaria vectors and on anaemia in children in the Gambia: a randomised controlled trial. Lancet. 2013;374:998–1009.
24. Njie M, Dilger E, Lindsay SW, Kirby MJ. Importance of eaves to house entry by anopheline, but not culicine, mosquitoes. J Med Entomol. 2009;46:505–10.
25. Ghebreyesus TA, Haile M, Witten KH, Getachew A, Yohannes M, Lindsay SW, et al. Household risk factors for malaria among children in the Ethiopian highlands. Trans R Soc Trop Med Hyg. 2000;94:17–21.
26. Tusting LS, Ippolito M, Willey B, Kleinschmidt I, Dorsey G, Gosling RD, et al. The evidence for improving housing to reduce malaria: a systematic review and meta-analysis. Malar J. 2015;14:209.
27. Kirby MJ, Bah P, Jones CO, Kelly AH, Jasseh M, Lindsay SW. Social acceptability and durability of two different house screening interventions against exposure to malaria vectors, plasmodium falciparum infection, and anemia in children in the Gambia, West Africa. Am J Trop Med Hyg. 2010;83:965–72.
28. Tusting LS, Rek J, Arinaitwe E, Staedke SG, Kamya MR, Cano J, et al. Why is malaria associated with poverty? Find Cohort Study in Rural Uganda Malar J. 2016;5:78.
29. Snow RW, Peshu N, Forster D, Bomu G, Mitsanze E, Ngumbao E, et al. Environmental and entomological risk factors for the development of clinical malaria among children on the Kenya coast. Trans R Soc Trop Med Hyg. 1998;92:381–5.
30. Pongvongsa T, Nonaka D, Iwagami M, Nakatsu M, Phongmany P, Nishimoto F, et al. Household clustering of asymptomatic malaria infections in Xepon district, Savannakhet province. Lao PDR Malar J. 2016;15:508.

6

Environmental factors associated with the distribution of visceral leishmaniasis in endemic areas of Bangladesh: modeling the ecological niche

Abu Yousuf Md Abdullah[1*], Ashraf Dewan[2], Md Rakibul Islam Shogib[1], Md Masudur Rahman[1] and Md Faruk Hossain[1]

Abstract

Background: Visceral leishmaniasis (VL) is a parasitic infection (also called kala-azar in South Asia) caused by *Leishmania donovani* that is a considerable threat to public health in the Indian subcontinent, including densely populated Bangladesh. The disease seriously affects the poorest subset of the population in the subcontinent. Despite the fact that the incidence of VL results in significant morbidity and mortality, its environmental determinants are relatively poorly understood, especially in Bangladesh. In this study, we have extracted a number of environmental variables obtained from a range of sources, along with human VL cases collected through several field visits, to model the distribution of disease which may then be used as a surrogate for determining the distribution of *Phlebotomus argentipes* vector, in hyperendemic and endemic areas of Mymensingh and Gazipur districts in Bangladesh. The analysis was carried out within an ecological niche model (ENM) framework using a maxent to explore the ecological requirements of the disease.

Results: The results suggest that VL in the study area can be predicted by precipitation during the warmest quarter of the year, land surface temperature (LST), and normalized difference water index (NDWI). As *P. argentipes* is the single proven vector of *L. donovani* in the study area, its distribution could reasonably be determined by the same environmental variables. The analysis further showed that the majority of VL cases were located in *mauzas* where the estimated probability of the disease occurrence was high. This may reflect the potential distribution of the disease and consequently *P. argentipes* in the study area.

Conclusions: The results of this study are expected to have important implications, particularly in vector control strategies and management of risk associated with this disease. Public health officials can use the results to prioritize their visits in specific areas. Further, the findings can be used as a baseline to model how the distribution of the disease caused by *P. argentipes* might change in the event of climatic and environmental changes that resulted from increased anthropogenic activities in Bangladesh and elsewhere.

Keywords: Ecological niche model (ENM), Visceral leishmaniasis (VL), Bangladesh, Environmental factors, Human VL cases, Disease modeling

* Correspondence: abuyousufabdullah@yahoo.com
[1]Department of Geography and Environment, University of Dhaka, University Road, Dhaka 1000, Bangladesh
Full list of author information is available at the end of the article

Background

Visceral leishmaniasis (hereafter, VL) caused by *Leishmania donovani* is transmitted to humans by the bite of the sand fly vector. Some of the prominent species include *Phlebotomus argentipes* [1], *Phlebotomus orientalis* in East African lowlands [2], *Phlebotomus papatasi* in Southwest Asia [3], and *Phlebotomus martini* in Kenya/Ethiopia [4]. The disease is endemic in 98 countries with an estimated global burden of 300 million people [5]. Annually, between 20,000 and 40,000 human fatalities are believed to be attributed to this disease worldwide [6], and the risk of insurgence/resurgence or spread into new areas is likely to increase with the changing climate [7].

Of the total global incidences of VL (also called kala-azar in South Asia), more than 67% of the cases are found in the Indian subcontinent, largely affecting the poorest in a population [6, 8]. The literature suggests that the number of people at risk in India, Bangladesh, and Nepal ranges from 200 to 300 million [9], and the annual economic impact is estimated to be US$350 million [10]. Because of the significant increase in VL cases in the Indian subcontinent, in 2005, India, Bangladesh, and Nepal undertook a program to eliminate the disease [11].

Environmental factors acquired from various sources, including geographic information and remotely sensed data, have been used to predict and elucidate the distribution of the disease caused by vectors. This approach has proven to be highly useful for disease prevention and has been used to forecast epidemics, which is imperative for the preparedness of health systems to cope with such outbreaks [3, 4, 7, 12–19]. For example, land surface temperature and vegetation index obtained from satellite data showed significant correlation with the occurrence of sand flies in East Africa [4]. An ecological niche model (hereinafter, ENM) showed that the distribution of the sand fly vector was strongly linked with land cover type in the Middle East [14]. *P. papatasi* was found to be associated with vegetation in Southwest Asia [3]. Using two predictive models, Nieto et al. [20] showed that the highest VL risk in the interior region of Brazil was linked with a semiarid and hot climate, while the coastal forest region was unsuitable for sand fly. Spatiotemporal dynamics of vector species and human dengue cases was investigated using the monthly normalized difference vegetation index from NOAA–AVHRR data together with surface properties and topographic index [17]. Their study revealed significant correspondence between predicted vector activity and human dengue cases in South America. Similarly, elevation, rainfall, temperature, and forest cover were found to be associated with the distribution of sand flies in France [13]. Therefore, Guernier et al. [21] emphasized that consideration of a combination of ecological and climatic factors could greatly enhance the understanding

about the distribution of human pathogens. All of the studies noted above have demonstrated the influence of environmental factors on the occurrence of disease and, consequently, potential distribution of vectors in various settings, which could support targeted interventions to tackle vector-borne diseases such as VL caused by sand fly.

Various modeling techniques are now available to integrate environmental layers with disease cases, which allow environmental factors to be isolated and potential vector distribution to be mapped. Among them, the ENM has played a vital role in determining the underlying factors that contribute to the spatial patterns of the disease [17]. It is a powerful tool because of its ability to predict the distribution of vectors in areas where detailed sampling is lacking [22], and has been utilized in various studies around the world to model dengue [23], malaria [24, 25], canine leishmaniasis [13], anthrax [15], visceral leishmaniasis [20, 26], leishmaniasis transmitted by *Lutzomyia* [27–29], Chagas disease [19], and Japanese encephalitis [16]. For example, using climatic variables together with topographic parameters in an ENM, González et al. [7] predicted that climate change will exacerbate the ecological risk of human exposure to leishmaniasis in North America.

Although the incidence of VL is not a new phenomenon in Bangladesh, the major resurgence after the 1990s was mainly attributed to the cessation of DDT (dichloro diphenyl trichloroethane) spraying, originally undertaken to control malaria vectors in South Asia [30, 31]. To date, a number of initiatives were taken into account to eliminate the disease from Bangladesh, of which the VL elimination program is the most recent and currently in place [32]. With the introduction of the program in 2005, there had been a sharp decrease in the number of cases [11, 33]. Environmental vector management was implemented as part of the elimination program, for instance in Mymensingh district, but its effectiveness showed mixed outcomes [34]. Le Rutte et al. [35] emphasized that such measures require additional intervention in highly endemic areas. Thornton et al. [36] emphasized that a "one size fits all" strategy may not be an appropriate approach because VL occurrence is a multifaceted problem. As noted by Joshi et al. [10], complete elimination may be difficult to achieve in South Asia due to a number of reasons, including shortcomings of disease surveillance systems and resource constraints. Because the natural environment is constantly disturbed by humans through agricultural development and/or deforestation due to the ever-increasing population in Bangladesh, minimizing "ecological risk" of VL spread [7] could be an important alternative to keep its occurrence at an acceptable level. The exact terrestrial habitat of the sand fly vector is largely unknown [37]; therefore, modeling the distribution of disease based on environmental conditions could provide the information required for the effective management of this fatal disease [38–40]. The outcome may then guide health officials in making informed decisions and targeted interventions.

Although a number of studies of the clinical manifestations, epidemiological features, and socioeconomic aspect of VL have been conducted in Bangladesh [9, 11, 33, 34, 41–55], very few studies have used VL cases together with environmental variables to investigate the disease occurrence and factors affecting its distribution, particularly in endemic areas of Bangladesh [56]. This study aims to fill this gap with an assumption that if the probability of the distribution of the disease can be modeled, then the occurrence of vectors could be determined since their geographical spread appears to be the same. Here, the human cases obtained from the field visits were used to model the distribution of VL. As sand flies are found to be distributed in and around infected households in endemic areas of Bangladesh [54, 56, 57], we believe that using human VL cases, in the absence of actual vector locations, could provide valuable insights into the likelihood of vectors over space and contribute to the understanding of the geographic ecology of the vectors.

In this work, first, we aimed to develop an ENM to predict the distribution of disease in endemic areas of Bangladesh by assuming that its distribution is likely to follow the incidence of its vectors. Second, we attempted to characterize the environmental and ecological conditions suitable for the occurrence of *P. argentipes*, which is important in formulating appropriate measures for effective health-care delivery.

Methods

Study area

In this study, we concentrated on two districts of Bangladesh: one is hyperendemic, and the other is relatively endemic [58]. Three *upazilas* (subdistricts), namely Fulbaria, Trishal, and Gaffargaon, in Mymensingh district and Sreepur *upazila* in Gazipur district constitute the study area, which lies between longitudes of 90.26°–90.54° E and latitudes of 24.19°–24.62° N (Fig. 1). Of the 15,850 VL cases reported in Bangladesh between 2008 and 2014, Fulbaria had 4858 cases (30.65%), Trishal had 4670 cases (29.47%), Gaffargaon had 1426 cases (9.0%), and Sreepur had 283 cases (1.8%) [59]. These four *upazilas* comprised 70.92% of the total number of VL cases reported in Bangladesh. Therefore, we believe the study area provides a unique opportunity to examine the correspondence between human VL cases and potential distribution of *P. argentipes*.

Environmental variables

The environmental data (Table 1) included 19 bioclimatic (bioclim) variables, six variables derived from

remotely sensed data, and four soil variables obtained from a public database. The bioclim variables were downloaded from the WorldClim website [60]. They have a nominal resolution of approximately 1 km^2 and were developed from monthly average climate data between 1950 and 2000 using observed data [61].

Six Landsat scenes, from 2010 to 2015 (11 Mar. 2010, 14 Mar. 2011, 16 Mar. 2012, 19 Mar. 2013, 30 Mar. 2014, 17 Mar. 2015), were downloaded from the USGS site [62]. Preprocessing of Landsat data included georeferencing, subsetting, and atmospheric correction [63]. A number of derivatives were then computed, including land surface temperature (LST), normalized difference vegetation index (NDVI) [64], and normalized difference water index (NDWI) [65]. A land use/land cover (LULC) map was also derived via maximum likelihood supervised classification [63, 66]. The major LULC categories were vegetation, human settlements, waterbodies, and cultivated land. To derive LST, the thermal band of each Landsat scene was converted to spectral radiance [67], which was corrected for emissivity [68]. The images were then converted to the Celsius unit. Mean annual LST, NDVI, and NDWI data were then computed from these images. A digital elevation model (DEM) was also downloaded from ASTER GDEM [62] and used to calculate the topographic wetness index (TWI) as well as elevation surface. The TWI was calculated using slope and flow accumulation data derived from DEM [69].

Apart from the bioclim and satellite-derived parameters, edaphic layers were retrieved from Bangladesh Agricultural Research Council (BARC) [70]. All the layers were then clipped to the study area and resampled to the same geographic extent. As the bioclim variables have a nominal resolution of 1 km^2, the Landsat-derived products and other variables were resampled to the same spatial resolution.

Human VL cases

Multitemporal human VL cases were obtained from kala-azar patient registry logbooks located in each *Upazila* Health Complex (UHC). The *union* (lowest administrative unit in Bangladesh) and village names were then extracted from logbooks against the *mauza* (village and *mauza* are synonymous but *mauza* is used in Bengali) names, obtained from a community series database provided by the Bangladesh Bureau of Statistics (BBS). This operation resulted in a total of 3671 cases from 2010 to 2015, whose residence was within the study area. In early 2016 (January–May), we conducted several field visits to obtain the geographic coordinates of infected VL cases, occurred between 2010 and 2015, and successfully located 333 households. A Global Positioning System (GPS) was used to obtain the precise coordinates of the individual

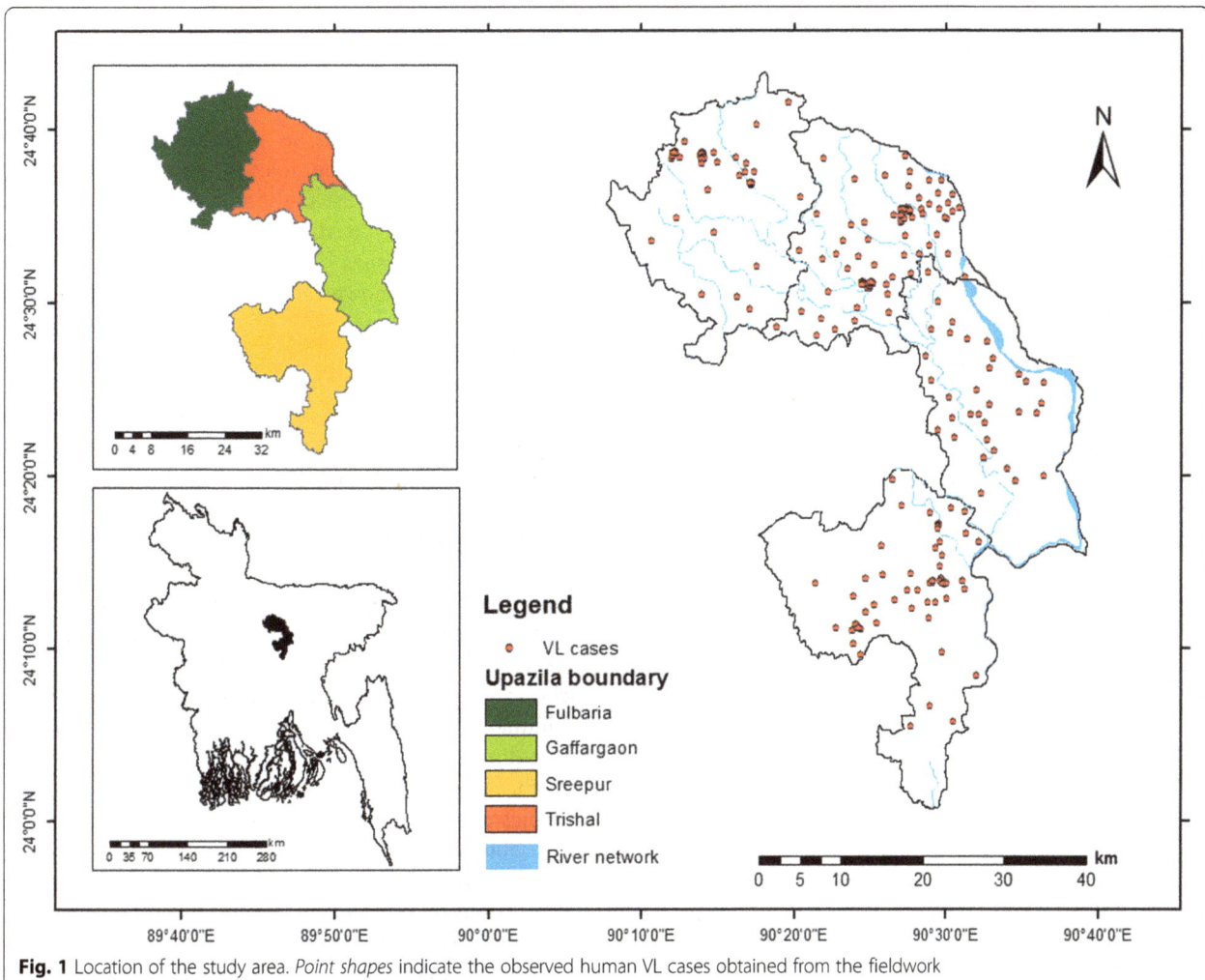

Fig. 1 Location of the study area. *Point shapes* indicate the observed human VL cases obtained from the fieldwork

households. Two handheld GPSs (Trimble Nomad 800GXE) were employed to record the absolute location of a case. If a household had multiple cases, we recorded only one point for that household to facilitate the dispersed distribution of cases over the area of interest. Because living with or near a person who had recently experienced VL has been identified as an important risk factor in Bangladesh [9, 49], we hypothesized that the use of multiple cases from the same household could lead to household clustering that may bias our model. During the fieldwork, each household was assigned a code in the database to uniquely identify its location related to *upazila*, *mauza*, and *union*. Besides, geotagged photographs of physical and cultural features were taken to facilitate this study. The location of the 333 VL cases is shown in Fig. 1.

Given the paucity of case locations, the spatially unique human VL cases obtained from the fieldwork were used as presence data in our effort to develop an ENM. Human cases have been used as presence data in a number of previous studies to develop ENMs for determining potential vector distribution in different settings [20, 71, 72].

Ecological niche modeling

There are two approaches to construct an ENM for modeling disease and the distribution of vectors [73]. The first approach involves modeling the species, with occurrence data, that participate in the transmission cycle [14, 16, 74] while the second approach analyzes the distribution of disease occurrence, as if it was a species, considering the entire transmission cycle and its ecological relationships [20, 71, 72]. In addition to this, *P. argentipes* has been shown to be the single proven vector of *L. donovani* in the study area [50]; thus, its distribution could reasonably be determined by the same environmental variables used to model the distribution of the disease.

In this study, we employed the second approach, using the maxent software to construct an ENM [75], which is based on a maximum entropy algorithm. This algorithm has been found to be robust in predicting vectors or species distribution from presence-only data [76, 77]. Sillero [22], however, observed that the use of presence-only data results in the identification of a "realized niche,"

Table 1 Environmental variables used in this study

Serial no.	Variable	Description of the variable	Source
1	Bio_1	Annual mean temperature	www.worldclim.org/current
2	Bio_2	Mean diurnal range (mean of monthly (max temp – min temp))	
3	Bio_3	Isothermality (Bio2/Bio7) (*100)	
4	Bio_4	Temperature seasonality (standard deviation*100)	
5	Bio_5	Max temperature of warmest month	
6	Bio_6	Min temperature of coldest month	
7	Bio_7	Temperature annual range (Bio5–Bio6)	
8	Bio_8	Mean temperature of wettest quarter	
9	Bio_9	Mean temperature of driest quarter	
10	Bio_10	Mean temperature of warmest quarter	
11	Bio_11	Mean temperature of coldest quarter	
12	Bio_12	Annual precipitation	
13	Bio_13	Precipitation of wettest month	
14	Bio_14	Precipitation of driest month	
15	Bio_15	Precipitation seasonality (coefficient of variation)	
16	Bio_16	Precipitation of wettest quarter	
17	Bio_17	Precipitation of driest quarter	
18	Bio_18	Precipitation of warmest quarter	
19	Bio_19	Precipitation of coldest quarter	
20	Drainage	Soil drainage	www.barc.gov.bd
21	GST	General soil type	
22	Soil moisture	Soil moisture	
23	Soil reaction	Soil reaction or soil pH	
24	LULC	Land use/land cover	Landsat images (https://earthexplorer.usgs.gov/)
25	NDVI	Normalized difference vegetation index	
26	NDWI	Normalized difference water index	
27	TWI	Topographic wetness index	
28	LST	Land surface temperature	
29	Dem	Elevation	ASTER GDEM

which is the area suitable in terms of biotic and abiotic factors. In contrast, Lobo et al. [78] noted that the use of absence or pseudo absence data increases the chance of error of estimation. In this work, we utilized field-derived VL case locations, as presence-only data to be used as input data. The maxent software computes niches by finding the distribution of probabilities closest to uniform, with the constraint that feature values match their empirical averages [79]. Based on the environmental conditions of known locations, maxent estimates a probability distribution map with a value between 0 and 1 for each cell, where 0 indicates the least suitable and 1 indicates the most suitable cell for disease or species occurrence [76]. The reasons for using maxent in this study were threefold: one, it is good at characterizing environments in a study area [80] and identifying potential niches of vectors [81]; two, the results are highly useful for regions where actual vector locations are missing or limited [76]; and three, the fact that the disease is both zoonotic and anthroponotic [82] means that a realized niche for *P. argentipes* is achievable, which is therefore a potential niche for VL and can readily become a realized niche for VL by the introduction of an infected animal or human. Hence, the second approach seems to be relevant to this work.

In this study, we used a wide range of environmental variables and developed 30 models, each with one of the 29 variables (Table 1) removed and one with none of the variables removed. The 30 models were run to evaluate the contribution of each variable to the modeling results. In each iteration, we recorded the best combination of variables by calculating the test area under the curve (AUC). High test AUC values indicate a good fit of the model to the testing data, implying high predictive power [83]. The excluded variables that caused the greatest decreases in AUC values were also recorded. This operation outputted a total of six variables, namely LST, NDWI, precipitation of the warmest quarter, precipitation seasonality, general soil type (GST), and drainage (Table 2). These variables were then used to construct an ENM to determine their influence on the likelihood of *P. argentipes* occurrence.

Out of the 333 VL case locations, 75% (248 presence points) were assigned randomly as training data and the remaining 25% (82 points) were used as testing points for model validation. Note that three duplicate points were removed by maxent during the model building. Both threshold-dependent and threshold-independent approaches were employed to evaluate the ENM. The AUC of the receiver operating characteristic (ROC) is a threshold-independent method that was used to calculate the total AUC of the sensitivity versus the fractional predicted area [77]. Models with AUC values from 0.75 to 0.90 are considered very useful, and >0.90 is considered highly accurate [72, 84]. The threshold-dependent measure was based on minimum training presence and used a one-tail binomial test. The null hypothesis was that the ENM does not predict the test/predicted presence points better than a random model. If the null hypothesis is rejected, then the ENM is a better predictor [14, 77].

To determine the variables that contributed most to the ENM construction, the percent contribution and the jackknife test of variable importance were used. The maxent algorithm measures the drop in the training AUC during permutation and expresses it as the percent contribution to the model. On the other hand, during the jackknife test, the model is developed using only one variable to find the increase in training gain and then with all variables while excluding that variable to determine the decrease in training gain [85, 86]. The variable that causes the highest gain when used in isolation encompasses the most useful information, and the one causing the highest decrease in gain contains the most unique information [83]. Therefore, we isolated the top three variables during the final ENM development based on the highest percent contribution and the two variables that produced the highest increase and decrease in training gain (when included and excluded alone). However, when a single variable was found in all three criteria, we extended our search based on the highest values of training gain, test gain, and test AUC in the jackknife test. The variables that produced the highest gains and test AUCs when used alone were considered as the most important variables [83]. The probability distribution map produced by maxent was then consulted to extract logistic probability values of each *mazua*, in order to determine suitable and unsuitable locations (based on the probability values) for the distribution of *P. argentipes*. A threshold value of 0.5 is commonly used [87] to identify moderate to high probable locations of the disease, consequently the vectors. The mean VL cases obtained from the UHC records were subsequently computed for each *mauza* and compared with the probability value. This comparison may be useful to understand the strength of the ENM developed here and the suitability of the disease distribution and, consequently, potential distribution of vectors in the study area.

Results

The results of 30 runs of the models, where each variable was excluded one at a time and once with all the variables included, are shown in Table 2. Only six variables produced test AUC values below 0.815, namely precipitation seasonality, precipitation during the warmest quarter, drainage, general soil type, NDWI, and LST.

These variables were considered to have contributed most to the model development.

In Fig. 2, sensitivity versus the fractional area graphs for the final ENM with LST, NDWI, precipitation of the warmest quarter, precipitation seasonality, general soil type, and drainage are shown for the training and test data. The AUC value for the training was 0.842 and the test AUC was 0.804 with a standard deviation of 0.030, indicating the performance of the model was highly satisfactory. Further, the test AUC was well above the random prediction AUC, suggesting that the ENM was much better at predicting the distribution of disease, hence the occurrence of *P. argentipes* than a random model. The narrow range of the standard deviation showed the high accuracy of the average output produced. The minimum training presence for a training point was 0.024; therefore, this value was used as the threshold in the model evaluation. The fractional predicted area was 0.977 with a test omission rate of 0.012. At this threshold, the null hypothesis was rejected because the constructed ENM performed significantly better than a random model ($p < 0.05$).

Table 3 shows that precipitation of the warmest quarter had the highest percent contribution, along with the highest increase and decrease in training gain in the jackknife test. As shown in Fig. 3, the jackknife test of variable importance revealed that both the test gain and test AUC were higher for LST, precipitation of the warmest quarter, and NDWI. These three variables had a total contribution of 70.2% to the model building (Table 3) and were possibly highly influential for disease occurrence. The specific probability values of these three variables showed that precipitation of the warmest quarter, which had a value of 1040 mm, was potentially suitable, while NDWI values from −0.35 to −0.10 and LSTs between 29.86 and 31.19 °C were estimated to be conducive. An LST of 29.9 °C and NDWI of −0.225 produced the highest probability of affecting the distribution of disease.

The probability distribution map of the disease produced by the ENM is shown in Fig. 4. The distribution map can be used to identify areas with high and low portability of the disease occurrence or potential of *P. argentipes* distribution at the *mauza* level. Intersection of this map with the *mauza* database indicated that out of 479 *mauzas*, four in Fulbaria, three in Gaffargaon, eight in Trishal, and seven in Sreepur *upazilas* exhibited moderate to high probability of disease occurrence (Table 4), consequently the potential of the distribution of *P. argentipes* in the study area.

Interestingly, of the 22 *mauzas* (27.5% of the study area), which were identified using a cutoff value of 0.5, 18 had the higher numbers of mean VL cases. This result suggests that the ENM performed well and

Table 2 Results of the 30 runs of the models with individual variables excluded in turn

Excluded variable	Test AUC	Standard deviation	% Contribution in model development 1st	Jackknife test (based on training gain) 2nd	3rd
None	0.819	0.0328	bio18	bio18	LST
Annual mean temperature (Bio_1)	0.818	0.0330	bio18	bio18	LST
Mean diurnal range (Bio_2)	0.820	0.0329	bio18	bio18	LST
Isothermality (Bio_3)	0.821	0.0327	bio18	bio18	LST
Temperature seasonality (Bio_4)	0.819	0.0331	bio18	bio18	LST
Max temperature of warmest month (Bio_5)	0.819	0.0330	bio18	bio18	NDWI
Min temperature of coldest month (Bio_6)	0.819	0.0332	bio18	bio18	LST
Temperature annual range (Bio_7)	0.820	0.0329	bio18	bio18	LST
Mean temperature of wettest quarter (Bio_8)	0.819	0.0329	bio18	bio18	LST
Mean temperature of driest quarter (Bio_9)	0.820	0.0328	bio18	bio18	LST
Mean temperature of warmest quarter (Bio_10)	0.819	0.0330	bio18	bio18	LST
Mean temperature of coldest quarter (Bio_11)	0.819	0.0329	bio18	bio18	LST
Annual precipitation (Bio_12)	0.820	0.0328	bio18	bio18	LST
Precipitation of wettest month (Bio_13)	0.818	0.0330	bio18	bio18	LST
Precipitation of driest month (Bio_14)	0.820	0.0325	bio18	bio18	LST
Precipitation seasonality (Bio_15)	*0.812*	*0.0337*	bio18	bio18	LST
Precipitation of wettest quarter (Bio_16)	0.820	0.0327	bio18	bio18	LST
Precipitation of driest quarter (Bio_17)	0.819	0.0329	bio18	bio18	LST
Precipitation of warmest quarter (Bio_18)	*0.814*	*0.0331*	GST	bio13	LST
Precipitation of coldest quarter (Bio_19)	0.819	0.0330	bio18	bio18	LST
Soil drainage	*0.814*	*0.033*	bio18	bio18	GST
General soil type (GST)	*0.811*	*0.0342*	bio18	bio18	LST
Soil moisture	0.820	0.0327	bio18	bio18	LST
Soil reaction	0.820	0.0327	bio18	bio18	NDWI
Land use/land cover category (LULC)	0.820	0.0328	bio18	bio18	LST
Normalized difference vegetation index (NDVI)	0.822	0.0321	bio18	bio18	NDWI
Normalized difference water index (NDWI)	*0.813*	*0.0334*	bio18	bio18	LST
Topographic wetness index (TWI)	0.819	0.0328	bio18	bio18	LST
Land surface temperature (LST)	*0.813*	*0.0328*	bio18	bio18	NDWI
Elevation	0.820	0.0327	bio18	bio18	LST

Italicized variables are considered to have contributed most to the model development

demonstrates the correspondence between known VL cases and potential distribution of vectors. In other words, if the probability of the disease occurrence itself is being modeled, one can expect that its incidence will follow the same. In addition, the ecological requirements of the disease as a result of *P. argentipes* abundance in these *mauzas* (Table 4) indicated positive relationships between observed human cases and precipitation during the warmest quarter of the year, LST, and NDWI. For instance, the mean LST (30.17 °C), mean NDWI (−0.24), and mean precipitation of the warmest quarter (1040.8 mm) were found to account for the high

VL occurrence in Kushmail *mauza* in Fulbaria *upazila*, as exemplified by the high probability of disease distribution. A somewhat similar association was found in Kakchar *mazua* in Trishal *upazila*. However, this association was not always true for every *mauza* investigated in this study. For instance, Achim Patuli *mauza* in Fulbaria *upazila* showed some non-linearity between mean VL cases and probability of the disease distribution.

Discussion

VL is a life-threatening disease that disproportionately affects the poorest subset of populations in the Indian

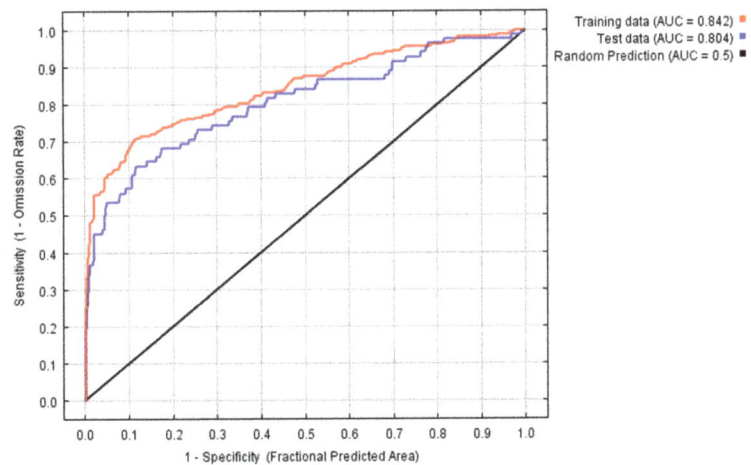

Fig. 2 Sensitivity versus specificity graphs for VL disease distribution using the final ENM

subcontinent and elsewhere [8]. We developed an ENM to demonstrate the correspondence between human VL cases and potential distribution of *P. argentipes* in endemic areas of Bangladesh. Ecological requirements of the disease occurrence caused by the sand fly vector were also determined. The analysis revealed that precipitation during the warmest quarter of the year (bio18), NDWI, and LST were the main environmental factors associated with the distribution and incidence of the disease. As *P. argentipes* is the single proven vector of *L. donovani* in the study area [50], its distribution is likely be determined by the same environmental variables. One highly likely explanation is the role of these environmental factors in regulating microclimates of the region, which potentially affect vector populations and the reservoir hosts.

Precipitation during the warmest quarter of the year appeared to be the main climatic factor influencing actual and probable incidences of the disease, which reinforces the general consensus that moist conditions are suitable for sand flies such as *P. argentipes*. High seasonality in the occurrence of the disease has been observed during the warm months in Bangladesh [9]. Therefore,

the influence of precipitation during this period is not surprising as sand fly populations and the proportion of gravid females are at their highest during this period [34]. The Irrigation Support Project for Asia and the Near East (ISPAN) [88] observed that adult sand flies usually emerge during early summer (March–May) in Bangladesh and continue to thrive until the monsoon period (June–September/October) as a result of increased humidity. It is, thus, reasonable to assume that moist conditions resulting from heavy rainfall lead to the occurrence of the disease and possibly support sand fly emergence and abundance, especially in the study area, because high humidity is a prerequisite for their survival [38, 89]. Humidity determines the extrinsic incubation and vector life cycle, and Bhunia et al. [90], for example, observed that the abundance of *P. argentipes* in Bihar was associated with high humidity and heavy rainfall. Our results differ slightly from those of similar studies in Iran [91], India [39, 89], and Sudan [38] in which annual rainfall, rather than precipitation during a certain period, was reported as an influential factor affecting the distribution of the disease. The difference between our findings and those of others may stem from local

Table 3 Identification of the top three variables based on percent contribution, and training and test gains

Variable	Percent contribution	Training gain (without variable)	Training gain (only variable)	Test gain (without variable)	Test gain (only variable)	Test AUC (without variable)	Test AUC (only variable)
LST	15.8	0.7247	0.2379	1.0048	0.4909	0.7891	0.6779
NDWI	22.8	0.676	0.2681	0.9771	0.4878	0.8048	0.7146
Precipitation seasonality	5.6	0.785	0.0975	1.066	0.1523	0.7873	0.6582
Precipitation of the warmest quarter	31.6	0.6261	0.293	0.9063	0.5081	0.7878	0.7322
Drainage	15.4	0.7819	0.135	1.1004	0.1171	0.7958	0.6489
GST	8.8	0.7527	0.0771	1.1058	0.0326	0.7914	0.572

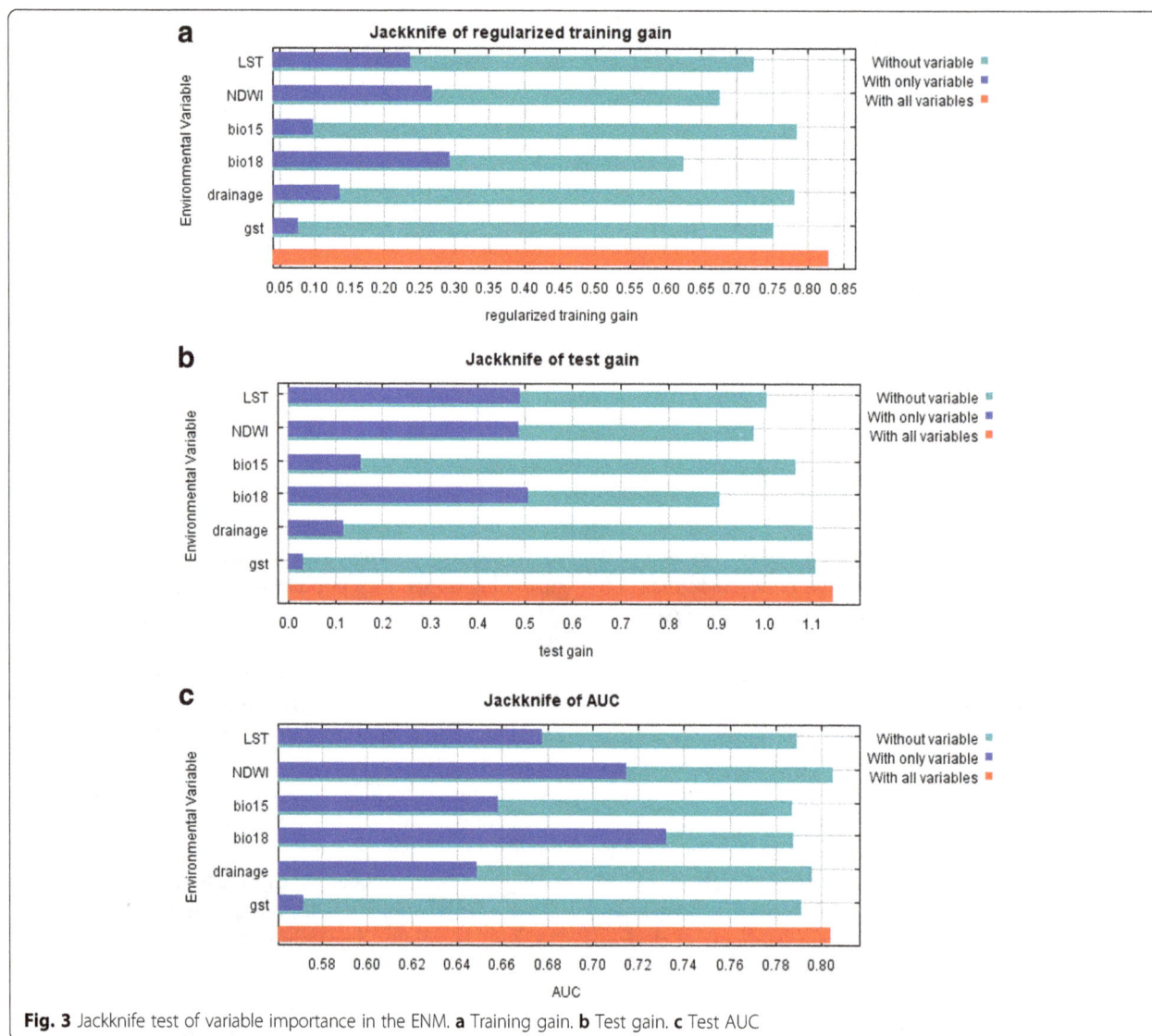

Fig. 3 Jackknife test of variable importance in the ENM. **a** Training gain. **b** Test gain. **c** Test AUC

physiographic and climatic characteristics of the study sites as well as differences in the methods used. Because the transmission of many parasitic diseases is confined to the summer season, changes in the lengths of rainy and dry seasons, together with changes in the intervals between seasons as a result of climatic changes, are likely to affect larvae and adult vector development and abundance [92]. Additional study is therefore warranted.

The NDWI is another important variable affecting the occurrence of the disease and potentially accountable for vector abundance in the study area. In an NDWI image derived from Landsat, negative values are a reflection of water features [65]. Over the study area, we found that water features ranged from −0.351 to 0.104, which may have contributed to the occurrence of *P. argentipes*. The presence of waterbodies, such as swamps, ponds, ephemeral canals, and marshy lands, is considered to

provide suitable vector breeding sites [93]. This result suggests that people living close to waterbodies may have elevated risk of infection. Case–control studies in India confirmed that rural households in close proximity to waterbodies were at greater risk of VL than those apart [40, 94]. Bhunia et al. [39, 90] examined the effect of waterbodies/NDWI derived from satellite data on VL cases and reported a strong association, which agrees with our finding. Their study further revealed that VL cases decreased with increased distance from waterbodies. In a recent study, Abedi-Astaneh et al. [95] showed that low-lying land provides a good ecological niche for the sand fly vector. Our study area is characterized by lowlands with widespread water features; therefore, higher transmission potential of *P. argentipes* is very likely. The role of waterbodies in supporting vector abundance in the study area may be

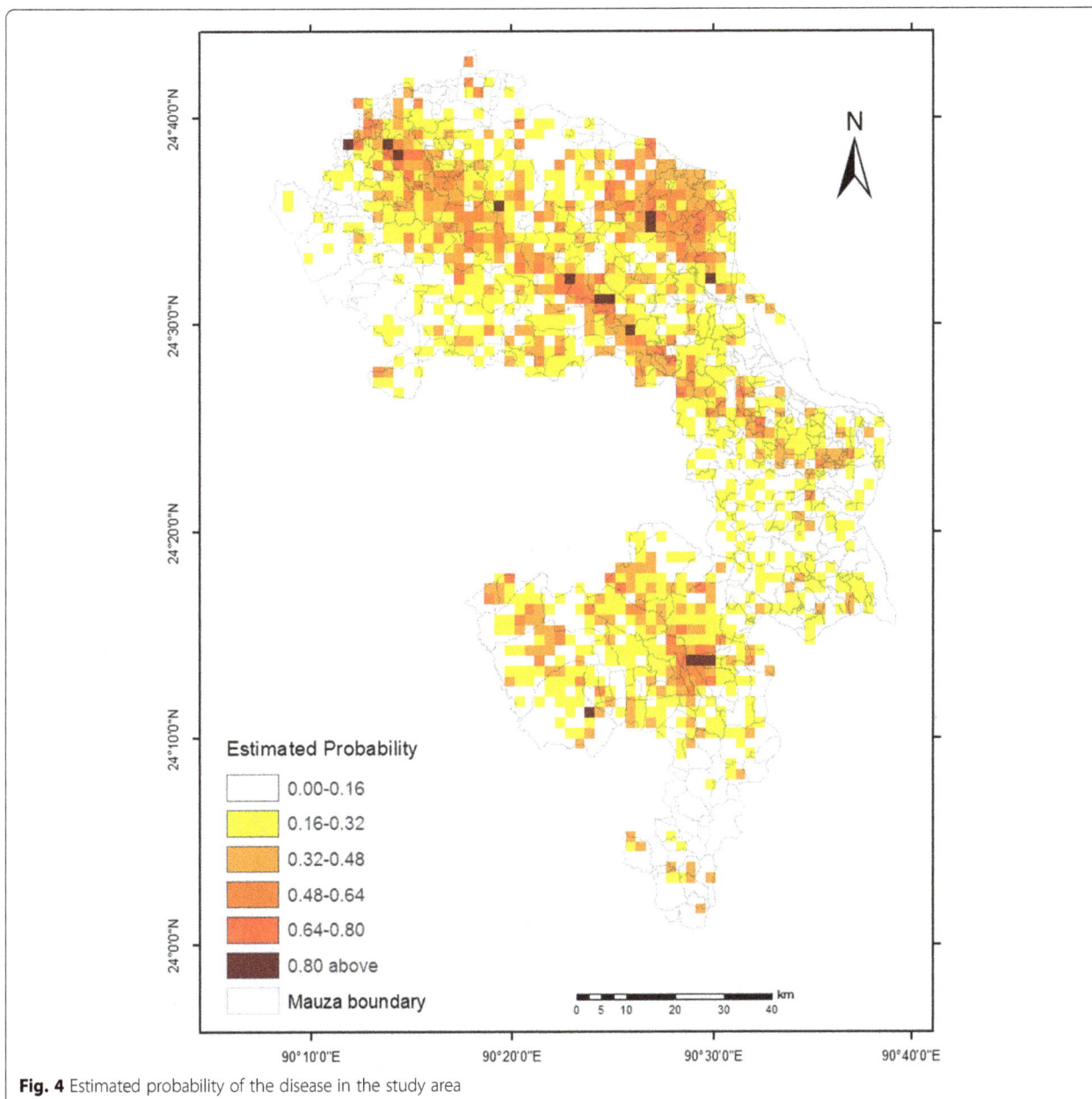

Fig. 4 Estimated probability of the disease in the study area

because they contribute significantly to maintaining moisture in the soil/subsoil, which suits the breeding and propagation of the immature stages of sand flies as well as provides resting habitats for the vector in adjoining domestic biotopes [40].

In addition to the presence of waterbodies in endemic areas, modification of the natural hydrological system through flood control, drainage, and/or irrigation may be equally responsible for the distribution of disease via enhanced vector activity. This was evidenced by Emch [53], who noticed that the incidence of VL cases in flood-controlled (e.g., embanked) areas of northwest Bangladesh was significantly higher than that in non-embanked areas, which he attributed to lack of seasonal

flooding within the embanked areas. Despite the mechanism being not fully clear, ISPAN [88] argued that floods can wash away organic matter and larvae sites, and this process is impeded by flood control works that evidently facilitate larval development and breeding of sand flies. The efficacy of flooding on immature stages of sand fly was also observed by Mukhopadhyay et al. [96] in India, suggesting that flooding beneficially removes vector breeding sites. Hence, environmental changes caused by population growth, agricultural intensification, and development activities (e.g., flood control works, road construction) may have resulted in an environment that is humid, a factor essential for sand fly larval development. In addition, widespread rainfall

Table 4 *Mauzas* showing moderate to high probabilities of the VL cases, caused by *P. argentipes* with corresponding mean value of environmental variables

	Union	Mauza	Mean cases	Probability	LST Mean (°C)	NDWI Mean	Precipitation of the warmest quarter Mean (mm)
Fulbaria	Kushmail	Kushmail	24	0.92	30.174	−0.244	1040.833
	Achim Patuli	Achim Patuli	18	0.65	30.223	−0.221	1027.950
	Putijana	Putijana	16	0.76	29.956	−0.276	1040.833
	Radhakanai	Radhakanai Dhurdhuri	14	0.51	30.135	−0.238	1050.540
Trishal	Rampur	Kakchar	41	0.97	30.135	−0.252	1064.750
	Kanihari	Kanihari	35	0.96	30.214	−0.232	1076.440
	Harirampur	Magurjora	29	0.96	30.364	−0.211	1044.500
	Kanihari	Barma	16	0.87	30.128	−0.233	1068.800
	Harirampur	Rargaon	13	0.81	30.211	−0.233	1041.643
	Trishal	Satra Para	10	0.88	30.343	−0.237	1045.500
	Bali Para	Bahadurpur	7	0.58	30.177	−0.245	1066.667
	Kanthal	Kanthal	6	0.54	30.041	−0.248	1073.609
Gafargaon	Raona	Raona	7	0.63	30.071	−0.250	1037.667
	Jessora	Jasara	5	0.60	30.295	−0.226	1046.636
	Gaffargaon	Autbaria	6	0.52	30.105	−0.253	1050.500
Sreepur	Maona	Maona	33	0.86	30.635	−0.223	990.160
	Maona	Bara Rathura	13	0.76	30.677	−0.231	986.286
	Ward No-04	Bhangahati	12	0.80	30.457	−0.217	995.500
	Barmi	Satkhamair	9	0.71	30.478	−0.248	1004.485
	Telihati	Tengra	9	0.64	30.532	−0.229	1002.200
	Rajabari	Noagaon	8	0.66	30.366	−0.240	976.670
	Ward No-01	Ujilaba Purbapara	4	0.51	30.183	−0.288	997.000

during summer in the study area could lead to artificial logging and/or riverine pools due to its low elevation, which appear to affect the ecological environment of the vectors [40]. Consequently, the population dynamics of disease-carrying insects or their breeding periods and reproduction may be affected, because the breeding success of sand flies is highly dependent on rainfall duration [97]. Furthermore, people in rural Bangladesh commonly interact with waterbodies for various reasons such as fishing, bathing, and/or irrigation. These types of activities may enhance transmission potential of VL to humans. The transmission dynamics of VL in relation to waterbodies, therefore, remains a very promising area for detailed investigation.

One of the most important factors in the distribution of sand fly is temperature because it affects its survival and the speed of development of the different stages in the life cycle [98]. A temperature range of 7–37 °C with a relative humidity of >70% is highly favorable for sand fly survival in India [99]. Our analysis indicated that mean annual LST in the range 29 to 31 °C was an important predictor of the distribution of the disease, which may be useful to understand the distribution of *P. argentipes* in the study area, since one can expect that the incidence of disease generally follows the occurrence of sand fly [49]. This finding supports an earlier observation by Kesari et al. [100], who demonstrated that mean and maximum LSTs were significantly associated with sand fly density in India. Thomson et al. [101] also found that mean annual maximum daily LST from 34 to 38 °C was one of the most important ecological determinants of *P. orientalis* distribution in Sudan. Similarly, Gebre-Michael et al. [4] reported that, in East Africa, seasonal and annual LSTs were one of the best ecological determinants of *P. martini* and *P. orientalis*. Another study in Sudan, however, reported a negative relationship between LST and VL occurrence but confirmed the role of annual mean maximum and minimum daily atmospheric temperatures in the distribution of vectors [98]. Kesari et al. [100] indicated that a dry season LST of 22.23 °C and a wet season LST of 23–34 °C could account for *P. argentipes* distribution; however, in our study, we found that an annual LST of 29–31 °C likely provided a suitable niche for the incidence of the disease, suggesting the potential of *P. argentipes* survival and abundance in the study area. Nevertheless, our study together with findings from previous work in India and East Africa clearly underscored the role of LST in the occurrence of the disease.

If temperatures increase and rainfall regimes change as a result of climate warming, there would be a significant effect on vector populations. Rainfall helps to increase relative humidity, and alterations of temperature could support longevity of the vector and transmission of the disease [102]. Therefore, the impact of probable climate changes on the spread of the disease caused by sand flies (e.g., *P. argentipes*) remains a very important research topic in South Asia and Bangladesh.

Based on the probability value of 0.5, our ENM differentiated *mauzas* that had moderate to high probability of the disease (Table 4, Fig. 4), suggesting the likelihood of vector presence over space. These *mauzas* were distributed in all four *upazilas* in the study area, and in these *mauzas*, the observed mean VL cases appeared to follow the likelihood of *P. argentipes* distribution. Although the human cases in this study were retrospective, this finding does not seem to have occurred at random, meaning that our modeling approach clearly coincides the potential vector distribution with observed VL cases. This finding is partially consistent with those of Bern et al. [9] and Chowdhury et al. [11], who found that Fulbaria and Trishal in Bangladesh were highly endemic to VL. Note that the slight disagreement between probability of disease distribution and mean VL cases of three *mauzas* (Achim Patulia in Fulbaria, Satra Para in Trishal, and Naogaon in Sreepur) may have resulted from the socioeconomic situation and cultural behavior of the inhabitants of the investigated *upazilas*. An ongoing study is expected to clarify this.

A number of improvements to this study are possible. First, ENMs, such as the one developed in this study, are based on limited numbers of historical human VL cases. Small samples of occurrence points could lead to sampling bias, which may affect the overall results [25], though maxent arguably produces accurate predictions [76]. Second, inclusion of absence points (if available) could help to identify reasons for unsuitable ecological conditions, though Ortega-Huerta and Peterson [103] have suggested that this issue has a negligible effect when the spatial scale of analysis is small. Third, ENM predictions are based on input variables that affect larval development and vector survival [16]. Since we used the location of human cases as an input variable, the modeling result may be interpreted as a proxy for the potential distribution of *P. argentipes*. Fourth, the use of too many environmental variables may lead to misrepresentations due to overfitting [104], which might have increased the model complexity [77]. Fifth, we used a grid-based

model to predict potential *P. argentipes* distribution based on human cases and environmental parameters as opposed to using biogeographic limits [15]. This could be another limitation. Since *P. argentipes* is the single proven vector accountable for disease transmission in the study area [50], this work did not consider other species that may be responsible for the transmission of VL in the study area. This might be another shortcoming of this work. Finally, VL case data obtained from UHCs were very poorly recorded and required very careful assimilation. Due to a shortage of funds and the sparse distribution of VL-affected households, we had to rely on a small sample size to develop the ENM. Future studies should include more samples from the endemic areas.

Despite the limitations described above, the major strengths of this study are the identification of a fine-scale regional map that shows potential distribution of the disease and the isolation of the factors affecting the occurrence of *P. argentipes*. Our modeling result could certainly be used as a proxy for potential distribution of vectors that influences sand fly distribution in the endemic areas of Bangladesh. We believe that this work may be of considerable value, especially since a recent study strongly emphasized the need for microenvironmental studies of factors that influence VL distribution in endemic areas of Bangladesh [56].

Conclusions

To the best of our knowledge, this is the first attempt to identify underlying environmental factors that are accountable for visceral leishmaniasis (VL) incidence in Bangladesh. We developed an ENM to model the distribution of the disease which can be used as a proxy for potential distribution of vectors in endemic areas. In addition, ecological niches of the disease were identified, based on a wide range of environmental variables.

The analysis demonstrated that precipitation during the warmest quarter, land surface temperature (LST), and normalized difference water index (NDWI) were the main environmental factors influencing the occurrence of the disease in the study area. The result of the ENM may also be used to determine potential distribution of *P. argentipes*, as it is the only proven vector in the study area. Further, the occurrence of the vectors is likely to be determined by these environmental variables. This model could be used as a stepping stone to improve vector surveillance and sand fly control efforts, which could then support mapping of at-risk households. This work can be used as a baseline to model how the disease as well as vector distribution might change in the event of global environmental changes. Awareness should be raised in regions with high probability of the disease occurrence to prevent its insurgence/resurgence since it is anthroponotic in and around Bangladesh. This ecological study could be used with other socioeconomic parameters to develop a holistic and foolproof policy for eradicating the disease. We believe that knowledge of the environmental requirements to predict the distribution of the disease and, consequently, the vectors over space could help to support targeted responses to tackle this lethal disease, which affects the poorest people in Bangladesh.

Abbreviations
AUC: Area under the curve; DEM: Digital elevation model; ENM: Ecological niche model; GPS: Global Positioning System; GST: General soil type; LST: Land surface temperature; NDVI: Normalized difference vegetation index; NDWI: Normalized difference water index; TWI: Topographic wetness index; VL: Visceral leishmaniasis

Acknowledgements
We gratefully thank the study households and the health officials at the UHCs in the study area.

Funding
Self-funded.

Authors' contributions
The work was conceived and designed by AD, AYMA, and MMR. The field study was performed by all the authors with AD, AYMA, MRIS, and MMR analyzing the data involved in the study. AD, AYMA, and MFH contributed to writing the paper. All authors read and approved the final manuscript.

Competing interests
The authors declare that they have no competing interests.

Author details
[1]Department of Geography and Environment, University of Dhaka, University Road, Dhaka 1000, Bangladesh. [2]Department of Spatial Sciences, Curtin University, Perth, Australia.

References
1. Dinesh DS, Das ML, Picado A, Roy L, Rijal S, Singh SP, et al. Insecticide susceptibility of Phlebotomus argentipes in visceral leishmaniasis endemic districts in India and Nepal. PLoS Negl Trop Dis. 2010;4:e859.

2. Elnaiem DEA. Ecology and control of the sand fly vectors of Leishmania donovani in East Africa, with special emphasis on Phlebotomus orientalis. J Vector Ecol. 2011;36:S23–31.

3. Cross ER, Newcomb WW, Tucker CJ. Use of weather data and remote sensing to predict the geographic and seasonal distribution of Phlebotomus papatasi in southwest Asia. Am J Trop Med Hyg. 1996;54:530–6.

4. Gebre-Michael T, Malone J, Balkew M, Ali A, Berhe N, Hailu A, et al. Mapping the potential distribution of Phlebotomus martini and P. orientalis (Diptera: Psychodidae), vectors of kala-azar in East Africa by use of geographic information systems. Acta Trop. 2004;90:73–86.

5. Yangzom T, Cruz I, Bern C, Argaw D, den Boer M, Vélez ID, et al. Endemic transmission of visceral leishmaniasis in Bhutan. Am J Trop Med Hyg. 2012;87:1028–37.

6. Alvar J, Vélez ID, Bern C, Herrero M, Desjeux P, Cano J, et al. Leishmaniasis worldwide and global estimates of its incidence. PLoS One. 2012;7:e35671.

7. González C, Wang O, Strutz SE, González-Salazar C, Sánchez-Cordero V, Sarkar S. Climate change and risk of leishmaniasis in North America: predictions from ecological niche models of vector and reservoir species. PLoS Negl Trop Dis. 2010;4:e585.

8. Boelaert M, Meheus F, Robays J, Lutumba P. Socio-economic aspects of neglected diseases: sleeping sickness and visceral leishmaniasis. Ann Trop Med Parasitol. 2010;104:535–42.

9. Bern C, Hightower AW, Chowdhury R, Ali M, Amann J, Wagatsuma Y, et al. Risk factors for kala-azar in Bangladesh. Emerg Infect Dis. 2005;11:655–62.

10. Joshi A, Narain J, Prasittisuk C, Bhatia R, Hashim G, Jorge A, et al. Can visceral leishmaniasis be eliminated from Asia? J Vector Borne Dis. 2008;45:105.

11. Chowdhury R, Mondal D, Chowdhury V, Faria S, Alvar J, Nabi SG, et al. How far are we from visceral leishmaniasis elimination in Bangladesh? An assessment of epidemiological surveillance data. PLoS Negl Trop Dis. 2014;8:e3020.

12. Ebi KL, Nealon J. Dengue in a changing climate. Environ Res. 2016;151:115–23.

13. Chamaillé L, Tran A, Meunier A, Bourdoiseau G, Ready P, Dedet J-P. Environmental risk mapping of canine leishmaniasis in France. Parasit Vectors. 2010;3:1.

14. Colacicco-Mayhugh MG, Masuoka PM, Grieco JP. Ecological niche model of Phlebotomus alexandri and P. papatasi (Diptera: Psychodidae) in the Middle East. Int J Health Geogr. 2010;9:1.

15. Mullins J, Lukhnova L, Aikimbayev A, Pazilov Y, Van Ert M, Blackburn JK. Ecological niche modelling of the Bacillus anthracis A1.a sub-lineage in Kazakhstan. BMC Ecol. 2011;11:32.

16. Miller RH, Masuoka P, Klein TA, Kim H-C, Somer T, Grieco J. Ecological niche modeling to estimate the distribution of Japanese encephalitis virus in Asia. PLoS Negl Trop Dis. 2012;6:e1678.

17. Peterson AT, Martínez-Campos C, Nakazawa Y, Martínez-Meyer E. Time-specific ecological niche modeling predicts spatial dynamics of vector insects and human dengue cases. Trans R Soc Trop Med Hyg. 2005;99:647–55.

18. Peterson AT, Pereira RS, Neves VFC. Using epidemiological survey data to infer geographic distributions of leishmaniasis vector species. Rev Soc Bras Med Trop. 2004;37:10–4.

19. Costa J, Peterson AT, Beard CB. Ecologic niche modeling and differentiation of populations of Triatoma brasiliensis neiva, 1911, the most important Chagas' disease vector in northeastern Brazil (hemiptera, reduviidae, triatominae). Am J Trop Med Hyg. 2002;67:516–20.

20. Nieto P, Malone JB, Bavia ME. Ecological niche modeling for visceral leishmaniasis in the state of Bahia, Brazil, using genetic algorithm for rule-set prediction and growing degree day-water budget analysis. Geospat Health. 2006;1:115–26.

21. Guernier V, Hochberg ME, Guégan J-F. Ecology drives the worldwide distribution of human diseases. PLoS Biol. 2004;2:e141.

22. Sillero N. What does ecological modelling model? A proposed classification of ecological niche models based on their underlying methods. Ecol Model. 2011;222:1343–6.

23. Campbell LP, Luther C, Moo-Llanes D, Ramsey JM, Danis-Lozano R, Peterson AT. Climate change influences on global distributions of dengue and chikungunya virus vectors. Phil Trans R Soc B. 2015;370:20140135.

24. Ayala D, Costantini C, Ose K, Kamdem GC, Antonio-Nkondjio C, Agbor J-P, et al. Habitat suitability and ecological niche profile of major malaria vectors in Cameroon. Malar J. 2009;8:307.

25. Neerinckx SB, Peterson AT, Gulinck H, Deckers J, Leirs H. Geographic distribution and ecological niche of plague in sub-Saharan Africa. Int J Health Geogr. 2008;7:54.

26. Hanafi-Bojd A, Rassi Y, Yaghoobi-Ershadi M, Haghdoost A, Akhavan A, Charrahy Z, et al. Predicted distribution of visceral leishmaniasis vectors (Diptera: Psychodidae; Phlebotominae) in Iran: a niche model study. Zoonoses Public Health. 2015;62:644–54.

27. González C, Paz A, Ferro C. Predicted altitudinal shifts and reduced spatial distribution of Leishmania infantum vector species under climate change scenarios in Colombia. Acta Trop. 2014;129:83–90.

28. Moo-Llanes D, Ibarra-Cerdeña CN, Rebollar-Téllez EA, Ibáñez-Bernal S, González A, Ramsey JM. Current and future niche of North and Central American sand flies (Diptera: Psychodidae) in climate change scenarios. PLoS Negl Trop Dis. 2013;7:e2421.

29. Carvalho BM, Rangel EF, Ready PD, Vale MM. Ecological niche modelling predicts southward expansion of Lutzomyia (Nyssomyia) flaviscutellata (Diptera: Psychodidae: Phlebotominae), vector of Leishmania (Leishmania) amazonensis in South America, under climate change. PLoS One. 2015;10:e0143282.

30. Mukhopadhyay A, Hati A, Chakraborty S, Saxena N. Effect of DDT on Phlebotomus sandflies in kala-azar endemic foci in West Bengal. J Commun Disord. 1996;28:171.

31. Birley M. An historical review of malaria, kala-azar and filariasis in Bangladesh in relation to the Flood Action Plan. Ann Trop Med Parasitol. 1993;87:319–34.

32. Medley GF, Hollingsworth TD, Olliaro PL, Adams ER. Health-seeking behaviour, diagnostics and transmission dynamics in the control of visceral leishmaniasis in the Indian subcontinent. Nature. 2015;528:S102–S8.

33. Ferdousi F, Alam MS, Hossain MS, Ma E, Itoh M, Mondal D, et al. Visceral leishmaniasis eradication is a reality: data from a community-based active surveillance in Bangladesh. Trop Med Health. 2012;40:133–9.

34. Chowdhury R, Dotson E, Blackstock AJ, McClintock S, Maheswary NP, Faria S, et al. Comparison of insecticide-treated nets and indoor residual spraying to control the vector of visceral leishmaniasis in Mymensingh District, Bangladesh. Am J Trop Med Hyg. 2011;84:662–7.

35. Le Rutte EA, Coffeng LE, Bontje DM, Hasker EC, Postigo JAR, Argaw D, et al. Feasibility of eliminating visceral leishmaniasis from the Indian subcontinent: explorations with a set of deterministic age-structured transmission models. Parasit Vectors. 2016;9:24.

36. Thornton SJ, Wasan KM, Piecuch A, Lynd LLD, Wasan EK. Barriers to treatment for visceral leishmaniasis in hyperendemic areas: India, Bangladesh, Nepal, Brazil and Sudan. Drug Dev Ind Pharm. 2010;36:1312–9.

37. Ready PD. Epidemiology of visceral leishmaniasis. Clin Epidemiol. 2014;6:147–54.

38. Elnaiem D-EA, Schorscher J, Bendall A, Obsomer V, Osman ME, Mekkawi AM, et al. Risk mapping of visceral leishmaniasis: the role of local variation in rainfall and altitude on the presence and incidence of kala-azar in eastern Sudan. Am J Trop Med Hyg. 2003;68:10–7.

39. Bhunia GS, Kesari S, Jeyaram A, Kumar V, Das P. Influence of topography on the endemicity of kala-azar: a study based on remote sensing and geographical information system. Geospat Health. 2010;4:155–65.

40. Sudhakar S, Srinivas T, Palit A, Kar S, Battacharya S. Mapping of risk prone areas of kala-azar (visceral leishmaniasis) in parts of Bihar state, India: an RS and GIS approach. J Vector Borne Dis. 2006;43:115–22.

41. Rahman KM, Islam S, Rahman MW, Kenah E, Galive CM, Zahid M, et al. Increasing incidence of post-kala-azar dermal leishmaniasis in a population-based study in Bangladesh. Clin Infect Dis. 2010;50:73–6.

42. Rahman KM, Samarawickrema IV, Harley D, Olsen A, Butler CD, Sumon SA, et al. Performance of kala-azar surveillance in Gaffargaon subdistrict of Mymensingh, Bangladesh. PLoS Negl Trop Dis. 2015;9:e0003531.

43. Khatun J, Huda MM, Hossain MS, Presber W, Ghosh D, Kroeger A, et al. Accelerated active case detection of visceral leishmaniasis patients in endemic villages of Bangladesh. PLoS One. 2014;9:e103678.

44. Huda MM, Chowdhury R, Ghosh D, Dash AP, Bhattacharya SK, Mondal D. Visceral leishmaniasis-associated mortality in Bangladesh: a retrospective cross-sectional study. BMJ Open. 2014;4:e005408.

45. Amin MR, Tareq SM, Rahman SH, Uddin MR. Effects of temperature, rainfall and relative humidity on visceral leishmaniasis prevalence at two highly affected upazilas in Bangladesh. Life Sci J. 2013;10:1440–6.

46. Stauch A, Sarkar RR, Picado A, Ostyn B, Sundar S, Rijal S, et al. Visceral leishmaniasis in the Indian subcontinent: modelling epidemiology and control. PLoS Negl Trop Dis. 2011;5:e1405.

47. Alam MS, Ghosh D, Khan MGM, Islam MF, Mondal D, Itoh M, et al. Survey of domestic cattle for anti-Leishmania antibodies and Leishmania DNA in a visceral leishmaniasis endemic area of Bangladesh. BMC Vet Res. 2011;7:27.

48. Bern C, Haque R, Chowdhury R, Ali M, Kurkjian KM, Vaz L, et al. The epidemiology of visceral leishmaniasis and asymptomatic leishmanial infection in a highly endemic Bangladeshi village. Am J Trop Med Hyg. 2007;76:909–14.

49. Bern C, Courtenay O, Alvar J. Of cattle, sand flies and men: a systematic review of risk factor analyses for South Asian visceral leishmaniasis and implications for elimination. PLoS Negl Trop Dis. 2010;4:e599.

50. Alam MS, Wagatsuma Y, Mondal D, Khanum H, Haque R. Relationship between sand fly fauna and kala-azar endemicity in Bangladesh. Acta Trop. 2009;112:23–5.

51. Anoopa Sharma D, Bern C, Varghese B, Chowdhury R, Haque R, Ali M, et al. The economic impact of visceral leishmaniasis on households in Bangladesh. Trop Med Int Health. 2006;11:757–64.

52. Ahluwalia IB, Bern C, Wagatsuma Y, Costa C, Chowdhury R, Ali M, et al. Visceral leishmaniasis: consequences to women in a Bangladeshi community. J Women's Health. 2004;13:360–4.

53. Emch M. Relationships between flood control, kala-azar, and diarrheal disease in Bangladesh. Environ Plan A. 2000;32:1051–63.

54. Elias M, Rahman A, Khan N. Visceral leishmaniasis and its control in Bangladesh. Bull World Health Organ. 1989;67:43.

55. Rahman K, Islam N. Resurgence of visceral leishmaniasis in Bangladesh. Bull World Health Organ. 1983;61:113.

56. Özbel Y, Sanjoba C, Matsumoto Y. Geographical distribution and ecological aspect of sand fly species in Bangladesh. In: E. Noiri TKJ, editor. Kala Azar in South Asia. 2 ed. Switzerland: Springer International Publishing; 2016. p. 199–209.

57. Bern C, Chowdhury R. The epidemiology of visceral leishmaniasis in Bangladesh: prospects for improved control. Indian J Med Res. 2006;123:275.

58. Hossain M, Jamil KM. Geographical distribution of kala-azar in South Asia. In: TKJ E. Noiri, editor. Kala Azar in South Asia. Dordrecht: Springer Netherlands; 2011. p. 3–9.

59. Dewan AM, Hashizume M, Rahman M, Abdullah AYM, Corner R, Rakibul S, et al. Environmental change and kala-azar with particular reference to Bangladesh. In: E. Noiri TKJ, editor. Kala Azar in South Asia. 2nd ed. Switzerland: Springer International Publishing; 2016. p. 223–47.

60. WorldClim. WorldClim—global climate data. http://www.worldclim.org/bioclim. Accessed 10 Aug 2016.

61. Hijmans RJ, Cameron SE, Parra JL, Jones PG, Jarvis A. Very high resolution interpolated climate surfaces for global land areas. Int J Climatol. 2005;25:1965–78.

62. USGS-EarthExplorer. USGS EarthExplorer. https://earthexplorer.usgs.gov/. Accessed 10 Aug 2016.

63. Jensen JR. Remote sensing of the environment: an earth resource perspective 2/e. India: Pearson Education India; 2009.

64. Tucker CJ. Red and photographic infrared linear combinations for monitoring vegetation. Remote Sens Environ. 1979;8:127–50.

65. McFeeters SK. The use of the normalized difference water index (NDWI) in the delineation of open water features. Int J Remote Sens. 1996;17:1425–32.

66. Jensen JR. Introductory digital image processing: a remote sensing perspective. Columbus: Univ. of South Carolina; 1986.

67. Chander G, Markham B. Revised Landsat-5 TM radiometric calibration procedures and postcalibration dynamic ranges. IEEE Trans Geosci Remote Sens. 2003;41:2674–7.

68. Nichol J. Remote sensing of urban heat islands by day and night. Photogramm Eng Remote Sens. 2005;71:613–21.

69. Qin C-Z, Zhu A-X, Pei T, Li B-L, Scholten T, Behrens T, et al. An approach to computing topographic wetness index based on maximum downslope gradient. Precis Agric. 2011;12:32–43.

70. Bangladesh Agricultural Research Council (BARC). http://maps.barcapps.gov.bd. Accessed 8 Aug 2016.

71. Mak S, Morshed M, Henry B. Ecological niche modeling of Lyme disease in British Columbia, Canada. J Med Entomol. 2010;47:99–105.

72. Lu L, Ren Z, Yue Y, Yu X, Lu S, Li G, et al. Niche modeling predictions of the potential distribution of Marmota himalayana, the host animal of plague in Yushu County of Qinghai. BMC Public Health. 2016;16:1.

73. Peterson AT. Ecological niches and geographic distributions (MPB-49). New Jersey: Princeton University Press; 2011.

74. Samy AM, Annajar BB, Dokhan MR, Boussaa S, Peterson AT. Coarse-resolution ecology of etiological agent, vector, and reservoirs of zoonotic cutaneous leishmaniasis in Libya. PLoS Negl Trop Dis. 2016;10:e0004381.

75. Maxent software for species habitat modeling. http://biodiversityinformatics.amnh.org/open_source/maxent/. Accessed 18 Sept 2016.

76. Phillips SJ, Anderson RP, Schapire RE. Maximum entropy modeling of species geographic distributions. Ecol Model. 2006;190:231–59.

77. Phillips SJ, Dudík M. Modeling of species distributions with Maxent: new extensions and a comprehensive evaluation. Ecography. 2008;31:161–75.

78. Lobo JM, Jiménez-Valverde A, Hortal J. The uncertain nature of absences and their importance in species distribution modelling. Ecography. 2010;33:103–14.

79. Phillips SJ, Dudík M, Schapire RE, editors. A maximum entropy approach to species distribution modeling. Proceedings of the twenty-first international conference on machine learning. USA: ACM; 2004.

80. Elith J, Leathwick JR. Species distribution models: ecological explanation and prediction across space and time. Annu Rev Ecol Evol Syst. 2009;40:677–97.

81. Townsend Peterson A, Papeş M, Eaton M. Transferability and model evaluation in ecological niche modeling: a comparison of GARP and Maxent. Ecography. 2007;30:550–60.

82. Connolly MA. Communicable disease control in emergencies: a field manual. Geneva: World Health Organization; 2005.

83. Phillips SJ. A brief tutorial on Maxent. New Jersey: AT&T Research; 2005.

84. Elith J. Quantitative methods for modeling species habitat: comparative performance and an application to Australian plants. Quantitative methods for conservation biology. New York: Springer New York; 2000. p. 39–58.

85. Pearson RG, Raxworthy CJ, Nakamura M, Townsend PA. Predicting species distributions from small numbers of occurrence records: a test case using cryptic geckos in Madagascar. J Biogeogr. 2007;34:102–17.

86. Wang X, Huang X, Jiang L, Qiao G. Predicting potential distribution of chestnut phylloxerid (Hemiptera: Phylloxeridae) based on GARP and Maxent ecological niche models. J Appl Entomol. 2010;134:45–54.

87. Pearce J, Ferrier S. Evaluating the predictive performance of habitat models developed using logistic regression. Ecol Model. 2000;133:225–45.

88. Irrigation Support Project for Asia and The Near East (ISPAN). The kala-azar epidemic in Bangladesh and its relationship to flood control embankments, Flood Action Plan 16, Dhaka. 1995.

89. Ranjan A, Sur D, Singh VP, Siddique NA, Manna B, Lal CS, et al. Risk factors for Indian kala-azar. Am J Trop Med Hyg. 2005;73:74–8.

90. Bhunia GS, Kesari S, Chatterjee N, Mandal R, Kumar V, Das P. Seasonal relationship between normalized difference vegetation index and abundance of the Phlebotomus kala-azar vector in an endemic focus in Bihar, India. Geospat Health. 2012;7:51–62.

91. Salahi-Moghaddam A, Mohebali M, Moshfae A, Habibi M. Ecological study and risk mapping of visceral leishmaniasis in an endemic area of Iran based on a geographical information systems approach. Geospat Health. 2010;5:71–7.

92. Patz JA, Campbell-Lendrum D, Holloway T, Foley JA. Impact of regional climate change on human health. Nature. 2005;438:310–7.

93. Kesari S, Bhunia GS, Kumar V, Jeyaram A, Ranjan A, Das P. Study of house-level risk factors associated in the transmission of Indian kala-azar. Parasit Vectors. 2010;3:94.

94. Saha S, Ramachandran R, Hutin YJ, Gupte MD. Visceral leishmaniasis is preventable in a highly endemic village in West Bengal, India. Trans R Soc Trop Med Hyg. 2009;103:737–42.

95. Abedi-Astaneh F, Akhavan AA, Shirzadi MR, Rassi Y, Yaghoobi-Ershadi MR, Hanafi-Bojd AA, et al. Species diversity of sand flies and ecological niche model of Phlebotomus papatasi in central Iran. Acta Trop. 2015;149:246–53.

96. Mukhopadhyay A, Rahaman S, Chakravarty A. Effect of flood on immature stages of sandflies in a flood-prone kala-azar endemic village of North Bihar, India. Effect of flood on immature stages of sandflies in a flood-prone kala-azar endemic village of North Bihar, India. 1990. p. 1–5.

97. Lysenko AJ. Distribution of leishmaniasis in the Old World. Bull World Health Organ. 1971;44:515.

98. Elnaiem D, Connor S, Thomson M, Hassan M, Hassan H, Aboud M, et al. Environmental determinants of the distribution of Phlebotomus orientalis in Sudan. Ann Trop Med Parasitol. 1998;92:877–87.

99. Napier LE. An epidemiological investigation of kala-azar in a rural area in Bengal. Indian J Med Res. 1931;19:295–341.

100. Kesari S, Bhunia GS, Chatterjee N, Kumar V, Mandal R, Das P. Appraisal of Phlebotomus argentipes habitat suitability using a remotely sensed index in the kala-azar endemic focus of Bihar, India. Mem Inst Oswaldo Cruz. 2013; 108:197–204.

101. Thomson M, Elnaiern D, Ashford R, Connor S. Towards a kala azar risk map for Sudan: mapping the potential distribution of Phlebotomus orientalis using digital data of environmental variables. Trop Med Int Health. 1999;4:105–13.

102. Dhiman RC, Pahwa S, Dhillon G, Dash AP. Climate change and threat of vector-borne diseases in India: are we prepared? Parasitol Res. 2010;106:763–73.

103. Ortega-Huerta MA, Peterson AT. Modeling ecological niches and predicting geographic distributions: a test of six presence-only methods. Rev Mex Biodivers. 2008;79:205–16.

104. Dupin M, Reynaud P, Jarošík V, Baker R, Brunel S, Eyre D, et al. Effects of the training dataset characteristics on the performance of nine species distribution models: application to Diabrotica virgifera virgifera. PLoS One. 2011;6:e20957.

7

Professional care delivery or traditional birth attendants? The impact of the type of care utilized by mothers on under-five mortality of their children

Choolwe Muzyamba[1,2*], Wim Groot[3,4], Milena Pavlova[3], Iryna Rud[4] and Sonila M. Tomini[1,5]

Abstract

Background: Because of the high under-five mortality rate, the government in Zambia has adopted the World Health Organization (WHO) policy on child delivery which insists on professional maternal care. However, there are scholars who criticize this policy by arguing that although built on good intentions, the policy to ban traditional birth attendants (TBAs) is out of touch with local reality in Zambia. There is lack of evidence to legitimize either of the two positions, nor how the outcome differs between women with HIV and those without HIV. Thus, the aim of this paper is to investigate the effect of using professional maternal care or TBA care by mothers (during antenatal, delivery, and postnatal) on under-five mortality of their children. We also compare these outcomes between HIV-positive and HIV-negative women.

Methods: By relying on data from the 2013–2014 Zambia Demographic Health Survey (ZDHS), we carried out propensity score matching (PSM) to investigate the effect of utilization of professional care or TBA during antenatal, childbirth, and postnatal on under-five mortality. This method allows us to estimate the average treatment effect on the treated (ATT).

Results: Our results show that the use of professional care as opposed to TBAs in all three stages of maternal care increases the probability of children surviving beyond 5 years old. Specifically for women with HIV, professional care usage during antenatal, at birth, and during postnatal periods increases probability of survival by 0.07 percentage points (p.p), 0.71 p.p, and 0.87 p.p respectively. Similarly, for HIV-negative women, professional care usage during antenatal, at birth, and during postnatal periods increases probability of survival by 0.71 p.p, 0.52 p.p, and 0.37 p.p respectively. However, although there is a positive impact when mothers choose professional care over TBAs, the differences at all three points of maternal care are small.

Conclusion: Given our findings, showing small differences in under-five child's mortality between utilizers of professional care and utilizers of TBAs, it may be questioned whether the government's intention of completely excluding TBAs (who despite being outlawed are still being used) without replacement by good quality professional care is the right decision.

* Correspondence: muzyamba@merit.unu.edu
[1]Maastricht Graduate School of Governance/UNU-Merit, Maastricht University, Maastricht, Netherlands
[2]Lusaka, Zambia
Full list of author information is available at the end of the article

Background

Following the western-influenced evidence-based bio-medical approach and the World Health Organization (WHO) policy on child delivery which insists on skilled delivery, most countries in Sub-Saharan Africa (SSA) have moved to exclude traditional birth attendants (TBAs) in preference for institutional care [1]. Nowhere else is this more evident than in Zambia where TBAs were officially excluded from the line of care in 2010 [2–4].

Proponents of institutional care argue that opportunistic infections such as malaria, tuberculosis, and delicate complications that mothers face during antenatal, child birth, and postnatal periods require the attention of trained personnel, especially for women with HIV. This is in order to ensure better management of postpartum hemorrhage, pre-eclampsia, and neonatal sepsis including prevention of mother to child transmission (PMTCT) [4, 5]. Scholars from this school of thought argue that the low utilization of skilled attendants in Zambia has led to unacceptably high maternal, neonatal, infant, and under-five mortality [6–9]. This is worsened by high HIV rates among women of reproductive age (15–49 years old) which currently stands at 16.1% in Zambia [6]. Evidence from Zambia indicates that children born from women with HIV are more likely to die before reaching the age of 5 than those born from HIV-negative mothers [7, 10, 11]. As an antidote to this predicament, proponents of institutional care have been calling for mandatory skilled attendance during antenatal, childbirth, and postnatal periods especially for women with HIV [12]. This is in order to ensure consistent uptake of antiretroviral treatment and any necessary surgical procedures to reduce the child's chances of dying before reaching age five.

There are however other scholars who criticize the Zambian government's policy on TBAs by suggesting that although built on good intentions, the policy to exclude TBAs is out of touch with reality in Zambia and contributes to high maternal, neonatal, infant, and under-five mortality rates in the country [2, 3, 13, 14]. Excluding TBAs who in most cases are the only feasible source of maternity care in preference for ideally better trained but unavailable professionals is counterproductive [2]. These scholars intimate that the Zambian health system is too weak to sustain the government's policy of strict institutional care. For example, Lukonga and Michelo [12] posit that Zambia has poorly equipped and overcrowded health institutions which lack sufficient numbers of technically skilled personnel. This makes professional care ideal but not practical. A combination of all these shortcomings compromises the care for pregnant women, and subsequently the survival of their children beyond the age of 5 [11]. This is why despite the government directive to exclude TBAs in preference for professional care, many women in Zambia have continued to utilize TBAs [2, 15].

Further, despite the forgoing two conflicting positions, there is a lack of evidence to legitimize either of the two positions [12, 16]. It is not yet known whether in the Zambian case, utilization of skilled professionals as opposed to TBAs during antenatal, childbirth, and postnatal periods significantly reduces under-five mortality [13]. It is also not yet known if on the basis of type of care, the resulting under-five mortality outcomes are similar for women with HIV and those who are HIV negative. There are no studies that specifically focus on comparing the differences in outcomes on the basis of utilizing skilled care or TBAs during the continuum of maternal care for women with HIV and those without HIV [5, 13, 17].

The expectation however is that in both HIV-negative women and women with HIV, skilled care along the continuum of maternal care would reduce the chances of under-five mortality [18]. It is expected that the impact will be higher for women with HIV [18]. This is because skilled care allows women with HIV (who are more vulnerable) to access life-saving antiretroviral treatment, cesarean birth, and continuation of antiretroviral treatment which promote PMTCT and ultimately reduce under-five mortality [19]. However, the extent to which this is evident in Zambia is still unclear [20]. It is vital to provide evidence on the causal nature of this relationship and clearly demonstrate how in the context of Zambia, utilization of skilled attendants affects under-five mortality for women with HIV and how this differs for HIV-negative women. This delineation will serve as a first step towards the formulation of context-specific and effective policy to reduce under-five mortality in Zambia [16]. Thus, the aim of this paper is to investigate and compare the effect of utilization of professional maternal care (or TBA care) during antenatal, delivery, and postnatal periods on under-five mortality in women with HIV and in HIV-negative women.

Methods

Data

We used the 2013–2014 Zambia Demographic Health Survey (ZDHS). The ZDHS included data demographic and health indicators for women who were aged between 15 and 49 years during the survey. Regarding HIV test results, the HIV data were obtained by collecting blood samples during interviews from consenting participants which were later tested for HIV. The HIV data were however not publicly available. The data were only availed to us after obtaining ethical clearance from the Zambia ethics board, the Ministry of Health of Zambia, and the ZDHS team. This was followed by signing a confidentiality form to treat the data with strict confidentiality. We then linked the HIV data to the rest of the ZDHS data based on unique IDs as instructed and recommended by the ZDHS team.

From the main ZDHS dataset on all women (aged 15 to 49), we selected a sub-sample of women who had stated that they had given birth at least once in the last 5 years preceding the survey and who consented to having an HIV test. If the respondents did not consent to testing using their sample, their HIV statuses were left unstated in the data and treated as missing [6]. The final sample and the associated data are shown in Table 1. These data enabled us to investigate the effect of utilizing professional maternal care (or TBAs) during antenatal, childbirth, and postnatal periods on under-five mortality of children for both women with HIV and those without HIV.

Estimation

Propensity score matching (PMS) was applied to investigate the effect of utilizing professional care or TBA during antenatal, childbirth, and postnatal periods on under-five mortality. This method allows us to calculate the average treatment effect on the treated (ATT). We do this at three different stages (antenatal, childbirth, and postnatal) for both women with HIV and HIV-negative women giving us six different PSM investigations.

More specifically, we investigated (a) the effect of utilizing either professional care or TBAs during *antenatal* among women with HIV (and those without HIV) on under-five mortality, (b) the effect of utilizing either professional care or TBAs during *childbirth* among women with HIV (and those without HIV) on under-five mortality, and (c) the effect of utilizing either professional care or TBAs during *postnatal* among women with HIV (and those without HIV) on under-five mortality.

The propensity score was estimated using a probit regression with the following confounders: age at the most recent birth of the woman, total number of children, mother's level of education, mother's employment status, household wealth, whether the woman resides in an urban or rural area, religion, ethnicity, distance to nearest health facility, and access to health insurance. The selection of variables was guided by theory and consensus in extant empirical literature regarding what factors are likely to influence women to access professional care [21, 22].

We generated the propensity scores by using STATA. This means we used PSM to enable us to statistically create a control group (women with HIV/HIV-negative women who utilize TBAs) by matching the observed characteristics of the treated participants (women with HIV/HIV-negative women who utilize skilled attendants) to the control group. This is done on the basis of similar values of the propensity score [23]. Heckman et al. [24] defined PSM as the probability of selection into the treated group, which in this case means the probability of utilizing professional care. It is also important to note that the "unbiased inference" which arises from propensity score matching is based on the assumption that the potential outcomes are independent of treatment assignment conditional on observable characteristics [25]. Another important condition is that there must exist a "common-support" region in the propensity score distributions comprising of participants from both the treatment and control groups [25].

To estimate the ATT, we used the nearest neighbor matching technique. The nearest neighbor matching method works by matching individuals in the control to the treated group and then discards individuals who are not selected as matches [23]. By using this technique, the individual from the comparison group is selected which then acts as a matching partner for the closest treated partner in terms of the propensity score [26, 27]. We make use of the 1:1 nearest neighbor matching technique which works by selecting for each individual in the treated group, the closest individual (in terms of propensity score) from the control group. The disadvantage of 1:1 nearest neighbor matching technique is that it discards a large number of observations which may reduce statistical power [28]. This is however not a concern for our study since we have enough observations in our sample to identify statistically significant effects.

The reliability of the estimated effect of either utilizing professional care or TBAs on under-five mortality when using PSM depends on selection of observables [25]. We thus checked to ensure that the common support assumption was satisfied. This was done by inspecting the propensity score distribution [29]. For the balancing test, several iterations of estimation of the propensity score were carried out in which variables were recoded to have satisfied the balancing property [30].

For robustness, we compare our ATT results obtained from the nearest neighbor matching method with two other matching techniques (see Appendix) to ensure that our findings are consistent, namely Kernel matching and stratification matching [26]. The Kernel matching uses weighted average of the

Table 1 Summary of characteristics (differences and similarities) between HIV-positive and HIV-negative populations

Variable (N = 12, 225)		Frequency		Valid percentage (%)		(t) and (χ^2)
		HIV+	HIV−	HIV+	HIV−	
Type of residence	Urban	1014	4752	48.66	47.85	103.151***
	Rural	1098	5359	51.34	52.15	17.117***
	Total	2113	10, 112			
Religion	Catholic	369	1792	17.47	17.72	17.011***
	Protestant	1722	8209	81.50	81.19	13.060***
	Muslim	10	50	0.45	0.49	1.251**
	Other	12	62	0.58	0.60	0.015***
	Total	2113	10,112			
Education	No education	165	1187	7.8	11.74	23.110***
	Primary	951	5747	45.54	56.83	9.463***
	Secondary	845	2811	40.50	27.80	16.717***
	Higher	128	404	6.11	4.01	76.701***
	Total	2113	10,112			
Wealth index	Poorest	374	1742	17.72	17.23	121.123***
	Poorer	364	1866	17.23	18.45	10.104***
	Middle	464	2154	21.50	21.24	12.330***
	Richer	467	2053	21.37	20.91	8.145***
	Richest	468	2225	22.17	22.18	109.204***
	Total	2113	10,112			
Age	Age 15–25	972	4045	46	40.61	111.020**
	Age 26–35	592	3235	28	32.26	20.511***
	Age 36–45	549	2732	26	27.14	0.500**
	Total	2113	10,112			
Health insurance	No health insurance	2066	9808	97.82	97.40	91.166**
	With health insurance	46	303	2.18	2.60	76.661***
	Total	2113	10,112			
Availability of drugs in facility	Big problem	586	4142	27.74	40.96	10.221***
	Not a big problem	1527	5970	72.26	59.04	12.770***
	Total	2113	10,112			
Distance to facilitates	Big problem	795	4348	37.64	43.95	2.091***
	Not a big problem	1318	5764	63.26	59.05	12.413**
	Total	2113	10,112			
Attitude of health professionals	Big problem	549	3369	26.40	33.32	8.543***
	Not a big problem	1564	6743	73.60	66.68	4.500***
	Total	2113	10,112			
Choice of care at antenatal	TBA	486	2375	23.00	23.49	0.828***
	Health professional	1527	7737	77.00	76.51	2.798***
	Total	2113	10,112			
Choice of care at birth	TBA	448	2124	21.10	21.00	16.223***
	Health professional	1665	7989	78.90	79.00	18.123***
	Total	2113	10,112			
Choice of care at postnatal	TBA	507	2395	24.01	23.68	13.352***

Table 1 Summary of characteristics (differences and similarities) between HIV-positive and HIV-negative populations *(Continued)*

Variable (N = 12, 225)		Frequency		Valid percentage (%)		(t) and (χ²)
		HIV+	HIV–	HIV+	HIV–	
	Health professional	1606	7718	75.09	76.32	19.113***
	Total	2113	10,112			
Child is still alive	Yes	1860	9696	88.02	95.89	103.991***
	No	253	416	11.98	4.11	11.441***
	Total	2113	10,112			

Reported *p* values are based on *t* tests of means for continuous variables and chi-squares for proportions/categorical variables
***$p < 0.01$
**$p < 0.05$
*$p < 0.10$

individuals in the control group to construct a counterfactual [25] whereas stratification matching works by partitioning the common support into different strata and after which impact is computed in each of those two strata [26].

Hidden bias and sensitivity test

The weakness with PSM is that it does not correct for bias due to unobserved characteristics. In order to overcome this bias, conducting sensitivity analysis of hidden bias is recommended. This is achieved by establishing the level of unobserved heterogeneity that would change the statistical significance of the treatment effects (ATT) [25]. Therefore, we adopt the technique proposed by Altonji et al. [31] to estimate how sensitive the estimates are to selection on unobservables. This technique links selection on observed factors to selection on unobserved factors. For this, we estimate a bivariate probit model and impose constraints on the correlation between unobserved factors that influence, on the one hand, the probability of being in the treatment group and, on the other, the outcome.

Results

By relying on PSM, we investigated the effect of utilizing professional care (or TBA care) by mothers during antenatal, delivery, and postnatal periods on under-five mortality of children. This was done for mothers with HIV and those without HIV. As recommended [26], the three steps of propensity score matching estimation were followed. Firstly, we ran probit models for the three stages of maternal care (antenatal, birth, and postnatal) in order to estimate the propensity score. After this, the estimated propensity scores were used to match a group of individuals who utilized professional care but were comparable to those that utilized TBAs in terms of propensity scores generated in the first step. The final step was to compare the under-five child's mortality outcomes of professional care and TBA-utilizers between women with HIV and HIV-negative women at the three different stages of maternal care, a process which enables us to estimate the ATT effects.

By checking the ATT result column in Table 2, we can see the effect of the mothers' choice of care (between professional and TBA care) on the survival of their children beyond 5 years.

In general, the results in Table 2 show that utilizing professional care (as opposed to TBAs) in all three stages of maternal care for both women with HIV and those without HIV slightly increases the probability of their children surviving beyond 5 years old.

For the specific stages in women with HIV, uptake of professional antenatal care (as opposed to TBAs) by women with HIV increased the probability of the child surviving beyond age five by 0.07 percentage points (p.p) representing a survival rate of 97.1% for professional care utilizers and 97.0% for TBA utilizers. Similarly, the uptake of professional care during

Table 2 Average treatment effect on the treated (ATT) results

Maternal health stage	Survival rate treated		Survival rate controls		ATT (percentage point increase in the probability of a child surviving beyond 5 years)	
	HIV+	HIV–	HIV+	HIV–	HIV+	HIV–
Antenatal	.971	.978	.970	.971	.000677***	.00713***
At birth	.972	.975	.965	.970	.007100***	.00518***
Postnatal	.977	.976	.968	.972	.008711***	.00373***

***$p < 0.01$
**$p < 0.05$
*$p < 0.10$

childbirth (as opposed to TBAs) by women with HIV increased the probability of the child surviving beyond age five by 0.71 p.p, representing a survival rate of 97.2% for professional care users and 96.5% for TBA users. At postnatal, the probability increases by 0.87 p.p. representing a survival rate of 97.7% for professional care utilizers and 96.8% for TBA-utilizers.

Similarly, for HIV-negative women, uptake of professional care (as opposed to TBAs) during antenatal, at birth, and postnatal period slightly increased the probability of the child surviving beyond age 5. For example, the probability of a child surviving beyond age increased by 0.71 p.p as a result of using professional care. This represents a survival rate of 97.8% for professional care utilizers and 97.1% for TBA utilizers. At birth, the uptake of professional care for HIV-negative women increased the probability of the child surviving beyond age 5 by 0.52 p.p representing a survival rate of 97.5% for professional care utilizers and 97.0% for TBA utilizers. During postnatal, it increased by 0.37p.p representing a survival rate of 97.6% for professional care utilizers and 97.2% for TBA utilizers.

Robustness checks for the ATT were done by the use of two alternative matching techniques, namely, Kernel matching and stratification matching (see Appendices 1 and 2). Both of the matching techniques produced similar ATT results in direction and magnitude for all the three stages. We further carried out the Altonji test to see if there was any bias resulting from the effect of unobservables. The Altonji sensitivity test indicates that our results are robust to selection on unobservables (see Appendix 3).

Discussion

The aim of this paper was to investigate the effect of utilization of professional maternal care or TBA care during antenatal, delivery, and postnatal period on under-five mortality for women with HIV and those who are HIV negative.

Our findings highlight the fact that, in general, children born from mothers who utilize professional care (as opposed to TBAs) have a slightly higher probability of surviving beyond the age of 5 regardless of the HIV status of the mother. However, despite these positive results in support of professional care, the differences, although statistically significant, are small in magnitude. From the forgoing, we make the following two conclusions: (a) for both HIV-negative women and those living with HIV, professional care at all the three stages of care leads to slightly higher probability of their children surviving beyond age 5; (b) although professional care appears to produce comparatively higher survival rates, the difference between those who utilize professional care and those who utilize TBAs is relatively small.

The slightly lower probability of under-five mortality resulting from professional care stands out as the most important finding of this paper, especially considering the fact that in the recent past, there has been an increased focus on the need to promote professional care during antenatal, at birth, and postnatal period, from the Zambian government and the WHO [15, 32]. Other studies have emphasized the importance of professional care as a means of reducing under-five mortality [5, 19]. In this regard, professional care is credited for helping to mitigate pregnancy-related complications, particularly pre-eclampsia, and also specifically for mothers with HIV, it helps in the promotion of PMTCT [33]. These studies have also demonstrated that professional care at all three stages is a practical platform through which any potential complications arising during birth can be effectively handled. This is especially important for women with HIV where ART and periodic monitoring by professionals can help in the promotion of PMTCT. This is why, according to Lincetto et al. [33], the WHO [32] and subsequently the government of Zambia disapproves of TBAs in preference for professional caregivers with the anticipation that professional caregivers could significantly reduce the probability of dying before age five [33].

However, our findings indicate that in both women with HIV and those without HIV, professional maternal care led to a slightly higher probability of surviving beyond age 5.

The WHO's notion of change that anchored on the assumption that professional care automatically and significantly leads to high reduction in under-five mortality has been challenged [34]. Some scholars have observed that the increased utilization of professional antenatal care has not significantly reduced under-five mortality in Zambia regardless of HIV status. This could, as other scholars have shown, be the result of poor standards of care under professional care in Zambia epitomized by inadequate medical supplies, equipment, and staff [11, 34]. We have shown that in the case of Zambia, there is a small difference in under-five mortality between professional care utilizers and TBA-utilizers for both HIV negative and women living with HIV. That notwithstanding, it seems legitimate to assume that when these results are combined with maternal mortality outcomes (which we did not investigate in this study), the effects of professional care utilization may even be greater. It was also evident that the effect of professional care does not differ much between HIV-negative women and those living with HIV.

Given these findings, important questions worth asking are (a) how good is the quality of professional care in Zambia? (b) and, similarly, how good is the care under TBAs?

Although professional care produces slightly better outcomes than TBAs, there is a lack of adequate health personnel in Zambia [4, 8, 35]. This observation is in line with what other studies from Zambia [1, 4, 36] have continued to highlight, which is that most professional maternal care stations in Zambia are crippled with a shortage of qualified medical personnel and medical equipment, shortage of life-saving antiretroviral drugs, overcrowding, and poor infrastructure especially in rural parts of Zambia [1, 2, 10, 36]. Further, whereas it appears logical to recommend improvement in the availability and quality of care in Zambia, such recommendations are frequently not achievable due to the high costs involved in implementing them. The government in Zambia has been reluctant and to some extent financially incapable of implementing these ideal, yet costly recommendations [10]. Given the small differences between professional care and TBAs in terms of probability of under-five mortality in our results, it seems legitimate to explore ways through which TBAs can be better involved to complement the weak health system in Zambia. Elsewhere within Sub-Saharan Africa, it has been demonstrated that training and incorporating TBAs in the line of care increases the availability of care and may improve maternal outcomes [37]. Similarly, another study in neighboring Malawi has shown that banning TBAs does not lead to a reduction in maternal mortality [38]. Thus, the decision to exclude TBAs in the line of care in Zambia without good quality professional care being available to replace it seems counterproductive especially considering that they are still being relied upon (albeit illegally) amidst an inefficient health system. In a country like Zambia, which is experiencing a critical shortage of professional health workers, relying on already established traditional and indigenous solutions such as TBAs may be necessary and useful. TBAs may also be trained, regulated, and given suitable functions within the line of maternal care. This might help complement professional attendants (who are in most cases inadequate or unavailable).

Limitations

A dominant limitation in this paper, like in many other studies that rely on household surveys, is the problem of recall bias. The quality of the survey normally depends on the respondent's ability to accurately recall events, which in some cases is very difficult to assure, and to deal with. We believe the probability of recalling such events is similar in the treatment group (i.e., utilizing professional care) and the control group (i.e., utilizing TBAs) and therefore PSM partly accounts for possible bias. Secondly, some women who did not consent to have their HIV status determined were excluded from the sample which might have affected the representativeness of the sample and hence external validity of the findings. Further, the HIV-positive population could have been underrepresented in the sample due to the fact that people who already know their HIV-positive status could have been less willing to participate in the study, which represents the so-called selection bias. Similarly, we also note that given the fact that TBAs are outlawed in Zambia, respondents are more inclined not to report usage of TBAs. These two biases are however difficult to address in the absence of quasi-experimental variation in the data [39]. That notwithstanding, our findings provide useful insights in understanding the impact of professional care on under-five mortality. Therefore, more studies must be undertaken in this area of research, preferably by addressing the stated above limitations, in order to substantiate the internal validity and the generalizability of our findings.

Conclusion

In this paper, we have demonstrated that in general, children born to mothers who utilize professional care have a slightly higher probability of surviving beyond the age of 5, regardless of the HIV status of the mother. However, although there is a positive impact when mothers choose professional care over TBAs, the difference at all the three points of maternal care is small (although it is possible that when this is combined with maternal mortality outcomes, the effects of professional care utilization may even be greater).

Given our findings, showing small differences in under-five child's mortality between utilizers of professional care and utilizers of TBAs, it may be questioned whether the government's intention of completely excluding TBAs (who despite being outlawed are still being used) without replacement by good quality professional care is the right decision. The idea of completely excluding TBAs in the line of care in Zambia may be counterproductive in a health system that lacks personnel and equipment and is highly inaccessible to the majority of the rural population. The current policy in Zambia might benefit from further investigation of professionalization of TBA's.

Appendix 1

Table 3 Matching using stratification method

Maternal health stage	Survival rate treated		Survival rate controls		ATT (percentage points increase in the probability of a child surviving beyond 5 years)	
	HIV+	HIV−	HIV+	HIV−	HIV+	HIV−
Antenatal	.970	.974	.970	.971	0.00031***	0.0032***
At birth	.977	.976	.965	.970	0.0045 ***	0.0064***
Postnatal	.972	.977	.968	.972	0.0042 ***	0.0052***

***$p < 0.01$
**$p < 0.05$
*$p < 0.10$

Appendix 2

Table 4 Matching using Kernel method

Maternal health stage	Survival rate treated		Survival rate controls		ATT (percentage points increase in the probability of a child surviving beyond 5 years)	
	HIV+	HIV−	HIV+	HIV−	HIV+	HIV−
Antenatal	.973	.976	.970	.971	0.0031***	0.005***
At birth	.971	.973	.965	.970	0.0061 ***	0.0034***
Postnatal	.973	.978	.968	.972	0.0052 ***	0.0061***

***$p < 0.01$
**$p < 0.05$
*$p < 0.10$

Appendix 3

Table 5 Appendix G: Atonji test (under-five mortality). Summary of p values from different r levels

Correlation level (r)	HIV+			HIV−		
	Antenatal	Birth	Postnatal	Antenatal	Birth	Postnatal
	p value	p value	p value	p value	p value	p value
0.05	0.00	0.00	0.00	0.00	0.00	0.00
0.10	0.00	0.00	0.00	0.00	0.00	0.00
0.15	0.02	0.04	0.04	0.02	0.08	0.07
0.20	0.06	0.09	0.08	0.07	0.11	0.15
0.25	0.11	0.23	0.18	0.12	0.54	0.48

Decision rule: significant results (seen by the p value) despite increasing correlation indicate robust results

To help us see the effect of unobservables on our outcome variable, we focus on the correlation between error terms which capture the extent to which unobservables affect the treatment and the outcome, in our case taking up professional care and eventually the probability of kids surviving beyond age 5. The Altonji test works by assigning different values of correlation (r) and estimating the probit model conditional on these r values. This allows us to see if the parameter changes significantly given the different r values. We allow our r values to range from 0 to 0.25 (by using 0.05 intervals). If the ATT remains significant despite increasing r, then our results are robust

By checking our p values from table above, we can see that even assuming relatively high selection on unobservables ($r = 0.15$), the effect of professional care on under-five mortality remains highly statistically significant. This therefore means that sensitivity analysis shows that our results are robust and unlikely to be affected by unobservables

Abbreviations
AIDS: Acquired immune deficiency syndrome; ART: Antiretroviral treatment; HIV: Human immunodeficiency virus; PMTCT: Prevention of mother to child transmission; SSA: Sub-Saharan Africa; TBA: Traditional birth attendants; WHO: World Health Organization

Acknowledgements
We would like to acknowledge the DHS team for their assistance in the collection and provision of the data.

Funding
The study was self-funded.

Authors' contributions
All authors collaborated and contributed in the formulation of objectives of the study and oversaw the development of the study concept and design, data collection, and analysis, including the drafting of the manuscript. All authors at every stage contributed to drafting, correcting, and perfecting the manuscript. CM was tasked with consolidating all the contributions to the manuscript and taking care of all correspondence. All authors read and approved the final manuscript.

Competing interests
The authors declare that they have no competing interests.

Author details
[1]Maastricht Graduate School of Governance/UNU-Merit, Maastricht University, Maastricht, Netherlands. [2]Lusaka, Zambia. [3]Department of Health Services Research, CAPHRI, Maastricht University Medical Center, Faculty of Health, Medicine and Life Sciences, Maastricht University, Maastricht, Netherlands. [4]Top Institute for Evidence-Based Education Research (TIER), Maastricht University, Maastricht, Netherlands. [5]Department of Economics, University of Liege, Liège, Belgium.

References
1. Sialubanje C, Massar K, Hamer DH, Ruiter RA. Reasons for home delivery and use of traditional birth attendants in rural Zambia: a qualitative study. BMC J Preg Childb. 2015;15(26)
2. Stekelenburg J, Kyanamina S, Mukelabai M, Wolffers I, van Roosmalen J. Waiting too long: low use of maternal health services in Kalabo, Zambia. Tropical Med Int Health. 2004;9:390–8.
3. Sialubanje C, Massar K, Hamer DH, Ruiter RA. Reasons for home delivery and use of traditional birth attendants in rural Zambia: a qualitative study. BMC Preg Childb. 2015;15(216)
4. Cheelo C, Nzala S, Zulu JM. Banning traditional birth attendants from conducting deliveries: experiences and effects of the ban in a rural district of Kazungula in Zambia. BMC Preg Childb. 2016;16(323)
5. Chi BH, Bolton-Moore MC, Holmes CB. Prevention of mother-to-child HIV transmission within the continuum of maternal, newborn, and child health services. Curr Opin HIV AIDS. 2013;8(5):498–503.
6. ZDHS. Zambia demographic and health survey. Lusaka: ZDS/CSO; 2014.
7. Vallely L, Ahmed Y, Murray SF. Postpartum maternal morbidity requiring hospital admission in Lusaka, Zambia—a descriptive study. BMC Preg Childb. 2005;5(1)
8. Banda PC. Status of maternal mortality in Zambia: use of routine data. Afr Popul Stud. 2015;29(2)
9. Catling C, Medley N, Foureur M, Ryan C, Leap NTAH. Group versus conventional antenatal care for pregnant women. Cochrane. 2015;2
10. Gartland MG, Chintu NT, Li MS, Lembalemba MK, Mulenga SN, Bweupe M, Musonda P, Stringer EM. Field effectiveness of combination antiretroviral prophylaxis for the prevention of mother-to-child HIV transmission in rural Zambia. AIDS. 2013;27(8)
11. Gill CJ. Effect of training traditional birth attendants on neonatal mortality (Lufwanyama Neonatal Survival Project): randomised controlled study. BMJ Glob Health J. 2011;342(346).
12. Lukonga E, Michelo C. Factors associated with neonatal mortality in the general population: evidence from the 2007 Zambia Demographic and Health Survey (ZDHS); a cross sectional study. Pan Afr Med J. 2064:2015.
13. Kendall T, Dane I, Cooper D, Dilmitis S, Kaida A. Eliminating preventable HIV-related maternal mortality in sub-Saharan Africa: what do we need to know? J Acq Immune Deficiency Syndrome. 2014;1(64):250–8.
14. Green-top-Guideline-No-39. Management of HIV in pregnancy. London: Royal College of Obstetricians and Gynaecologists; 2010.
15. Bolu O, Anand A, Swartzendruber A, Hladik W, Marum L, Sheikh A. Utility of antenatal HIV surveillance data to evaluate prevention of mother-to-child HIV transmission programs in resource-limited settings. Am J Obstetr Gynecol. 2007;197:17–25.
16. Kendall T, Langer A. Critical maternal health knowledge gaps in low- and middle-income countries for the post-2015 era. Reprod Health. 2015;12(55):1–4.
17. Kuhn L, Aldrovandi GM, Sinkala M, Kankasa C, Mwiya M, Thea DM. Potential impact of new World Health Organization criteria for antiretroviral treatment for prevention of mother-to-child HIV transmission. AIDS. 2010; 24(9):1374–7.
18. WHO. Child health and development. Geneva: WHO; 2015.
19. Avert. Prevention of mother-to-child transmission (Pmtct) of HIV. London: Avert; 2016.
20. Tarekegn SM, Lieberman LS, Giedraitis V. Determinants of maternal health service utilization in Ethiopia: analysis of the 2011 Ethiopian Demographic and Health Survey. BMC Preg Childb. 2014;14(161)
21. Andersen R. Revisiting the behavioral model and access to medical care: does it matter? J Health Soc Behav. 1995;36(1):1–10.
22. Ansari Z, Carson N, Ackland M, Vaughan L, Serraglio A. A public health model of the social determinants of health. J Prev Med. 2003;48(4):242–51.
23. Rosenbaum P. Observational studies. New York: Springer; 2002.
24. Heckman JJ, Ichimura H, Todd P. Matching as an Econometric Evaluation Estimator. Rev Econ Stud. 1998;65(2):261–94
25. Caliendo M, Bonn I, Kopeinig S. Some practical guidance on how to implement propensity score matching. Köln: University of Cologne; 2008.
26. S. R. Khanker, G. B. Koowal and H. A. Samad, Handbook on impact evaluation: quantitative methods, world bank, 2010.
27. DiPrete T, Gangl M. Assessing bias in the estimation of causal effects: Rosenbaum bounds on matching estimators and instrumental variables estimation with imperfect instruments. Sociol Methodol. 2004;34(1):271–310.
28. Huber M, Lechner M, Steinmayr A. RADIUSMATCH: Stata module to perform distance-weighted radius matching with bias adjustment. Boston: ideas; 2012.
29. Rosenbaum P, Rubin D. The central role of the propensity score in observational. Biometrika. 1983;70(1):41–5.
30. Garrido MM, Kelley AS, Paris J, Roza K, Meier DE, Morrison RS. Methods for constructing and assessing propensity scores. Health Serv Res. 2014; 49(5):1701–20.
31. Altonji JG, Elder TE, Taber CR. Selection on Observed and Unobserved Variables: Assessing the Effectiveness of Catholic Schools. J Polit Econ. 2005;113(1)
32. WHO. World health statistics 2013. Geneva: WHO; 2013.
33. Lincetto O, Mothebesoane-Anoh S, Gomez P, Munjanja S. Antenatal care. Geneva: WHO; 2010.
34. Kyei NNA, Chansa C, Gabrysch S. Quality of antenatal care in Zambia: a national assessment. BMC Preg Childb. 2012;12(151).
35. Graham W, Varghese B. Quality, quality, quality: gaps in the continuum of care. Lancet. 2012;379:5–6.
36. van den Broek N, Graham W. Quality of care for maternal and newborn health: the neglected agenda. BJOG Int J Obstet Gynaecol. 2009;116(1):18–21.
37. Chileshe M. ARV treatment in ZAMBIA: current issues. Lusaka: Institute of Economic and Social Research, University of Zambia; 2014.
38. Wilson A, Gallos ID, Plana N, Lissaue D, Khan KS, Zamora J, MacArthur C. Effectiveness of strategies incorporating training and support of traditional birth attendants on perinatal and maternal mortality: meta-analysis. Br Med J. 2011;343(7102)
39. Godlonton S, Okeke EN. Does a ban on informal health providers save lives? Evidence from Malawi. J Dev Econ. 2016;1(118):112–32.

8

The burden of dengue, source reduction measures, and serotype patterns in Myanmar, 2011 to 2015–R2

Pwint Mon Oo[1*], Khin Thet Wai[2], Anthony D. Harries[3,4], Hemant Deepak Shewade[5], Tin Oo[2], Aung Thi[1] and Zaw Lin[1]

Abstract

Background: Myanmar is currently classified as a high burden dengue country in the Asian Pacific region. The Myanmar vector-borne diseases control (VBDC) program has collected data on dengue and source reduction measures since 1970, and there is a pressing need to collate, analyze, and interpret this information. The aim of this study was to describe the burden of hospital-based dengue disease, dengue control measures, and serotype patterns in Myanmar between 2011 and 2015.

Methods: This was a cross-sectional study using annual records from the Dengue Fever/Dengue Hemorrhagic Fever Prevention and Control Project in Myanmar.

Results: Between 2011 and 2015, there were a total of 89,832 cases and 393 deaths in hospitals, with 97% of cases being in children. In 2013 and 2015, there was an increased number of cases, respectively at 21,942 and 42,913, while during the other 3 years, numbers ranged from 4738 to 13,806. The distribution of dengue deaths each year mirrored the distribution of cases. Most cases (84%) occurred in the wet season and 54% occurred in the delta/lowlands. Case fatality rate (CFR) was highest in 2014 at 7 per 1000 dengue cases, while in the other years, it ranged from 3 to 5 per 1000 cases. High CFR per 1000 were also observed in infants < 1 year (CFR = 8), adults ≥ 15 years (CFR = 7), those with disease severity grade IV (CFR = 17), and those residing in hilly regions (CFR = 9). Implementation and coverage of dengue source reduction measures, including larval control, space spraying, and health education, all increased between 2012 and 2015, although there was low coverage of these interventions in households and schools and for water containers. In the 2013 outbreak, dengue virus serotype 1 predominated, while in the 2015 outbreak, serotypes 1, 2, and 4 were those mainly in circulation.

Conclusion: Dengue is a serious public health disease burden in Myanmar. More attention is needed to improve monitoring, recording, and reporting of cases, deaths, and vector control activities, and more investment is needed for programmatic research.

Keywords: Children, Dengue, Dengue hemorrhagic fever, Dengue case fatality, Dengue virus serotypes, Health education, Larval control measures, Myanmar, Space spraying

* Correspondence: pwintmonoo@gmail.com
[1]Central Vector Borne Disease Control Programme, Department of Public Health, Ministry of Health and Sport, Nay Pyi Taw, Myanmar
Full list of author information is available at the end of the article

Background

Dengue fever is a mosquito-borne tropical disease that usually lasts 2 to 7 days and is caused by the dengue virus [1, 2]. In a small proportion of cases, the disease develops into (a) life-threatening dengue hemorrhagic fever (DHF) or (b) dengue shock syndrome (DSS). There are no specific drugs for the treatment of dengue, which is merely supportive. The infection is spread by two species of *Aedes* mosquito, *Aedes aegypti* (the principal vector) and *Aedes albopictus*. The virus has four distinct, but closely related, serotypes. Recovery from infection by one serotype provides lifelong immunity against that particular serotype. Cross-immunity to the other serotypes occurs, but this is only partial and temporary, and subsequent infections by other serotypes increase the risk of that person developing severe dengue complications such as DHF or DSS. A novel vaccine (Dengvaxia) has been developed and has been shown to be effective [3–5], but, although it is licensed and in use, it is not yet fully deployed. Thus, prevention is currently focused on reducing the mosquito habitats and limiting human exposure to mosquito bites.

The incidence of dengue has grown dramatically around the world in recent decades, with a 30-fold increase in estimated cases in the last 50 years. On the basis of population data and geostatistical models, the burden of dengue infections globally is estimated at 390 million infections per year, with 96 million of those presenting clinically with mild, moderate, or severe disease [6, 7]. Further modeling suggests that 3.9 billion people living in 128 countries are at risk of infection with dengue viruses [7]. In the World Health Organization (WHO) South-East Asia region and Western Pacific Region, some 1.8 billion people (more than 70% of the population) are at risk of dengue, and this poses a substantial economic and disease burden on these countries [1, 8].

To combat this growing problem in the region, the Asia Pacific Dengue Strategic Plan (2008–2015) was developed with the goal of reversing the rising trend of dengue cases by enhancing preparedness to detect, characterize, and contain outbreaks rapidly and to stop the spread of the virus to new areas [9]. Progress is being made with implementation combined with operational and surveillance response research [10].

Myanmar has seen an escalating number of cases of dengue in the last 10 years, despite vector control efforts, and is currently classified as a high burden dengue country in the Asian Pacific region [8]. There is a prevention and treatment program which works as follows. Patients with dengue are diagnosed in hospitals of all States/Regions of Myanmar, with the diagnosis mainly based on clinical criteria according to 2011 WHO guidelines [11]. Rapid diagnostic test kits for dengue are available, but these are in limited supply and are rarely used. Serotype confirmation can be carried out, but this requires polymerase chain reaction (PCR), which is available at the National Health Laboratory under the Department of Public Health and the Department of Medical Research. PCR is done mainly through research and surveillance in response to outbreaks, but each year, children with dengue are also asked to provide specimens so that information can be obtained about circulating serotypes [12, 13]. Once patients are notified with dengue, source reduction measures (mainly control of mosquito larvae and adult mosquitoes) are implemented along with health education and social mobilization [14].

The Myanmar vector-borne diseases control (VBDC) program has collected data on dengue cases, dengue deaths, and vector control measures since 1970, but there is a pressing need to collate, analyze, and interpret this information and, particularly, to generate location-specific spot maps of the burden of dengue in the country. For a resource-constrained country like Myanmar, this information will enhance cost-effective mitigation strategies and help to promote community engagement for dengue control. The aim of this study, therefore, was to describe the burden of dengue disease, dengue control measures, and serotype patterns in Myanmar over a 5-year period between 2011 and 2015. Specific objectives were to describe for each year: (i) public hospital-reported cases of dengue and deaths, stratified by age, gender, urban/rural residence, disease severity grade, season, and geographical ecology; (ii) dengue vector control measures, including mass larval control, space spraying (fogging), and health education; and (iii) serotype patterns of dengue virus from selected states/regions that were identified in the National Health Laboratory.

Methods

Study design

This was a cross-sectional descriptive study using annual records from the Dengue Fever/Dengue Hemorrhagic Fever (DF/DHF) Prevention and Control Project in Myanmar.

Setting

General setting

Myanmar is located in the Southeast Asia Region, bordering the Republic of China on the north and northeast, Laos on the east, Thailand on the southeast, Bangladesh on the west, and India on the northwest. The country is divided administratively into the Nay Pyi Taw Council Territory and 14 states and regions and consists of 74 districts, 330 townships, 398 towns, 3065 wards, 13,619 village tracts, and 64,134 villages. The main geographical features of the country are the delta region and the central plain surrounded by hills and mountains. Myanmar enjoys a tropical climate with three distinct seasons: hot (February to

April), wet (May to September), and cool (October to January) [15]. Myanmar has a population of 51 million people with an urban-rural population ratio of 30:70. It has an area of 0.6 million square kilometer and a population density of 76 per km^2 [15].

Myanmar DF/DHF prevention and control project

In Myanmar, the DF/DHF surveillance program was launched in 1964 and dengue fever was made a notifiable disease in 1966. In 1968, the National Committee on DHF was formed and the *Aedes* Mosquito Control Unit was established. In 1969, sporadic cases of DHF were recorded in Yangon. The first epidemic of DHF in Myanmar was recorded in 1970. At that time, the disease was confined to the Yangon Division only. From 1974 onwards, DHF began to spread to other states and divisions and the disease is now endemic in all states and regions (divisions) except Chin State.

The current National DHF Control Strategy has followed the Asian Pacific Regional Dengue Strategic Plan (2008–2015) [9]. The major goal is to reduce the incidence rates of DF and DHF. The main components of the plan are (i) effective disease and vector surveillance systems based on reliable laboratory and health information; (ii) disease prevention through selective, stratified, and integrated vector control with community education and engagement; (iii) emergency preparedness to prevent and control outbreaks with appropriate contingency plans; (iv) prompt case management of DF/DHF including early recognition of signs and symptoms to prevent mortality; (v) increased awareness of the community about DF/DHF prevention, control, and management through information, education, and communication; and (vi) improved management and technical support systems and strengthened health facilities for health sector development.

Dengue case surveillance Cases that are admitted to hospital and diagnosed with possible dengue [dengue fever (DF) and DHF/DSS] based on WHO criteria [11] are notified to the health department that then introduces dengue source reduction measures as described below. Case records are kept at the hospital and a focal person from the VBDC team collects these data on a weekly basis through fax, electronic mail, and phone calls. It is estimated that data are collected from 90% or more of public hospitals in the country. During dengue outbreaks, the reporting is daily rather than weekly. These daily or weekly data are collated by focal persons of the VBDC team with data being transferred upwards from township to district to state/region and finally to the Central VBDC Programme at the Department of Public Health. The Central Programme also reports weekly to the Ministry of Health and Sports. From the Ministry of

Health and Sports, the reports are sent to WHO SEARO through the WHO Country Office of Myanmar.

Dengue vector control measures When a new dengue patient has been identified in an urban ward, the following measures take place within a 100-m radius from the patient's house within 1 week of diagnosis: (i) larval control: insecticide granules (Temephos) are placed into domestic and peri-domestic water containers every 3 months in the wet season to kill mosquito larvae; (ii) mosquito control: space spraying (thermal fogging) using malathion insecticide; and (iii) health education from the VBDC teams by conducting health education sessions, distributing pamphlets, posters, and vinyl printed materials to the general public and transmitting information through mass media channels.

Dengue serotypes During an outbreak of dengue, the National Health Laboratory requests hospitals at selected regions such as Yangon, Mandalay, Sagaing, Nay Pyi Taw, Mon, and Tanintharyi to send specimens from patients with severe complications. Serology was performed assessing for dengue viral-specific antibodies using the PAMBIO™ Dengue duo IgM and IgG rapid strip tests. Conventional PCR was then carried out on samples testing seropositive to determine the different serotypes according to the laboratory guidelines. This process is also carried out every year in children from the selected regions.

Study sample and population

The study includes all patients diagnosed with dengue in public hospitals in Myanmar between 2011 and 2015. The study also includes information on dengue source reduction measures during the same time period as well as the pattern of dengue serotypes from patients residing in selected states/regions.

Variables, data sources, and data collection

Data variables for the study included the following: For hospital-reported cases of dengue and deaths—year, month, age group, gender, urban/rural residence, disease severity grade, season, and ecological area of the country [16] for each case. The source of data was the VBDC electronic EXCEL database for aggregate data. For dengue vector control measures: (i) larval control—year, state/region, and coverage in townships, wards, households, and water containers; (ii) space spraying—year, state/region, and coverage in townships, wards, households, and schools; and (iii) health education—year, number of health education sessions, and number of people attending health education sessions. The source of data was the VBDC electronic EXCEL database for aggregate data from selected states/regions. For dengue serotypes—year, samples tested, samples seropositive, pattern of serotypes (1, 2, 3, or 4). The source of data was the National Health Laboratory electronic EXCEL database. The operational definitions for the study variables are explained in Table 1.

Analysis and statistics

Data were extracted and cleaned in the EXCEL File and then exported to EpiData software for analysis (version 2.2.2.183, EpiData Association, Odense, Denmark). A descriptive analysis was performed using frequencies and proportions. Absolute numbers of dengue cases and deaths per year were determined and case rates per 100,000 people and dengue case fatality rates per 1000 cases were calculated. Cases and deaths were also analyzed in relation to age group, gender, urban/rural residence, disease severity grade, season, and ecological area of the country. Nationwide spot maps of dengue cases and deaths across 5 years (2011–2015) by ecological regions were generated through a geographical information system using Quantum GIS software (version 2.18.3, Open source Geospatial Foundation Project).

Table 1 Operational definitions of study variables

SN	Variables	Operational definitions
1	Ecological regions:	
1.1	Delta and lowland (heavy rainfall more than 2500 mm)	Ayeyarwady, Yangon, and Bago regions; Mon and Kayin states
1.2	Hills (moderate to heavy rainfall)	Kachin, Kayah, Chin, and Shan states
1.3	Coastal (heavy rainfall more than 2500 mm)	Rakhine state and Taninthayi regions
1.4	Plains (uneven topography and rainfall less than 1000 mm)	Magway, Mandalay, Sagaing, and Nay Pyi Taw regions
2	Disease severity grade: (WHO grading of severity of DHF)	
2.1	DF	Fever with two of the following: headache, retro-orbital pain, myalgia, bone pain, rash, and hemorrhagic manifestations (No evidence of plasma leakage)
2.2	DHF grade I	Fever and hemorrhagic manifestation (positive tourniquet test) and evidence of plasma leakage
2.3	DHF grade II	As in grade I plus spontaneous bleeding
2.4	DHF grade III	As in grade I or II plus circulatory failure (weak pulse, narrow pulse pressure (≤ 20 mmHg), hypotension, restlessness)
2.5	DHF grade IV	As in grade III plus profound shock with undetectable blood pressure and pulse

WHO World Health Organization, *DF* dengue fever, *DHF* dengue hemorrhagic fever

Results
Hospital-reported cases of dengue and dengue deaths

The annual number of hospital-reported cases of dengue and associated deaths are shown in Figs. 1 and 2. During the five-year period, there were a total of 89,832 cases and 393 deaths. In 2013 and 2015, there was an increase in number of cases at 21,942 and 42,913, respectively, while during the other 3 years the number of cases ranged from 4738 to 13,806. The distribution of dengue deaths each year mirrored the distribution of cases. The case fatality rate was highest in 2014 at 7 per 1000 dengue cases, while in the other years, this ranged between 3 and 5 per 1000 cases.

The demographic and clinical characteristics of all the hospital-related dengue cases and deaths between 2011 and 2015 are shown in Table 2. Over 95% of all cases were in children, with those aged 5–9 years being the predominant age group affected. High case fatality rates were observed in infants < 1 year and adults ≥ 15 years. No differences were found in cases or deaths between males and females or those residing in urban versus rural settings. The commonest disease severity grade was DF plus DHF grade 1 (42%), although the majority of deaths and the highest case fatality occurred in those with disease severity grade IV.

The seasonal changes and ecological distribution of hospital-related dengue cases and deaths between 2011 and 2015 are shown in Table 3. The majority of cases and deaths, with the highest case fatality rates, occurred in the wet season from May to September. The majority of cases (85%) and deaths (82%) also occurred in persons living in the delta region and the plains, although case fatality was highest in the hills. Figs. 3 and 4 show dengue cases and deaths in relation to the four ecological regions of the country. The five main hot spots for cases were Mon state and the four regions of Yangon, Ayeyarwady, Mandalay, and Sagaing, and the main hot spots for death were Yangon followed by Ayeyarwady region.

Dengue vector control measures and health education

The implementation of dengue vector control measures in townships, wards, households, and water containers is shown in Table 4. The implementation of larval control measures varied from year to year, although coverage progressively increased at township, ward, and household levels between 2013 and 2015 (Table 4). The proportion of water containers for which there were appropriate larval control measures was low at < 10% coverage in the last 2 years. The implementation of space spraying as a chemical control measure, especially during outbreaks progressively increased in townships and wards between 2012 and 2015, although coverage at the household and school levels was low, often at < 1%

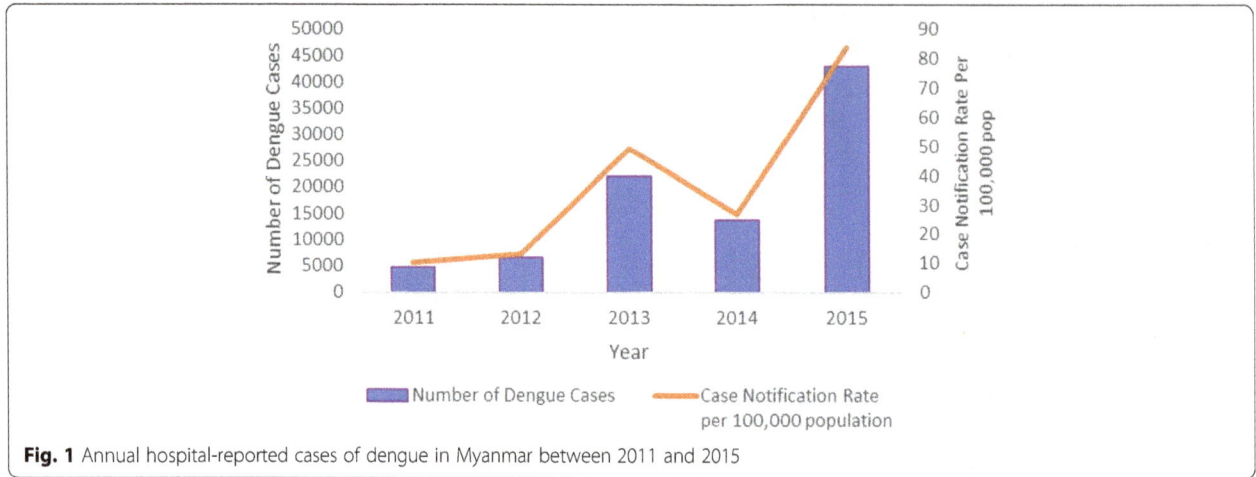

Fig. 1 Annual hospital-reported cases of dengue in Myanmar between 2011 and 2015

(Table 4). Health education sessions for the general public on dengue prevention and control along with numbers attending each year are shown in Table 5, the main findings being a large increase in education sessions and persons attending these sessions, particularly in 2014 and 2015.

Dengue serotype patterns

Dengue serotype patterns between 2013 and 2015 are shown in Table 6. In the 2013 outbreak, serotype 1 predominated, while in the 2015 outbreak, serotypes 1, 2, and 4 predominated.

Discussion

This is the first published study from Myanmar assessing the national burden and characteristics of hospital-reported dengue cases and deaths over a 5-year period, describing dengue vector control measures and health education in the community and reporting national health laboratory data on serotypes. There were some interesting findings.

The burden of hospital-recorded cases was high and mostly concentrated in children. In two of the five years (2013 and 2015), there were dengue outbreaks, which are variably defined, but in this context equate to case numbers that were significantly increased compared with the previous 5 years [2]. The annual pattern of dengue deaths mirrored that of cases, although, interestingly, case fatality was highest in the 2014, the year between the two outbreaks. The reasons for this are not completely clear, but may relate to the national census being carried out in 2014 providing more accurate population data and a shift to dengue virus serotypes 2 and 4 (which were more common in the 2015 outbreak) and which may be linked to secondary infections and more severe disease [17].

With the 5-year data combined, the highest case fatality was observed in infants and adults (aged 15 years and above). Unfortunately, in the adult population, the national information systems only capture those aged 15 years and above with no further stratification, so we

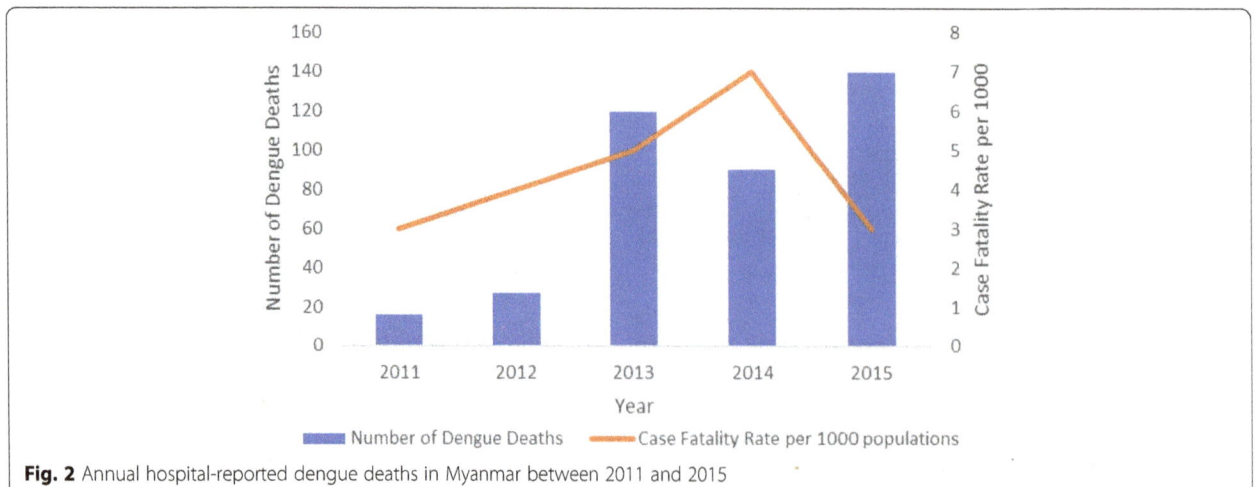

Fig. 2 Annual hospital-reported dengue deaths in Myanmar between 2011 and 2015

Table 2 Demographic and clinical characteristics in relation to all hospital-reported dengue cases and dengue deaths in Myanmar between 2011 and 2015

Characteristics	Dengue cases		Dengue deaths		Case fatality per 1000
	n	(%)	n	(%)	
Total	89,832	(100)	393	(100)	4
Age group in years					
< 1	5049	(6)	42	(11)	8
1–4	22,613	(25)	100	(25)	4
5–9	42,186	(47)	187	(48)	4
10–14	17,146	(19)	45	(11)	3
≥ 15	2838	(3)	19	(5)	7
Gender					
Male	43,875	(49)	180	(46)	4
Female	45,957	(51)	213	(54)	5
Residence					
Urban	43,282	(48)	194	(49)	5
Rural	46,550	(52)	199	(51)	4
Disease severity grade					
DF and DHF grade I	37,771	(42)	16	(4)	0
DHF grade II	19,244	(21)	20	(5)	1
DHF grade III	14,285	(16)	44	(11)	3
DHF grade IV	18,532	(21)	313	(80)	17

DF dengue fever, *DHF* dengue hemorrhagic fever

do not know which of the older age groups are mainly at risk. A recent systematic review highlighted the importance of old age and non-communicable diseases, such as diabetes mellitus, respiratory disease, and renal failure as risk factors for severe forms of dengue [18], so older adults may particularly be susceptible to DHF and DSS.

Not surprisingly, disease grade 4 accounted for the majority of deaths and was associated with the highest case

Table 3 Seasonal changes and the ecological distribution of hospital-reported dengue cases and dengue deaths in Myanmar between 2011 and 2015

Characteristics	Dengue cases		Dengue deaths		Case fatality per 1000
	n	(%)	n	(%)	
Total	89,832	(100)	393	(100)	4
Season:					
Hot (February to April)	4424	(5)	12	(3)	3
Wet (May to September)	75,171	(84)	330	(84)	4
Cool (October to January)	10,237	(11)	51	(13)	1
Ecological region:					
Delta and lowland	48,412	(54)	205	(52)	4
Hills	5732	(6)	49	(12)	9
Coastal	8327	(9)	24	(6)	3
Plains	27,361	(31)	115	(30)	4

fatality. The vascular permeability, thrombocytopenia, liver pathology, complement activation, and altered hemostasis in severe dengue have been well characterized through autopsy studies on children dying of dengue in Myanmar [19], but to date, treatment is still supportive effectively with no specific antiviral agents available for targeted therapy.

The finding that dengue cases were more common in the wet season and in the delta and lowland regions concurs with current knowledge about seasonal transmission. High temperatures, relative humidity, heavy rainfall in the wet season, and poor drainage not only assist the main vector, *Aedes aegypti*, to multiply and adapt to its urban environment, but these factors also favor the propagation of dengue viruses in the mosquito itself [20–23] Case fatality was higher in the hills, and this may relate to health facilities being not as well equipped in these areas, health staff less experienced in the diagnosis and management of dengue, and poor immunity of these populations to the dengue virus [2].

It was encouraging to see the progressive increase in implementation of larval control measures and space spraying in townships and wards, particularly from 2013 to 2015, and this was accompanied by a similar increase in dengue health education sessions and the number of people who attended these sessions. Why there was a decrease in vector control measures between 2011 and 2012 is not clear, but may have been due to poor community participation and engagement at this time. Despite the increases in vector control measures in the most recent years, the implementation coverage of larval control measures in households and for water containers that reflected community participation was still low at less than 25% and space spraying at households and at schools was even lower at less than 10%. We do not know whether this reflects the true picture or is an indicator of weak monitoring systems, but clearly, the intensive vector control efforts over the last few years did not prevent the dengue outbreak of 2015.

Finally, the serotype data show that dengue serotype 1 predominated in the 2013 outbreak, with all four serotypes participating in the 2015 outbreak. These findings accord with previous published studies confirming the predominance of serotype 1 and the lack of correlation between serotypes and clinical severity in the 2013 outbreak [24] and the circulation of all four serotypes in the 2015 outbreak [25].

The strengths of this study are the large data set of hospital-recorded cases and deaths from 90% or more of public hospitals in the country and dengue source control measures from selected states/regions, which make the findings representative of what is happening in the country. The conduct and reporting of this observational study are also in line with internationally recommended

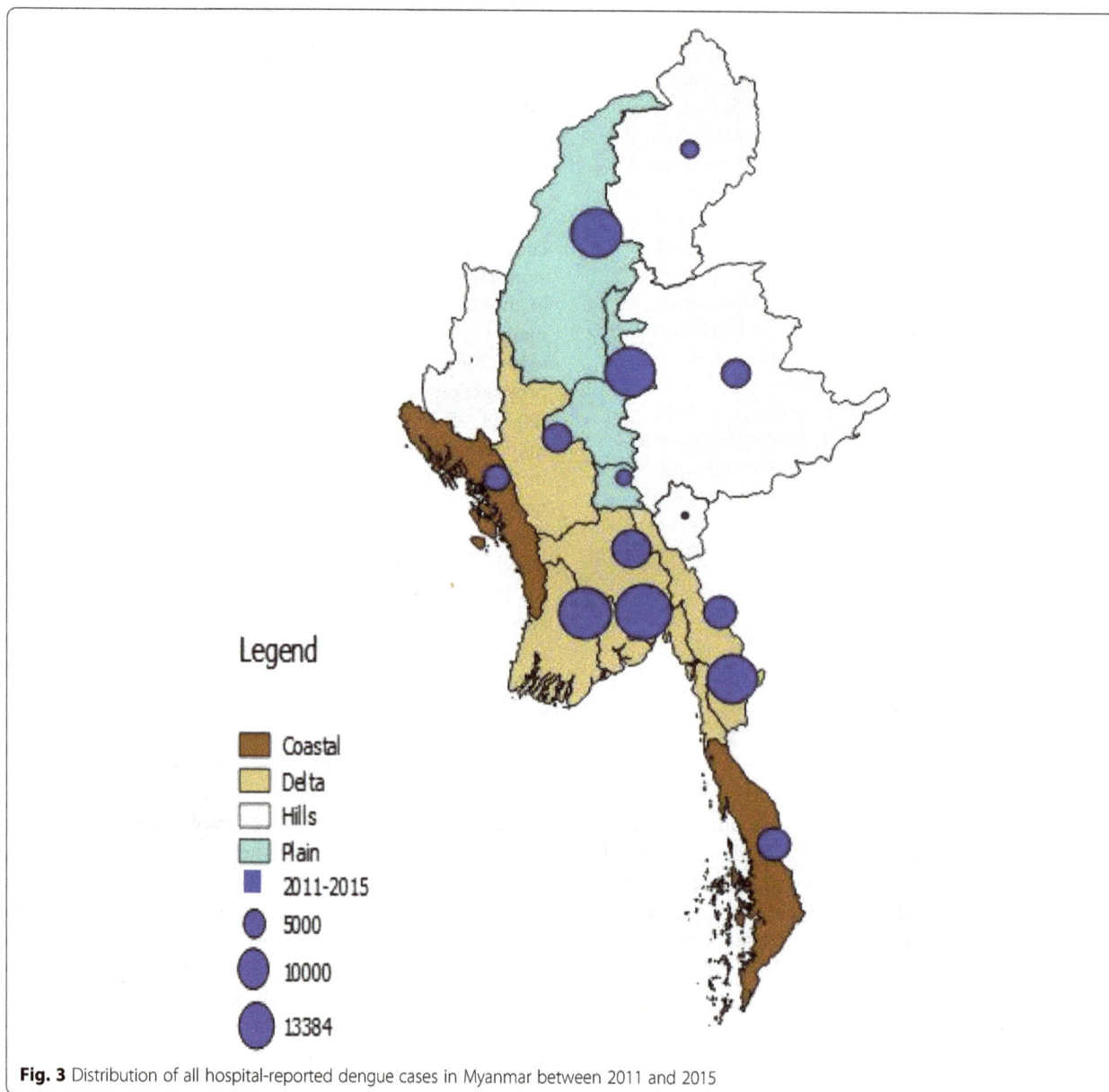

Fig. 3 Distribution of all hospital-reported dengue cases in Myanmar between 2011 and 2015

STROBE guidelines [26]. However, there are a number of limitations. First, the cases and deaths were all health facility based, we do not know from the records whether the dengue cases were based on admission or discharge diagnoses, and there is no information in our study about the community burden of dengue or about the burden of asymptomatic infections. Lack of information on asymptomatic infections is an important epidemiological gap as a recent study has shown that people with asymptomatic infections not only infect mosquitoes, but are more infectious to mosquitoes than those with dengue symptoms [27]. Second, we were unable in dengue cases classified as grade I to differentiate between DF and DHF. Third, we do not know (as stated earlier) whether the low implementation coverage of larval

control or space spraying measures in households and schools or in water containers is a true reflection of what is happening or whether this relates to weak monitoring, recording, and reporting. Finally, the data used in the study were all secondary and collected through the routine systems, so we have no means of checking accuracy or validity.

Despite these limitations, there are three important programmatic implications from this study. First, the health facility-based reporting of dengue cases and deaths needs to be revisited to ensure there is functionality at full capacity, the data are collected and transmitted in a timely way, and through regular supervision, the data are quality assured. It is also important for the program to collect a more detailed age-breakdown for those aged 15 years and

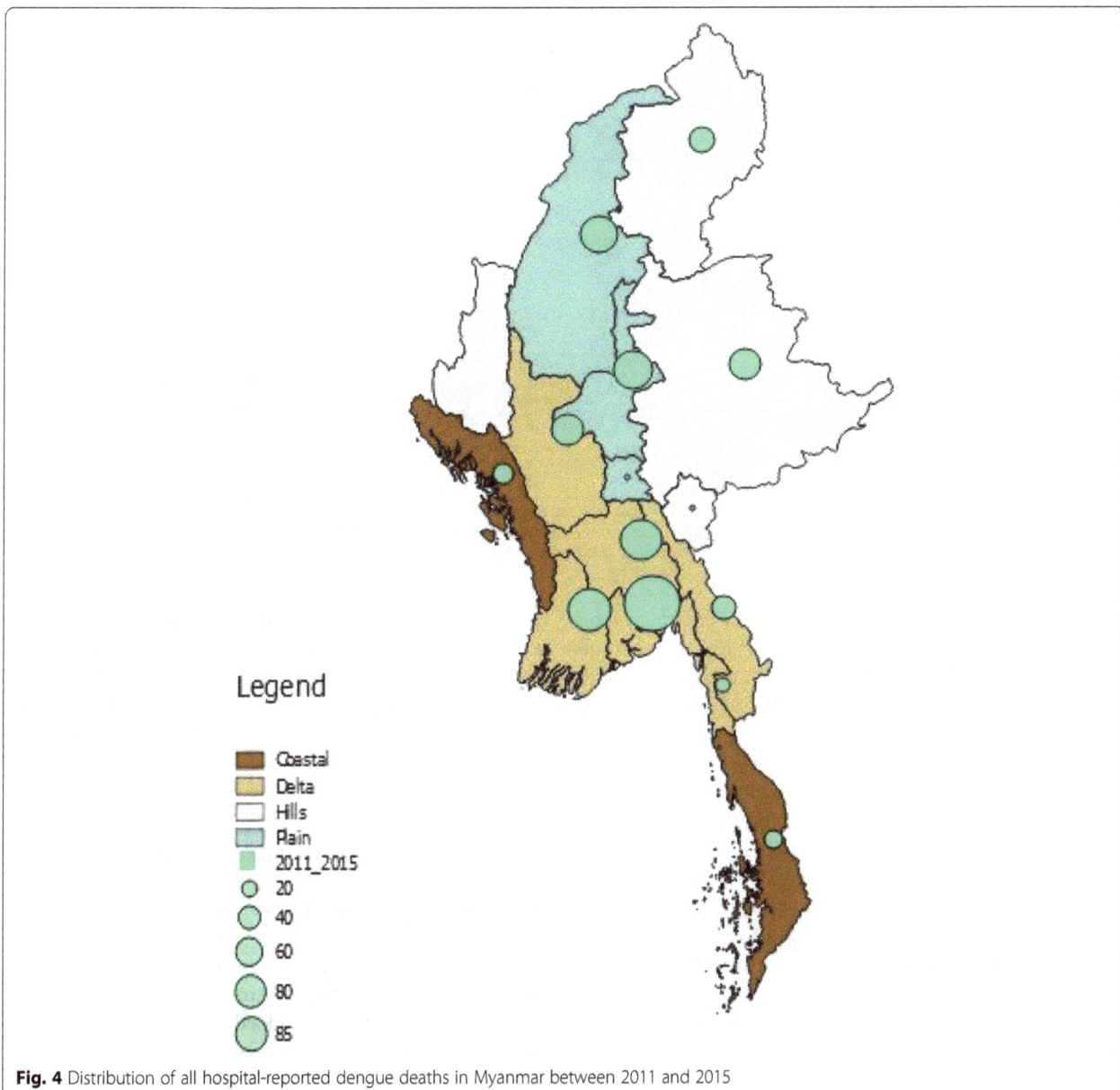

Fig. 4 Distribution of all hospital-reported dengue deaths in Myanmar between 2011 and 2015

above and to divide disease severity grade I into DF and DHF. Whether monitoring can extend to community-level disease and asymptomatic infection needs further discussion, but more accurate measurements and estimates of disease burden will be essential for planning vaccination campaigns. Vaccination, in combination with vector control, is seen as a promising tool in the fight against dengue. Currently, there are three candidate live-attenuated vaccines in phase 2/3 (NIH TV003/TV005 and Takeda TDV vaccines) or phase 4 (Sanofi Dengvaxia) trials, although there are many challenges to overcome before efficacy and safety are assured [28].

Second, there is need to strengthen (a) the monitoring and (b) recording of vector control measures,

particularly for households, schools, and water containers. Vector control represents a substantial portion of government dengue-related costs, and it is important to note that control of *Aedes aegypti* is likely to impact not only on dengue but also on chikungunya and *Zika* viruses. The chikungunya virus has been detected in Myanmar [29, 30], but due to overlap in the clinical presentation with dengue and cross-reactivity of the serological tests, the burden of disease in the country has not been determined. *Zika* virus was first detected in a foreign national in Myanmar in 2016 [31], but to date, there are no published reports of the burden of *Zika* virus in the country.

Third, basic science research is crucial to understand more about the virus (serotypes, genotypes, and

Table 4 Annual implementation of dengue vector control measures in Myanmar between 2011 and 2015

	Total number[a]	2011		2012		2013		2014		2015	
		n	(%)	n	(%)	n	(%)	n	(%)	n	(%)
A: larval control measures											
Implementation of larval control measures at:											
Townships	330	277	(84)	81	(25)	68	(21)	157	(48)	152	(46)
Wards	3065	2655	(87)	931	(30)	1364	(45)	1716	(56)	2026	(66)
Households	10,889,348	2,753,002	(25)	2,191,259	(20)	1,790,151	(16)	2,729,804	(25)	3,447,524	(32)
Water containers[b]	51,400,000	29,666,676	(58)	5,420,553	(11)	6,755,019	(13)	4,497,076	(9)	10,954,867	(21)
B: space spraying measures											
Implementation of space spraying measures at:											
Townships	330	120	(36)	15	(5)	68	(21)	84	(25)	158	(48)
Wards	3065	855	(28)	28	(< 1)	478	(16)	1206	(39)	2026	(66)
Households	10,889,348	31,455	(< 1)	39,169	(< 1)	26,293	(< 1)	43,744	(< 1)	410,117	(< 1)
Schools	41,000	305	(< 1)	441	(1)	139	(< 1)	1797	(4)	2568	(6)

[a]Total number = total number in the country and is the denominator against which the percentages are calculated
[b]The estimated total number of water containers in Myanmar was based on one container per person living in Myanmar. Previous unpublished surveys have suggested that each resident in the country has one or slightly more than one container with the types of container being drums, cement tanks, ceramic jars, flower vases, car tires, tins, and coconut shells

strains), the immune responses, the immune correlates of protection and risk, and the development of dengue vaccines. National programs, however, would do well to work in partnership with non-governmental organizations, local community-based organizations, and self-help groups to ensure better case management, develop and use point-of-care diagnostics, undertake timely and accurate surveillance/monitoring and reporting, to better engage with the community, to respond to outbreaks, and to implement source reduction measures in households as well as in public spaces [28, 32, 33]. More attention also needs to be given to novel biological, genetic, and behavioral approaches that target mosquitoes such as the use of Wolbachia bacteria strains that infect *Aedes aegypti* mosquitoes [34] and genetically modified mosquitoes carrying lethal genes [35].

Conclusions
In conclusion, this study has described the large burden of hospital-recorded dengue in Myanmar between 2011 and 2015, which was concentrated predominately in children and which included two outbreaks in 2013 and

2015. Case fatality was particularly high in infants aged less than 1 year, adults aged 15 years or more, patients with grade IV disease, and those residing in hilly regions of the country. Implementation and coverage of dengue vector control measures, including larval control, space spraying, and health education, all increased between 2012 and 2015, although there are concerns about low coverage of these interventions in households and schools. Dengue virus serotype 1 predominated in the 2013 outbreak, while all four serotypes circulated in the 2015 outbreak. Dengue is a serious public health disease burden in Myanmar. More attention is needed to improve the monitoring, recording, and reporting of cases, deaths, and vector control activities, and to avoid misclassification bias in reporting hospitalized dengue cases, the notification systems must just report the discharge diagnosis. Finally, more investment needed for programmatic research.

Table 5 Annual number of health education sessions about dengue control measures and numbers attending these sessions in Myanmar between 2011 and 2015

	2011	2012	2013	2014	2015
	n	n	n	n	n
Health education sessions	17,928	16,139	6005	72,045	93,664
Persons attending health education sessions	2,608,181	1,793,324	2,254,388	3,137,995	4,841,742

Table 6 Dengue serotypes identified each year in Myanmar between 2011 and 2015

Dengue serum samples and serotypes	2013		2014		2015	
	n	(%)[a]	n	(%)[a]	n	(%)[a]
Total serum samples tested:	230		21		37	
Samples seronegative	148		20		1	
Samples seropositive:	82		1		36	
Serotype 1	44	(54)	–		9	(25)
Serotype 2	4	(5)	–		11	(31)
Serotype 3	11	(13)	1	(100)	4	(11)
Serotype 4	23	(28)	–		12	(33)

[a]Numbers in percentages are column percentages and refer to serum samples seropositive

Abbreviations

DF/DHF: Dengue Fever/Dengue Hemorrhagic Fever; DSS: Dengue shock syndrome; VBDC: Vector-borne disease control; WHO: World Health Organization

Acknowledgements

This research was conducted through the Structured Operational Research and Training Initiative (SORT IT), a global partnership led by the Special Programme for Research and Training in Tropical Diseases at the World Health Organization (WHO/TDR). The model is based on a course developed jointly by the International Union Against Tuberculosis and Lung Disease (The Union) and Medécins sans Frontières (MSF/Doctors Without Borders). The specific SORT IT program which resulted in this publication was jointly organized and implemented by The Centre for Operational Research, The Union, Paris, France; The Department of Medical Research, Ministry of Health and Sports, Myanmar; The Department of Public Health, Ministry of Health and Sports, Myanmar; The Union Country Office, Mandalay, Myanmar; The Union South-East Asia Office, New Delhi, India; the Operational Research Unit (LUXOR), MSF Brussels Operational Center, Luxembourg; and Burnet Institute, Australia.

Funding

The training program, within which this paper was developed, and the open access publication costs were funded by the Department for International Development (DFID), UK, and La Fondation Veuve Emile Metz-Tesch (Luxembourg). The funders had no role in study design, data collection and analysis, decision to publish, or preparation of the manuscript.

Authors' contributions

PMO designed the study, collected and analyzed data, and wrote the first draft. KTW, ADH, and HDS participated in the design of the study, data analysis, and manuscript writing. All authors participated in data interpretation and preparation of the manuscript, and all authors read and approved the final manuscript.

Competing interests

The authors declare that they have no competing interests.

Author details

[1]Central Vector Borne Disease Control Programme, Department of Public Health, Ministry of Health and Sport, Nay Pyi Taw, Myanmar. [2]Department of Medical Research, Yangon, Myanmar. [3]International Union against Tuberculosis and Lung Disease, Paris, France. [4]London School of Hygiene and Tropical Medicine, London, UK. [5]International Union against Tuberculosis and Lung Disease (The Union), South-East Asia Office, New Delhi, India.

References

1. World Health Organization. Dengue and severe dengue. Fact Sheet. Updated July 2016. WHO, Geneva, Switzerland. Available: http://www.who.int/mediacentre/factsheets/fs117/en/. Accessed 29 May 2017.

2. Castro MC, Wilson ME, Bloom DE. Dengue 1. Disease and economic burdens of dengue. Lancet Infect Dis. 2017;17:e70–8. Available: http://dx.doi.org/10.1016/S1473-3099(16)30545-X. Accessed 29 May 2017

3. Khetarpal N, Khanna I. Dengue fever: causes, complications and vaccine strategies. J Immunonol Res. 2016;2016:6803098. doi:10.1155/2016/6803098. Available: https://www.hindawi.com/journals/jir/. Accessed 29 May 2017

4. Nealon J, Taurel AF, Capeding MR, et al. Symptomatic dengue disease in five South-East Asian countries; epidemiological evidence from a dengue vaccine trial. PLoS Negl Trop Dis. 2016;10:e0004918.

5. Pang T, Mak TK, Gubler DJ. Dengue 2. Prevention and control of dengue—the light at the end of the tunnel. Lancet Infect Dis. 2017;17: e79–87. Available: http://dx.doi.org/ 10.1016/ S1473-3099(16)30471-6. Accessed 29 May 2017

6. Bhatt S, Gething PW, Brady OJ, et al. The global distribution and burden of dengue. Nature. 2013;496:504–7.

7. Brady OJ, Gething PW, Bhatt S, et al. Refining the global spatial limits of dengue virus transmission by evidence-based consensus. PLoS Negl Trop Dis. 2012;6:e1760.

8. Shepard DS, Undurraga EA, Halasa YA. Economic and disease burden of dengue in South East Asia. PLoS Negl Trop Dis. 2013;7:e2055.

9. World Health Organization. The dengue strategic plan for the Asia Pacific Region 2008–2015. WHO Western Pacific Region, Manila, Philippines. Available: www.wpro.who.int/mvp/Dengue_Strategic_Plan. pdf. Accessed 29 May 2017

10. Tambo E, Chen JH, Zhou XN, Khater EIM. Outwitting dengue threat and epidemics resurgence in Asia-Pacific countries: strengthening integrated dengue surveillance, monitoring and response systems. Infect Dis Poverty. 2016;5:56.

11. World Health Organization. Comprehensive guidelines for prevention and control of dengue and dengue hemorrhagic fever, revised and expanded edition. New Delhi. WHO, South East Asia Regional Office 2011. Available: www.searo.who.int/entity/vector_borne_tropical_diseases/documents/.../en/. Accessed 29 May 2017.

12. Thu HM, Lowry K, Myint TT, et al. Myanmar dengue outbreak associated with displacement of serotypes 2, 3 and 4 by dengue 1. Emerg Infect Dis. 2004;10:593–7.

13. Myat TW, Thu HM, Kyaw YM, et al. Identification of dengue virus serotypes in children with dengue infection admitted to Yangon Children's Hospital in 2014. Myanmar Health Sci Res J. 2016;28:1–5. Available: www.myanmarhsrj. com/. Accessed 29 May 2017

14. Department of Health, Ministry of Health, Myanmar. Annual Report of Vector Borne Diseases Control Programme, Nay Pyi Taw, 2013. Available: www.moh.gov.mm/. Accessed 29 May 2017.

15. Ministry of Health. Health in Myanmar 2014. The Republic of the Union of Myanmar. Available: www.moh.gov.mm/. Accessed 29 May 2017.

16. Tun A, Myat SM, Gabrielli AF, Montresor A. Control of soil-transmitted helminthiasis in Myanmar: results of 7 years of deworming. Tropical Med Int Health. 2013;18:1017–20.

17. Gupta BP, Singh S, Kurmi R, Molla R, Sreekumar E, Manandhar KD. Reemergence of dengue virus serotype 2 strains in the 2013 outbreak in Nepal. Indian J Med Res. 2015;142(supplement):1–6. doi:10.4103/0971-5916.176564.

18. Toledo J, George L, Martinez E, et al. Relevance of non-communicable comorbidities for the development of the severe forms of dengue: a systematic literature review. PLoS Negl Trop Dis. 2016;10:e0004284.

19. Aye KS, Charngkaew K, Win N, et al. Pathologic highlights of dengue hemorrhagic fever in 13 autopsy cases from Myanmar. Hum Pathol. 2014;45:1221–33.

20. Thu HM, Aye KM, Thein S. The effect of temperature and humidity on dengue virus propagation in Aedes aegypti mosquitos. Southeast Asian J Trop Med Public Health. 1998;29:280–4.

21. Wai KT, Arunachalam N, Tana S, et al. Estimating dengue vector abundance in the wet and dry season: implications for targeted vector control in urban and peri-urban Asia. Pathog Glob Health. 2012;106:436–45.

22. Liu-Helmersson J, Stenlund H, Wilder-Smith A, Rocklov J. Vectorial capacity of Aedes aegypti: effects of temperature and implications for global dengue epidemic potential. PLoS One. 2014;9:e89783.

23. Heinen LBS, Zuchi N, Cardoso BF, et al. Dengue outbreak in Mato Grosso State, Midwestern Brazil. Rev Inst Med Trop Sao Paulo. 2015;57:489–96.

24. Ngwe Tun MM, Kyaw AK, Makki N, et al. Characterization of the 2013 dengue epidemic in Myanmar with dengue virus 1 as the dominant serotype. Infect Genet Evol. 2016;43:31–7.

25. Kyaw AK, Ngwe Tun MM, Moi ML, et al. Clinical, virological and epidemiological characterization of dengue outbreak in Myanmar, 2015. Epidemiol Infect. 2017:1–12. doi:10.1017/S0950268817000735.

26. Von Elm E, Altman DG, Egger M, et al. The Strengthening the Reporting of Observational Studies in Epidemiology (STROBE) Statement: guidelines for reporting observational studies. Lancet. 2007;370:1453–7.

27. Duong V, Lambrechts L, Paul RE, et al. Asymptomatic humans transmit dengue virus to mosquitoes. Proc Natl Acad Sci U S A. 2015;112:14688–93.

28. Katzelnick LC, Coloma J, Harris E. Dengue 3. Dengue: knowledge gaps, unmet needs, and research priorities. Lancet Infect Dis. 2017;17:e88–e100.

29. Tun MM, Thant KZ, Inoue S, et al. Detection of east/central/south African genotype of chikungunya virus in Myanmar, 2010. Emerg Infect Dis. 2014;20:1378–81.

30. Furuya-Kanamori L, Liang S, Milinovich G, et al. Co-distribution and co-infection of chikungunya and dengue viruses. BMC Infect Dis. 2016;16:84.

31. World Health Organization. First case of Zika virus infection detected in Myanmar; mosquito control measures must be at the forefront of the fight against vector-borne diseases. October 2016. Available: www.searo.who.int/myanmar/areas/zika_firstcaseinmyanmar/en/. Accessed 30 May 2017].

32. Arunachalam N, Tana S, Espino F, et al. Eco-bio-social determinants of dengue vector breeding: a multi-country study in urban and periurban Asia. Bull World Health Organ. 2010;88:173–84.

33. Wai KT, Htun PT, Tin O, et al. Community-centred eco-bio-social approach to control dengue vectors: an intervention study from Myanmar. Pathog Glob Health. 2012;106:461–8.

34. Hoffmann AA, Montgomery BL, Popovici J, et al. Successful establishment of wolbachia in Aedes populations to suppress dengue transmission. Nature. 2011;476:454–7.

35. Carvalho DO, McKemey AR, Garziera L, et al. Suppression of a field population of *Aedes aegypti* in Brazil by sustained release of transgenic male mosquitoes. PLoS Negl Trop Dis. 2015;9:e0003864.

9

Self-medication practice and associated factors among pregnant women in Addis Ababa, Ethiopia

Kidanemariam G/Michael Beyene[1*] and Solomon Worku Beza[2]

Abstract

Background: Self-medication which is the act of obtaining and using one or more medicines without medical supervision is a common practice among pregnant women. Unless proper caution is taken, it may result in maternal and fetal adverse outcomes. In Ethiopia, information on self-medication practice during pregnancy is scanty. Hence, this study aimed to assess self-medication practice and associated factors among pregnant women in government health centers in Addis Ababa.

Methods: An institution-based mixed study design using a sequential explanatory approach was employed among 617 pregnant women and nine key informants in Addis Ababa from May 8, 2017, to June 30, 2017. Multi-stage sampling technique was used to select study participants, and purposive sampling technique was used to select the key informants. The quantitative data were collected using a structured interview questionnaire and analyzed using Statistical Product and Service Solutions (SPSS) version 23.0 whereas semi-structured questionnaire was used for in-depth interviews. Binary logistic regression was used for quantitative data analysis, and thematic analysis method was used for qualitative data.

Results: The prevalence of self-medication practice was 26.6%. Previous medication use (Adjusted odds ratio (AOR) = 4.20, 95% CI 2.70–6.53), gestational period (AOR = 0.63, 95% CI 0.41–0.98), education on self-medication (AOR = 0.36, 95% CI 0.21–0.62), previous pregnancy and delivery related problems (AOR = 1.71, 95% CI 1.06–2.76), and knowledge about risk of self-medication (AOR = 0.64, 95% CI 0.42–0.97) were significantly associated with self-medication practice. Lack of attention and priority of program designers, absence of strategies and guidelines; weak screening mechanisms, and regulatory enforcement were cited by the key informants as contributing factors for self-medication practices.

Conclusions: Considerable proportion of pregnant women practiced self-medication, including medicines categorized to have high risks. Gestational period, previous medication use, education on self-medication, previous pregnancy- and delivery-related problems, and knowledge were significantly associated with self-medication practice. In addition, there are correctable gaps in program designing, screening of pregnant women, regulatory enforcement, and strategies and guidelines. Hence, necessary measures at all levels must be taken to reduce risks of self-medication during pregnancy.

Keywords: Self-medication practice, Pregnant women, Antenatal care, Health centers, Binary logistic regression, Addis Ababa, Ethiopia

* Correspondence: kidanemar4@gmail.com
[1]Ethiopian Food, Medicine and Healthcare Administration and Control Authority, Addis Ababa, Ethiopia
Full list of author information is available at the end of the article

Background

Maternal and child health is a priority agenda of the global community [1, 2] and must be addressed using consistent and coordinated policies and programs [1, 3, 4]. Pregnancy is a period of great physiological changes to the mother and fetus [5]. During this period, a pregnant woman may take medication to alleviate pregnancy-related symptoms [6]. Medication use during pregnancy has been a concern both for the mother and fetus since the discovery of birth defects resulting from thalidomide crisis in early pregnancy in 1960s and teratogenic effects discovered related to use of diethylstilboestrol in 1971 [7–10].This necessitates critical evaluation of the risk level of medicines during pregnancy [11].

According to the United States Food and Drug Administration (USFDA) risk classification of medicines during pregnancy, medicines under category A show no risks in controlled studies and those medicines in category B have no evidence of human risk in controlled studies. Medicines in category C may have potential risks to the fetus. The risks cannot be ruled out but the medicines under category C should be used only if the potential benefits justify the potential risks to the fetus. Medicines in category D have positive evidence of human fetal risk, and those in category X are totally contraindicated in pregnancy because they have proven fetal risks [11].

Self-medication is defined as the act of using medications by patients or individuals to treat self-diagnosed disorders or symptoms on their own initiative [12, 13]. It is a behavior in which the individual attempts to solve his/her health problem without professional knowledge or advice [13]. An unauthorized purchase of medicines for self-medication use from nearby medicine retail outlets and other sources are increasing. It becomes the most common form of self-care [7, 14] though the irrational practices must be intervened and discouraged [15, 16].

When practiced properly, self-medication has a positive impact on individuals and health care systems. It needs health professional advices and access to appropriate information. In most developing countries in which the health system is inefficient and people access medicines easily from retail outlets, there may be an increased risk of self-medication during pregnancy [6].

Self-medication may cause serious structural and functional adverse effects on the fetus [17–19] including fetal toxicity, malformations, teratogen effects, and other potential harms [5, 8, 17, 20, 21]. Furthermore, it may cause low birth weight, premature birth, feeding problems; and respiratory problems in the fetus and affect the health of mother [8, 17, 21]. For many commonly used medicines, evidences of safe use in pregnant women have not been established. This is because medication safety information for pregnant women is limited due to the fact that pregnant women are often excluded from clinical trials of medicines [8, 22–24]. The limited medicine information has considerable contribution to maternal and neonatal mortality and morbidity, and fetal death [17, 25]. Despite this, studies showed that there is a high level of self-medication use among pregnant women [22, 24].

Globally, self-medication practice during pregnancy has been increasing and found to be high in many regions of the world, especially in developing countries [22, 26, 27]. The type, extent, and reasons for its practice however vary. Studies showed that both modern and herbal medicines are commonly used for self-medication in developing countries. This is due to easy access to medicines [6, 16, 28, 29]. Herbal medicine use poses potential risks to the mother and fetus due to the fact that the composition and safety parameters of these products are unknown [27].

There are different reasons for self-medication among pregnant women in different countries. It is associated with factors such as age, income, education level, knowledge, access to medicines, time [14, 16], perception towards risk of self-medication [26, 30–32], previous medication use, gestational age, and occupation [33, 34]. Studies found that self-medication practice is high during pregnancy in Europe (Western, Northern, and Eastern); North and South America and Australia (66.9%); Yazd, Iran (> 35%); Ahvaz, south Iran (30.6%); Hyderabad, Pakistan (37.9%); and Paraná, Brazil (94.67%) [34–37]. However, low prevalence rates of self-medication were reported in Peru (10.2%), Portugal (1.3%), the Netherlands (12.5%), Brazil (16.4%), and Arak city, Iran (12%) [18, 38–41].

In Africa, both modern and herbal medicines are commonly used for self-medication. Studies conducted in different parts of Nigeria revealed that 72.4% in Uyo, 31.5% in Ado-Ekiti, 63.8% in Ibadan, and 85% in Jos of pregnant women practiced self-medication [19, 29, 33, 42]. A study conducted in the Democratic Republic of Congo found that 59.9% of pregnant women used self-medication [6]. In Ethiopia, an institution-based study conducted in governmental health centers in Bahirdar showed that 25% of pregnant women reported self-medication [27]. A hospital-based study conducted among pregnant women in Jimma University specialized hospital showed that the prevalence of self-medication was 20.1% (16). A similar institution-based study conducted in hospitals in Mekelle showed 9.5 and 2% self-utilized modern and herbal medicines respectively [43].

Maternal and child health is one of the major priority agendas of the government of Ethiopia [44] even though there is a remarkable achievement observed in the reduction of under-five mortality rates. The reduction in mortality and morbidity in neonatal age groups however is not impressive. Prematurity is the most common cause of neonatal mortality [44]. Preventing pregnancy- and delivery-related problems associated with self-medication practice helps to protect the health of the mother and fetus [17, 25]. Identifying the extent and determinants of self-medication among pregnant women may contribute in achieving the targets of Sustainable Development Goal (SDG).

However, in Ethiopia despite the potential risks of self-medication, researches on the extent and determinants of self-medication during pregnancy are scanty. The findings of this study will provide information for policy makers and relevant stakeholders to develop strategies and appropriate interventions to prevent the risks associated with self-medication practice during pregnancy.

Hence, this study aimed to assess self-medication practice and associated factors among pregnant women attending antenatal care in government health centers in Addis Ababa, Ethiopia.

Methods

Study design and setting
An institution-based cross-sectional mixed study method was employed with a sequential explanatory design to triangulate the quantitative data with the qualitative data. Data were collected from May 08 to June 30, 2017, in Addis Ababa.

Addis Ababa is the diplomatic capital of the African Union and capital city of Ethiopia, located about 2500 m above sea level. It has ten sub-cities and 116 woredas [45]. The city has an estimated population of 3.2 million of which 52.6% are female [46]. During the study period, there were 92 functional government health centers, 378 pharmacies, 278 drug shops, and 777 different types of clinics in Addis Ababa [46].

Study participants
The study participants were pregnant women attending antenatal care (ANC) in selected government health centers in Addis Ababa during the study period. The key informants for the in-depth interviews were directors, team leaders, ANC program coordinators, and ANC case team leaders in their current position.

Sample size and sampling procedure
The sample size was determined by using the single population proportion formula for the prevalence of self-medication practice and double population proportion formula for predictor variables assuming 25% prevalence of self-medication practice during pregnancy from a study conducted in Bahirdar [27] at 95% confidence level, 5% marginal error and design effect of two. Anticipating 10% non-response rate, the final sample size was 634 pregnant women. The sample size for the qualitative study was guided by the degree of information saturation based on preliminary analysis during data collection. Accordingly, a total of nine key informants were purposively selected and interviewed in order to gather more explanatory opinions and deepen information complementing the quantitative findings.

Multi-stage sampling technique was employed to select the study participants. There were a total of 92 functional government health centers in Addis Ababa. The lists of the health centers were obtained from Addis Ababa Health Bureau. All health centers were listed, and table of random numbers was employed to randomly draw the required number of health centers. Eighteen health centers (20% of the total health centers) were selected using simple random sampling technique. Proportional numbers of pregnant women were assigned to each health center based on the flow of pregnant women per month taking one previous year antenatal care records. Then, systematic random sampling technique with fixed sampling interval was used to draw 634 pregnant women attending antenatal care in the selected health centers. For the qualitative study, purposive sampling technique was used. The key informants were from the Ministry of Health; Addis Ababa Health Bureau (AAHB); Ethiopian Food, Medicine and Healthcare Administration and Control Authority; and health centers.

Data collection tools, procedures, and quality assurance
Quantitative data were collected using an interviewer-administered structured questionnaire. The structured interview questionnaire was adapted from previous studies [27, 29, 35, 47] and modified to fit the current study. The questionnaire was originally prepared in English, translated to Amharic language, and then back translated to English to validate consistency of meaning. Before the commencement of the actual data collection, the questionnaire was pretested on 5% randomly selected pregnant women attending antenatal care in government health centers who were later excluded from the study. Accordingly, the questionnaire was slightly modified.

The questionnaire consisted of questions related to socio-demographic factors, obstetric factors, previous medication use, education and counseling, and knowledge about risk of self-medication practices. To assess knowledge about risk of self-medication practice of the pregnant women, 12 questions in a five Likert scales (0–4 scale) were used and each question was coded and computed, and scores were dichotomized into good knowledge (Participants who scored ≥75% on knowledge based questions) and poor knowledge (Participants who scored < 75% on knowledge based questions). The collected data were checked for its consistency and completeness before any attempt to enter code and analyze it.

Finally, Epi-Info version 7.2.1.0 was used to control and manage errors resulting from the data entry process.

One-on-one, face-to-face, in-depth interviews were carried out with key informants using semi-structured, open-ended interview questionnaire with flexible probing techniques to elaborate original responses of the interviewee. The interview questions were classified into two sections. The first section focused on personal and professional information such as age, professional background, work experience, and educational background. The second section was designed to explore the stakeholders view on self-medication practice, screening mechanisms, education on self-medication, regulatory enforcements, reasons for self-medication, and availability of strategies, guidelines and charts or forms.

The interviews were conducted by principal investigators. The interviews were audio recorded and notes were taken properly. The participants were interviewed at the time and location of their choice. The average duration of the interviews was approximately 35 min.

Data management and analysis

The collected quantitative data were entered into Epi-Info version 7.2.1.0 and analyzed using SPSS version 23.0. Participants' socio-demographic characteristics, obstetric factors, previous medication use, education and counseling, and knowledge about risk of self-medication were presented using relevant descriptive statistics. Univariate analysis was done at 25% level of significance to screen out potentially significant independent variables. Multivariable logistic regression was performed by using the relevant independent variables. The association between the dependent variable and independent variables were assessed using binary logistic regression. Hosmer and Lemeshow goodness-of-fit test was used to check the adequacy of the final model and the model fitted to the data well (p value = 0.434). Results were expressed as crudes, adjusted odds ratio, and 95% confidence interval. Variables with p value < 0.05 were considered as statistically significant.

For the qualitative study, the audio records and notes of the interviews were transcribed using a verbatim transcription technique. The transcribed scripts were intensively read, and the data were categorized into themes. Thematic analysis method was used to analyze the data. The analysis was facilitated using OpenCode version 4.0.2.3 software. To check the accuracy of the translation, one of the recordings was translated and transcribed by a bi-lingual expert and compared with the primary work. In reporting the findings, codes were used to maintain anonymity of the key informants. Furthermore, the findings of the study were communicated to five of the key informants for authenticity of the transcripts and interpretations.

Results

Socio-demographic characteristics

Out of the 634 study participants, 617 pregnant women participated in the study making the response rate of 97.3%. The majority of the respondents, 251 (40.7%), were in the age group of 25–29 years, and 199 (32.3%) participants had completed secondary school (grade 9–12). Two hundred and twenty nine (37.1%) of the respondents were housewives, and 273 (44.2%) had a monthly average family income of 3000–5999 ETB (Table 1).

Obstetric factors

Out of 617 respondents, 268 (43.4%) were in the second trimester. Most of the pregnant women were multigravida (363/617, 58.8%) and were nulliparous (296/617; 48%). At the time of interview, 273 (44.2%) of pregnant women were on the first ANC visit (Table 2).

One hundred and thirty nine pregnant women (139/617; 22.5%) had encountered previous pregnancy- and delivery-related problems of which 82 (82/139; 59%) had encountered abortion (Fig. 1).

Maternal health education and counseling

Four hundred and eighty-nine (79.3%) of the pregnant women attended maternal health education provided by the health centers during the antenatal care follow-up. More than half (338/617, 54.8%) of them had received an education on risk of self-medication, and 341 (55.3%)

Table 1 Socio-demographic characteristics of the study participants, Addis Ababa, 2017 ($n = 617$)

Variables		n (%)
Age in year	18–24	194 (31.4)
	25–29	251 (40.7)
	30–34	110 (17.8)
	> 34	62 (10)
Education	No formal education	61 (9.9)
	Primary school (grades 1–8)	168 (27.2)
	Secondary school (grades 9–12)	199 (32.3)
	Certificate or diploma	133 (21.6)
	First degree and above	56 (9.1)
Employment	Housewife	229 (37.1)
	Government employee	127 (20.6)
	Private employee	170 (27.6)
	Merchant	55 (8.9)
	Housemaid	36 (5.8)
Average family monthly income in ETB	< 3000 ETB	189 (30.6)
	3000–5999 ETB	273 (44.2)
	> 6000 ETB	155 (25.1)

Table 2 Obstetric factors of pregnant women, Addis Ababa, 2017 ($n = 617$)

Variables		n (%)
Gestational period	First trimester	92 (14.9)
	Second trimester	268 (43.4)
	Third trimester	257 (41.7)
Previous pregnancy and delivery related problems	Yes	139 (22.5)
	No	478 (77.5)
Gravidity	Primigravida (1)	254 (41.2)
	Multigravida (> 1)	363 (58.8)
Parity	Nulliparous (0)	296 (48)
	Primiparous (1)	191 (31)
	Multiparous (> 1)	130 (21)
ANC Visit	First visit	273 (44.2)
	Second visit	186 (30.1)
	Third visit	99 (16)
	Four and above visit	59 (9.6)

of them had received counseling services about risk of self-medication.

Regarding the source of information about the risks of self-medication, majority (281/617, 45.5%) of the pregnant women obtained information from health professionals and 71 (11.5%) never obtained information from any sources (Fig. 2).

Self-medication practice during pregnancy

The study participants used both modern and herbal medicines during the current pregnancy. Among the 617 pregnant women, 296 (48%) of them had previous self-medication experience and 164 (26.6%) practiced self-medication during the current pregnancy. From these

who used medicines by themselves, 112 (18.2%) of them reported use of at least one modern medication while 67 (10.9%) of them took at least one herbal medicine. Fifteen (2.43%) participants took both modern and herbal medicines.

Among the 112 pregnant women who took modern medicines, the major reasons reported for self-medication were easy access to medicines without prescription from pharmacies or drug shops (80/112; 71.4%), thought that their disease was not serious (61/112; 54.5%) and said to save time (30/112; 26.8%). The sources of modern medicines for self-medication were pharmacies or drug shops (86/112, 76.8%), left-over medicines (21/112, 18.8%), and shared with family, friends or neighbors (11/112, 9.8%). Majority, 72 (64.3%) of the pregnant women decided by themselves to choose the modern medicines whereas 33 (29.5%) of the decision was made by their husband, family or neighbors (Table 3).

Among the 67 pregnant women who used herbal medicines, the reasons reported for self-medication were easily available herbal medicines (46/67; 68.7%), the disease was not serious (35/67; 52.2%), and believing that herbal medicines carry less risk than modern medicines (17/67; 25.4%). The sources of herbal medicines were homemade remedies (33, 49.3%), neighbors (23, 34.3%), and market or shops (7, 10.4%). The suggestions for herbal medicine use were made by the husband, family, or neighbors (35, 52.2%) and the pregnant women themselves (28, 41.8%) (Table 4).

In the present study, paracetamol (55/112; 49.1%) and amoxicillin (26/112; 23.2%) were the most commonly used medications for self-medication during pregnancy. Concerning the therapeutic category of the medicines, 76 (67.86%) were analgesics, 37 (33%) were antibiotics, and 17 (15.2%) were anthelmintics. As per US FDA

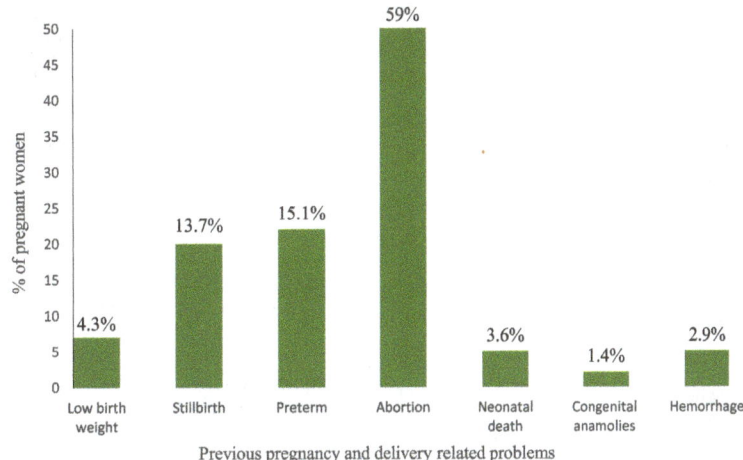

Fig. 1 Previous pregnancy- and delivery-related problems encountered among pregnant women attending antenatal care in government health centers, Addis Ababa, 2017 ($n = 139$)

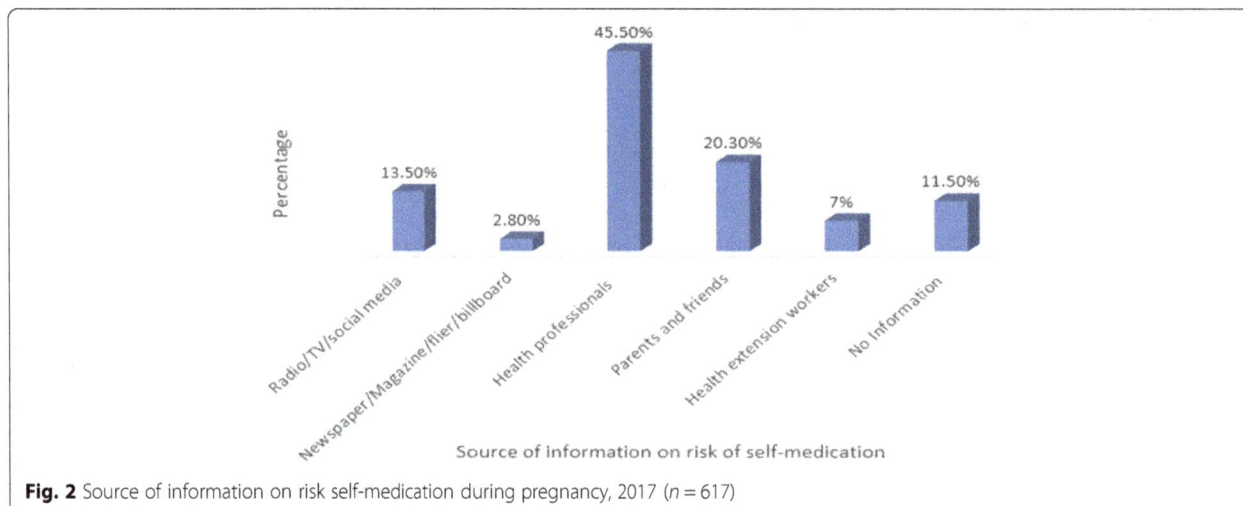

Fig. 2 Source of information on risk self-medication during pregnancy, 2017 (*n* = 617)

pregnancy risk classification, 91 (81.25%) of the modern medicines used by the pregnant women were from category B; 24 (21.43%) were from category C; 19 (16.96%) were from category D; and 1 (0.89%) was from category X (Table 5).

Table 3 Reasons for use, source of modern medication, and recommendation for self-medication of the pregnant women, Addis Ababa, 2017 (*n* = 112)

Variables		n (%)
Reasons for self-medication*	Time saving	30 (26.8)
	Obtaining medicines easily	80 (71.4)
	Disease not serious	61 (54.5)
	Self-medication is cheaper	20 (17.9)
	Previous medication experience	23 (20.5)
	Being embarrassed to tell about the disease	2 (1.8)
	High cost of visiting doctors and health service	5 (4.5)
	Poor health service provision	1 (0.9)
	Poor ethics of health professionals	1 (0.9)
	Long waiting time for health services	22 (19.6)
Source of modern medication*	Sharing with family, friends or neighbors	11 (9.8)
	Pharmacy or drug store	86 (76.8)
	Health facilities	1 (0.9)
	Left-over medicines	21 (18.8)
Recommended for self-medication by*	My Self	72 (64.3)
	My husband, family or neighbors	33 (29.5)
	Pharmacist or druggist	8 (7.14)
	Nurse	3 (2.7)

*More than one choice can be made by a pregnant woman

In this study, basil (47/67; 70.2%), rue (15/67; 22.4%), garlic (7/67; 10.5%), and ginger (5/67; 7.5%) were the commonly used herbal medicines for self-medication by the pregnant women (Table 6).

Knowledge about risk of self-medication

From the total study participants, more than half (327/617, 53%) of the pregnant women had a good knowledge about risk of self-medication during pregnancy, and 290 (47%) had poor knowledge.

Table 4 Reasons for use, source of herbal medication, and recommendation for herbal medication of the pregnant women, Addis Ababa, 2017 (*n* = 67)

Variables		n (%)*
Reasons for herbal medication*	Time saving	9 (13.4)
	Easily available herbal medicines	46 (68.7)
	Disease not serious	35 (52.2)
	Less risk of herbal medicines than modern medicines	17 (25.4)
	High cost of visiting health professionals and health service	3 (4.5)
	Long waiting time for health services	4 (6)
Source of herbal medications*	Family	5 (7.5)
	Homemade remedies	33 (49.3)
	Neighbors	23 (34.3)
	Market or shop	7 (10.4)
	Traditional healer	1 (1.5)
Recommended for herbal medication by*	My Self	28 (41.8)
	My husband, family or neighbors	35 (52.2)
	Traditional healer	2 (3)
	Traditional birth attendant	5 (7.5)

*More than one choice can made by a pregnant woman

Table 5 Modern medicines used for self-medication by pregnant women by trimester and US FDA pregnancy risk classification, Addis Ababa, 2017 (n = 112)

Medicines used	n (%)*	Trimester, n			US FDA risk category
		1st	2nd	3rd	
Paracetamol	55 (49.1)	27	22	6	B
Amoxicillin	26 (23.2)	12	14		B
Tinidazole	5 (4.5)	2	2	1	C
Metronidazole	4 (3.6)	1	2	1	B
Ibuprofen	6 (5.4)	2	4		C
Albendazole	6 (5.4)	4	2		C
Panadol	7 (6.3)	3	4		D
Diclofenac	5 (4.5)	1	3	1	C
Mebendazole	2 (1.8)	1	1		C
Augmentin (amoxicillin + clavulanate)	1(0.9)			1	B
Azithromycin	1 (0.9)		1		B
Tetracycline	3 (2.7)		3		D
Magnesium trisilicate	2 (1.8)	1	1		B
Ciprofloxacin	4 (3.6)	1	3		D
Aspirin	3 (2.7)	1	1	1	D
Bactrim (sulfamethoxazole + trimethoprim)	2 (1.8)	2			D
Ampicillin	2 (1.8)		2		B
Depo-provera (medroxyprogesterone)	1 (0.9)	1			X
Unknown medicines	3 (2.7)	2	1		

*More than one medicine could be used by a pregnant woman

Factors associated with self-medication practice during pregnancy

In univariate analysis, age, employment status, average monthly family income, gestational period, maternal education, education on self-medication, counseling, previous pregnancy- and delivery-related problems,

Table 6 Herbal medicines used for self-medication by the pregnant women by trimester, Addis Ababa, 2017 (n = 67)

Herbal medicines	n (%)[a]	Trimester, n		
		1st	2nd	3rd
Zingiber officinale (ginger)	5 (7.5%)	2	2	1
Allium sativum (garlic)	7 (10.5%)	6	1	
Ocimum lamiifolium (basil or damakasie)	47 (70.2%)	26	18	3
Hagenia abyssinica (koso)	1 (1.5%)	1		
Taverniera abyssinica (emergency herb)	1 (1.5%)	1		
Ruta chalepensis (rue or tena adam)	15 (22.4%)	10	3	2
Lepidium sativum (peppergrass or feto)	4 (6%)	2	2	
Coffea arabica linn (altet)	2 (3%)	1	1	
Eucalyptus globulus (eucalyptus leaf)	1 (1.5%)		1	
Brassica nigra (mustard seed)	1 (1.5%)		1	
Others*	3 (4.5%)	2	1	

Others*, dign, shikukonina and roots
[a]More than one herbal medicine could be used by a pregnant woman

previous medication use, and knowledge about risk of self-medication were significantly associated with self-medication practice. However, in multivariable logistic regression analysis, only gestational period, previous pregnancy- and delivery-related problems, previous medication use, education on self-medication, and knowledge about risk of self-medication were found to be significantly associated with self-medication practice during the current pregnancy.

In this study, the gestational period was significantly associated with self-medication practice. The odds of self-medication practice among women in their second trimester of pregnancy were 0.63 times the odds of those in their third trimester (AOR = 0.63, 95% CI 0.406–0.984).

Previous medication use was strongly associated with self-medication practice. Pregnant women who used medications before the current pregnancy were about four times more likely to practice self-medication during the current pregnancy as compared to those who did not use medications (AOR = 4.20, 95% CI 2.695–6.534). In addition, pregnant women who encountered previous pregnancy- and delivery-related problems were 1.7 times more likely to practice self-medication than those who did not encounter (AOR = 1.71, 95% CI 1.060–2.761).

Education on self-medication was also strongly associated with self-medication practice. The odds of self-medication practice among pregnant women who were educated about self-medication consequences were 0.36 times the odds of those who were not (AOR = 0.36, 95% CI 0.209–0.617). Moreover, the odds of self-medication practice among pregnant women who had good knowledge about risk of self-medication practice were 0.64 times the odds of those who had poor knowledge (AOR = 0.64, 95% CI 0.419–0.973) (Table 7).

Qualitative findings

A total of nine in-depth interviews were conducted with the key informants. The key informants were two pharmacists, two health officers, three midwives, and two nurses all with a bachelor degree and assumed roles as directors, team leaders, ANC program coordinators, or ANC case team leaders. Their age ranges from 25 to 37 years with 2 to 10 years of work experiences in various organizations.

The key informants were asked about the overall situations, guidance, and policies of self-medication practice among pregnant women. Key themes emerged from the analysis were (i) self-medication practices; (ii) regulatory enforcement; (iii) education and counseling on self-medication; (iv) strategies, guidelines, and forms related; and (v) reasons for self-medication. Analysis of the qualitative data from interviews with key informants is presented in detail as follows.

Self-medication practice

The participants thought that pregnant women were cautious not to use medicines without consulting health professionals. The majority of the participants believed that the trends of using medicines by the pregnant women were decreasing. However, they mentioned that since medicine retail outlets sale medicines without prescription, the pregnant women might use medicines without prescription. This was supported by one of the participant that:

"..... Although the pregnant women feel that self-medications are risky for them and the fetus, they [the pregnant] believe the recommendations from families or friends and this has encouraged them to use medicines by themselves" (SMP01).

Another participant also reinforced the ease of obtaining medicines without prescription from pharmacies or drug shops as follows:

"....... If a pregnant woman asks for a medicine, including antibiotics from pharmacies or drug shops, she can obtain the medicine easily. I feel that the dispensing practice is not as per the regulatory requirements and the regulatory body has not been controlling selling of prescription medicines without prescription" (SMP03).

One of the participants, however, was uncertain on whether self-medication practice among the pregnant women is increasing or decreasing. She pointed out that:

".........The trend of using medicines without prescription among pregnant women seems to decrease, but there is an increase in dispensing of medicines including antibiotics without prescription by pharmacies or drug shops. Hence, the cumulative effect of medicine sale to pregnant women without prescription might be higher or lower" (SMP02).

Reasons for self-medication practice

The participants argued that there are situations where pregnant women practice self-medication and different reasons were identified for such practices. Advice from families or friends or neighbors, inconsistent maternal education including risk of self-medication, poor awareness on risk of self-medication, time saving, feeling that the disease is minor, lack of attention and priorities of program designers, communication gap between pregnant women and health care providers, impairment of continuous assessment of women during pregnancy for self-medication, and weak regulatory enforcement were the major reasons for self-medication practice.

Weak regulatory enforcements

Weak regulation and enforcement on restricting non-prescription medicine sale to pregnant women was mentioned as one of the reasons for self-medication. One of the respondents indicated that unethical dispensing of medicines without prescription may not be due to the lack of knowledge about its consequences for pregnant women but it is due to lack of strong regulatory enforcements. One of the participants mentioned that:

"....These times it is easy to buy any medicine without a prescription from the retail outlets. This is due to the weak regulatory enforcement and I think this weak regulatory system is the main reason for the sale of medicines without prescription" (SMP04).

The respondents suggested the need for enforcing the regulation so as to protect the pregnant women from access to prescription medicines for self-medication. Moreover, the respondents said that even though the health professionals did not have a knowledge gap about the risk of self-medication, they emphasized the need to continuously update on the extent and burden of self-medication. One of the participants supplemented that:

Table 7 Univariate and multivariable analysis of factors associated with self-medication practice among pregnant women in Addis Ababa, 2017 ($n = 617$)

Variables	Self-medication practice		COR (95% CI)	AOR (95% CI)	p value
	Yes	No			
Age in years					
18–24	46	148	0.64 (0.381–1.072)	0.81 (0.446–1.475)	0.492
25–29	60	191	0.65 (0.395–1.057)	0.72 (0.419–1.246)	0.242
30–34	36	74	1.00	1.00	
> 34	22	40	1.13 (0.587–2.177)	1.002 (0.474–2.118)	0.996
Employment					
Housewife	55	174	0.69 (0.425–1.113)	0.82 (0.464–1.448)	0.494
Government employee	40	87	1.00	1.00	
Private employee	47	123	0.83 (0.503–1.375)	0.91 (0.514–1.622)	0.756
Merchant	13	42	0.67 (0.326–1.391)	0.68 (0.304–1.513)	0.343
Others*	9	27	0.73 (0.312–1.683)	0.61 (0.229–1.627)	0.324
Average monthly family income					
< 3000 ETB	54	135	1.00	1.00	
3000–5999 ETB	63	210	0.75 (0.491–1.145)	0.83 (0.517–1.334)	0.442
> 6000 ETB	47	108	1.09 (0.683–1.733)	1.47 (0.831–2.598)	0.185
Gestational Period					
First trimester	21	71	0.67 (0.383–1.160)	0.61 (0.326–1.128)	0.114
Second trimester	64	204	0.71 (0.480–1.040)	0.63 (0.406–0.984)	0.042*
Third trimester	79	178	1.00	1.00	
Maternal Education					
Yes	115	374	0.50 (0.328–0.479)	1.08 (0.631–1.851)	0.777
No	49	79	1.00	1.00	
Education on self-medication					
Yes	56	282	0.31 (0.216–0.457)	0.36 (0.209–0.617)	< 0.001*
No	108	171	1.00	1.00	
Counseling					
Yes	69	272	0.48 (0.336–0.693)	1.28 (0.706–2.321)	0.416
No	95	181	1.00	1.00	
Previous medication					
Yes	121	175	4.47 (3.008–6.642)	4.20 (2.695–6.534)	< 0.001*
No	43	278	1.00	1.00	
Previous pregnancy- and delivery-related problems					
Yes	51	88	1.87 (1.249–2.805)	1.71 (1.06–2.76)	0.028*
No	113	365	1.00	1.00	
Knowledge					
Poor knowledge	96	194	1.00	1.00	
Good knowledge	68	259	0.53 (0.369–0.762)	0.64 (0.419–0.973)	0.037*

AOR adjusted odds ratio, *COR* crude odds ratio, *CI* confidence interval
*Statistically significant ($p < 0.05$)

".......... Dispensers may know the consequence of self-medication. But, I don't think they are well aware of its burden. Hence, they should be well oriented on the impact of self-medication during pregnancy" (SMP05).

Strategies, guidelines, and forms or charts

The respondents stated that there is no written strategy or guidelines, including charts that articulate self-medication practice during pregnancy. As claimed by the participants, there is no guidance on self-medication. However, there is a strategy about maternal and reproductive health including antenatal care programs. But, this strategy does not address self-medication practices and its interventions. One of the respondents elaborated it in that the strategy fails to address risks of self-medication practices. They stated that it looks either the problem is not so well known or there is lack of priority and attention to the matter among policy makers and program designers.

Another important finding was that the ANC follow-up records missed to include a section for documenting self-medication which would have reminded ANC service providers to receive history and counseled pregnant women on taking caution on self-medication. One of the respondents highlighted as follows:

"......... The client screening chart used in the health center is not designed to have spaces where ANC providers write their concern of self-medication history" (SMP06).

The findings indicated that most of the screening activities for self-medication has been triggered when the pregnant women explained that she was sick and treated for her ailments. There is no procedure to ask the mother about self-medication and no guidance documents about risk of self-medication. This hinders recording of self-medication history of pregnant women during her follow-up.

Education and counseling

The majority of the respondents reported that maternal education, including education on self-medication is expected to be given to the pregnant women. However, this has been done inconsistently. This is because the education and counseling packages focus on danger signs and symptoms of pregnancy. It does not include risk of self-medication practice as a program. This results in poor awareness of the pregnant women on risk of self-medication. If a pregnant woman found a medicine effective based on her previous medication history, she will use the medicine during the current pregnancy. This was augmented by one of the respondents as follows:

"...... Pregnant women may request a medicine from a pharmacy or drug shop based on the effectiveness of their previous treatment experiences. They confidently request for a medicine if they feel the symptom of a disease seems the same as before. This is due to the knowledge gap on risks of using medicines to the fetus as well as her health" (SMP04).

The limited education and counseling of the pregnant women on risk of self-medication depends on the awareness and in-service training of the ANC service providers and other health professionals. Some respondents agreed that there were trainings on maternal and child health components to health professionals but the concept of risk of self-medication was missed. They also echoed that most of the providers at the health centers are junior staff and are less experienced. This exacerbated the limited focus to risk of self-medication. One of the respondents alluded that:

"......... I have never taken a training on medicine use risks including risks of self-medication during pregnancy. I have also never encountered national guidance documents on risk of self-medication which I may look up in my practice" (SMP07).

The other issue raised by one of the respondents was about the need for standardized self-medication related guidance. This was highlighted as shown below:

"........National guidance documents on risk of self-medication are necessary to protect the health of the pregnant women and fetus. Moreover, continuous follow up and in-service trainings are important for the betterment of the ANC services and health of the pregnant women" (SMP06).

Discussion

The present study assessed self-medication practice and associated factors among pregnant women in government health centers in Addis Ababa, Ethiopia. This study found out that a considerable proportion of pregnant women practiced self-medication with at least one modern and/or herbal medicine during the current pregnancy without consultation of health professionals. These findings were almost similar compared to studies conducted in the Democratic Republic of Congo, Nigeria, and south west part of Ethiopia [6, 16, 29]. More than a quarter (26.6%) of pregnant women practiced self-medication during their current pregnancy. The prevalence of self-medication practice in our study was higher when compared to reports in Iran, Pakistan, and Brazil [34–36] and lower than reports in Peru, Portugal, the Netherlands, Brazil, and Iran [18, 34, 38–41]. The possible reasons for the difference might be due to differences in study methods, health care settings, and restriction policies of dispensing practices.

The reasons why pregnant women practiced self-medication were easy access to medicines from pharmacies or drug shops without prescription followed by time saving, long waiting time for provision of health services, feeling that illness was not serious, and self-medication is cheaper. The easy access to medicines without prescription might be due to inadequate regulatory enforcements of dispensing practices and the imbalance between medicine trade and professional ethical standards among dispensers. This is supported by the qualitative findings, which showed that there is a gap in regulatory enforcements and lack of attention and priorities of policy makers and program designers on the burden of self-medication risks. This finding was similar to other studies conducted in Peru, Europe (Western, Northern and Eastern), North and South America and Australia, the Democratic Republic of Congo, and Ethiopia [6, 16, 37, 38].

Analgesics, antibiotics, and anthelmintics were the most commonly used classes of medicine for self-medication by the pregnant women, whereas paracetamol and amoxicillin were the most frequently used modern medicines. Studies from the Democratic Republic of Congo and south west part of Ethiopia had reported similar findings [6, 16]. Mainly, those medicines were obtained from pharmacies or drug shops. The reason for antibiotic medicines dispensing without prescription might be due to the weak enforcement of regulation and less strict dispensing policies. This may result in increased treatment costs, adverse effects, and the emergence of antimicrobial resistance.

Left-over medicines are other sources of modern medicines for self-medication by the pregnant women. This was found to be consistent with a study done in Peru [38]. As left-over medicines might be expired, inadequate in dosage, or contraindicated during pregnancy, such kind of practice should be discouraged. Sharing of medications is another source of modern medicines which was similar to a study done in Bahirdar, Ethiopia [27]. This indicated that families and friends have an influence on self-medication. This might be due to poor awareness about risk of self-medication, risk of sharing, and using left-over medicines.

The most worrisome issue in our findings is that pregnant women used herbal medicines which may be risky for the fetus. For instance, *Zingiber officinale* is known for its abortifacient, emmenagogue, and mutagenic effects [27, 48]. The reasons for self-medication of herbal medicines were easily available herbal medicines, feeling that the illness was not serious, perception of herbal medicines is less risk than modern medicines, and time saving. This finding was supported by other studies in Nigeria and Sudan [29, 32]. Furthermore, the sources of the herbal medications reported by the pregnant women were homemade remedies and neighbors. This could be due to family influences and sharing as a socio-cultural support for using and suggesting herbal medicines.

The findings of this study revealed that gestational period was significantly associated with self-medication practice. This is similar to a study conducted in Southern Iran [14]. The odds of self-medication practice among women in their second trimester of pregnancy were 0.63 times the odds of those in their third trimester. This might be due to the fact that initial discomforts associated with new pregnancy and most symptoms of pregnancy-related illness are during the first stage of pregnancy. Moreover, pregnant women might be less careful in the last trimesters due to the assumptions of the maturity of the fetus.

Pregnant women who had a history of self-medication practice before the current pregnancy were about fourfold more likely to practice self-medication during the current pregnancy as compared to those who had not. This might be due to the presence of chronic diseases, previous exposure to medicines, pregnancy- and delivery-related problems, and poor awareness on risk of self-medications. Another possible reason could be that commonly used medicines outside pregnancy might create the impression that over-the-counter medicines are safe to use during pregnancy. This study was in congruence with studies done in Iran, the Democratic Republic of Congo, Nigeria, and Jimma, Ethiopia [6, 14, 16, 29].

Pregnant women who encountered pregnancy- and delivery-related problems before were nearly twice more likely to practice self-medication than those who did not encounter. The possible reasons might be because the previous experience in using medication to treat problems related to pregnancy and delivery adverse outcomes and considered the medicines used were safe. These findings are almost similar to studies conducted in the Democratic Republic of Congo [6].

Pregnant women who were not educated about self-medication consequences were more prone to self-medication practices. The odds of self-medication practice among pregnant women who were educated about self-medication consequences during pregnancy were 0.36 times the odds of those who were not educated. This was augmented by the qualitative findings. Pregnant women who did not attend their regular ANC follow-up and maternal education on the consequences of self-medication had practiced self-medication. Lack of awareness on potential risks of self-medication and a communication gap between pregnant women and health care providers might be the possible reasons. This was complemented with other studies conducted in India and Sudan [22, 32, 34].

Moreover, the odds of self-medication practice among pregnant women who had good knowledge about risk of self-medication practice were 0.64 times the odds of those who had poor knowledge. The possible reasons could be poor awareness on risk of self-medications during pregnancy and the pregnant women believed the advices of their families, relatives or friends. The study showed, for example, some pregnant women believed that self-medication during pregnancy saved lives of many unborn babies than harm; it is better for the fetus that the mother uses medicines by herself and get well than to have an untreated illness during pregnancy; self-medication during pregnancy do more good than harm; pregnant women should not consult health professionals before taking herbal medicines; and herbal medicines use during pregnancy are safer than modern medicines. This finding was comparable to other studies done in Saudi, Western India, and Sudan [22, 30, 32].

Self-medication practice is one of the most common public health concerns during pregnancy. Unless necessary care is provided by responsible health professionals, it may lead to high risk, including maternal and neonatal mortality and morbidity [3, 27, 29]. In this study, more than one third (40%) of the pregnant women had self-medicated with medicines from category C, D, and X which are thought to cause possible fetal harm and high risk to the fetus and women. This indicated that some pregnant women were potentially at higher risk. For instance, aspirin and ibuprofen cause premature closure of ductus arteriosus during the third trimester, miscarriage, cardiac malformation, fetal renal impairment, pulmonary hypertension, and delayed onset of labor and prolongation of bleeding time in mother; paracetamol, the commonest non-steroidal anti-inflammatory drugs (NSAIDs), may also cause a risk of attention deficit hyperactivity in babies and reduced implantation sites at any time of pregnancy. Antihelmentics such as albendazole, mebendazole, metronidazole, and tinidazole cause incidence of fetal mortality, fetotoxicity, embryotoxicity, and skeletal malformations.

Furthermore, the use of medroxyprogesterone causes teratogenicity, fetotoxicity, fetal malformation, low birth weight, and neonatal death, and the use of tetracycline causes permanent discoloration of teeth, enamel hyperplasia, and impaired fetal skeletal growth [11].

Pregnant women should not only be cautious about modern medicines during pregnancy, they should also be cautious about commonly used herbal medicines. Since those herbs are understudied specially in pregnancy and their compositions are not well known, some of them cause serious risks [49]. For example, *Ocimum lamiifolium* (basil) contains eugenol and estragol with anticonvulsant and sedative antispasmodic effects; *Allium sativum* (garlic) has uterine stimulant effect; and *Ruta chalepensis* (rue) contains furanocumarins and is embryo toxic causing implantation failure and abortion. *Lepidium sativum* (peppergrass) contains sodium benzylisothiocyanate which induced low fetal and placental weights [27, 29, 48, 50, 51].

Strengths and limitations
The strengths of the study were that the quantitative data were triangulated with qualitative findings. Furthermore, the study considered factors such as knowledge, education on self-medication, counseling, previous pregnancy- and delivery-related problems, and policy- and program-related matters such as screening mechanisms for self-medication practice and adequacy of regulatory enforcements. The study had some limitations as well. Recall bias among pregnant women due to the fact that they were expected to recall information from their past experiences might affect the study findings. The other limitation of the study was that pregnant women might be confused or embarrassed to report the use of medicines during data collection since the study was institutional. In addition, the study might had response bias among key informants.

Conclusions
A considerable proportion of pregnant women attending antenatal care in government health centers in Addis Ababa practiced self-medication with at least one modern and/or herbal medicines. Gestational period; previous medication use; education on self-medication; previous pregnancy- and delivery-related problems; and knowledge about risk of self-medication were significantly associated with self-medication practice during the current pregnancy.

There is lack of attention among policy makers and program designers on addressing the risk of self-medication. There were no guidelines and recommendations on self-medication during pregnancy that ANC providers can use and there was no screening mechanisms for history of medication. There was also weak regulation enforcement on medicine retail outlets as they were good sources of medicines for self-medication. In addition, the pregnant women have limited awareness on self-medication, and they believe the advices of their families and friends.

The ANC follow-up records do not trigger health care providers to write and follow histories of self-medication of the pregnant women. For this reason, necessary measures at all levels must be taken to reduce the risks of self-medication during pregnancy.

Therefore, it is important to aware the pregnant women with risks of self-medication and train health care providers on how to help pregnant women stay safe from self-medication. Moreover, concerted efforts need to be exerted to strengthen regulatory enforcements and routinely screen pregnant women. It is also important to formulate and/or revise maternal and child health including ANC program-related strategies, guidelines, and ANC charts or forms to address risk of self-medication practices.

We recommend further research to assess the consequences of self-medication practice on pregnancy outcomes and community-based studies to identify factors for self-medication practice.

Abbreviations
AAHB: Addis Ababa Health Bureau; ANC: Antenatal Care; ETB: Ethiopian Birr; SDG: Sustainable Development Goal; SPSS: Statistical Product and Service Solutions

Acknowledgements
The authors would like to thank the data collectors for their collaboration during the data collection. We would also like to thank study participants and Woinshet Tassew who played a great role in the coordination of the data collection process.

Funding
The authors received no funding for this work.

Authors' contributions
KG conceived the idea, designed the study, involved in the supervision of the data collection process, did the data entry and analysis, and finally write up the manuscript. SW approved the proposal with some revisions, participated in the data analysis, and reviewed the manuscript. Both authors approved the final manuscript and agreed to be accountable for all aspects of the work in ensuring that questions related to the accuracy or integrity of any part of the work are appropriately investigated and resolved.

Authors' information
KG is Senior Advisor in Ethiopian Food, Medicine and Healthcare Administration and Control Authority. KG has Bachelor Degree in pharmacy, Masters of Business Administration specialization in Leadership and Masters Degree in Public Health.
SW is an assistant professor of public health at GAMBY Medical College. SW has degree of Doctor of Medicine and International Masters Degree in Public Health.

Ethics approval and consent to participate
The study was approved by GAMBY College of Medical Sciences (GAMBY, IRERC, 2017) and Addis Ababa Health Bureau (Ref. No: AAHB/6191/227) research ethics review committees. Supportive letter was obtained from Addis Ababa Health Bureau. Furthermore, prior to data collection permission was obtained from all sub-cities of Addis Ababa, all health centers and organizations selected for this study. Written consent was taken from study participants and the key informants after telling the objective of the study. Participants were informed that participation is voluntary and they could withdraw from the study at any time. The privacy of participants was fully respected during data collection and personal identifiers were not used to ensure anonymity. Finally, the collected data and audio records as well as transcripts were kept in a safe place and were accessible only to the research team.

Competing interests
The authors declared that they have no competing interests.

Author details
[1]Ethiopian Food, Medicine and Healthcare Administration and Control Authority, Addis Ababa, Ethiopia. [2]GAMBY College of Medical Sciences, Addis Ababa, Ethiopia.

References
1. WHO, UNICEF, UNFPA, World Bank, UNPD. Trends in maternal mortality 1990–2015. Geneva: WHO; 2015.
2. Kuruvilla S, Schweitzer J, Bishai D, Chowdhury S, Caramani D, Frost L, et al. Success factors for reducing maternal and child mortality. Bull World Health Organ. 2014;92(7):533–44.
3. Adeusi S, Adekeye O, Ebere L. Predictors of maternal health as perceived by pregnant women in Eti-Osa, Lagos state, Nigeria. Journal of Education and Practice. 2014;5(18):125–31.
4. Ahmed S, Rawal L, Chowdhury S, Murray J, Arscott-Mills S, Jack S, et al. Cross-country analysis of strategies for achieving progress towards global goals for women's and children's health. Bulletin of the World Health Organ. 2016;94(5):351–61.
5. Asfaw F, Bekele M, Temam S, Kelel M. Drug utilization pattern during pregnancy in Nekemte referral hospital: a cross sectional study. International Journal of Scientific Reports. 2016;2(8):201–6.
6. Mbarambara P, Songa P, Wansubi L, Mututa P, Minga B, Bisangamo C. Self-medication practice among pregnant women attending antenatal care at health centers in Bukavu, Eastern DR Congo. Int J Innov Appl Stud. 2016; 16(1):38.
7. Gebreegziabher T, Berhe D, Gutema G, Kabtyimer B. Drug utilization pattern and potential teratogenesity risk among pregnant women; the case of ayder referral hospital. Tigray, Ethiopia. Int J Pharm Sci Res. 2012;3(5):1371.
8. Yang T, Walker M, Krewski D, Yang Q, Nimrod C, Garner P, et al. Maternal characteristics associated with pregnancy exposure to FDA category C, D, and X drugs in a Canadian population. Pharmacoepidemiol Drug Saf. 2008; 17(3):270–7.
9. Kennedy D. Classifying drugs in pregnancy. Aust Prescr. 2014;37:38–40.
10. Wondesen A, Satessa G, Gelaw B. Drug use pattern among pregnant women in Adama hospital medical college, South East Shewa, Ethiopia. International journal of pharma sciences. 2016;6(2):1426–35.
11. Drugs.com. FDA pregnancy categories: FDA pregnancy risk information: an update 2000–2017 [cited 2017 March 18]. Available from: https://www. drugs.com/pregnancy-categories.html.
12. World Health Organization. Role of pharmacists in self-care and self-medication [cited 2017 January 25]. Available from: http://apps.who.int/ medicinedocs/pdf/whozip32e/whozip32e.pdf.
13. Azami-Aghdash S, Mohseni M, Etemadi M, Royani S, Moosavi A, Nakhaee M. Prevalence and cause of self-medication in Iran: a systematic review and meta-analysis article. Iranian journal of public health. 2015;44(12):1580.
14. Afshary P, Mohammadi S, Najar S, Pajohideh Z, Tabesh H. Prevalence and causes of self-medication in pregnant women referring to health centers in southern of Iran. Int J Pharm Sci Res. 2015;6(2):612.
15. Mohamed Saleem T, Dilip C, Azeem A. Self-medication with over the counter drugs: a questionnaire based study. Pharm Lett. 2011;3(1):91–8.
16. Befekadu A, Dhekama N, Mohammed M. Self-medication and contributing factors among pregnant women attending antenatal care in Ethiopia: the case of Jimma University specialized hospital. Medicine Science. 2014;3:1.
17. Creanga A, Sabel J, Ko J, Wasserman C, Shapiro-Mendoza C, Taylor P, et al. Maternal drug use and its effect on neonates: a population-based study in Washington State. Obstet Gynecol. 2012;119(5):924–33.
18. Verstappen G, Smolders E, Munster J, Aarnoudse J, Hak E. Prevalence and predictors of over-the-counter medication use among pregnant women: a cross-sectional study in the Netherlands. BMC Public Health. 2013;13(1):185.
19. Adanikin A, Awoleke J. Antenatal drug consumption: the burden of self-medication in a developing world setting. Trop Dr. 2016;0(0):1–5.
20. Wacha J, Szijarto A. Probiotics and pregnancy. Orv Hetil. 2011;152(11):420–6.
21. Pogliani L, Falvella F, Cattaneo D, Pileri P, Moscatielio A, Cheli S, et al. Pharmacokinetics and pharmacogenetics of selective serotonin reuptake inhibtors (SSRIs) during pregnancy: an observational study. Ther Drug Monit. 2017;39(2):197–201.
22. Kureshee N, Dhande P. Awareness of mothers and doctors about drug utilization pattern for illnesses encountered during pregnancy. Journal of clinical and diagnostic research : JCDR. 2013;7(11):2470–4.
23. Stephansson O, Granath F, Svensson T, Haglund B, Ekbom A, Kieler H. Drug use during pregnancy in Sweden—assessed by the prescribed drug register and the medical birth register. Clinical epidemiology. 2011;3:43.
24. Irvine L, Flynn R, Libby G, Crombie I, Evans J. Drugs dispensed in primary care during pregnancy. Drug Saf. 2010;33(7):593–604.
25. Smolina K, Hanley G, Mintzes B, Oberlander T, Morgan S. Trends and determinants of prescription drug use during pregnancy and postpartum in British Columbia, 2002–2011: a population-based cohort study. PLoS One. 2015;10(5):e0128312.
26. Mohammed A, Ahmed J, Bushra A, Aljadhey H. Medications use among pregnant women in Ethiopia: a cross sectional study. Journal of Applied Pharmaceutical Science. 2013;3(4):116–23.
27. Abeje G, Admasie C, Wasie B. Factors associated with self medication practice among pregnant mothers attending antenatal care at governmental health centers in Bahir Dar city administration, Northwest Ethiopia, a cross sectional study. The Pan African medical journal. 2015;20:276.

28. Kulkarni P, Khan M, Chandrasekhar A. Self medication practices among urban slum dwellers in South Indian city. Int J Pharm Bio Sci. 2012;3(3):81–7.

29. Emmanuel A, Achema G, Afoi B, Maroof K. Self medication practice among pregnant women attending antenatal clinic in selected hospitals in Jos, Nigeria. Inter J Nurs Health Sci. 2014;1(6):55–9.

30. Zaki N, Albarraq A. Use, attitudes and knowledge of medications among pregnant women: a Saudi study. Saudi Pharmaceutical Journal. 2014;22(5): 419–28.

31. Nordeng H, Koren G, Einarson A. Pregnant women's beliefs about medications—a study among 866 Norwegian women. Ann Pharmacother. 2010;44(9):1478–84.

32. Ahmed S, Siraj N, Yousif M. Pregnant women's awareness and perception about medicines. Lat Am J Pharm. 2015;34(5):869–74.

33. Yusuff K, Omarusehe L. Determinants of self medication practices among pregnant women in Ibadan, Nigeria. Int J Clin Pharm. 2011;33(5):868.

34. Bohio R, Brohi Z, Bohio F. Utilization of over the counter medication among pregnant women; a cross-sectional study conducted at Isra University Hospital, Hyderabad. The Journal of the Pakistan Medical Association. 2016; 66(1):68–71.

35. Baghianimoghadam M. Attitude and practice of pregnant women regarding self-medication in Yazd, Iran. Archives of Iranian Medicine. 2013; 16(10):580.

36. Kassada D, Miasso A, Waidman M, Marcon S. Prevalence and factors associated with drug use in pregnant women assisted in primary care. Texto & Contexto-Enfermagem. 2015;24(3):713–21.

37. Lupattelli A, Spigset O, Twigg M, Zagorodnikova K, Mardby A, Moretti M, et al. Medication use in pregnancy: a cross-sectional, multinational web-based study. BMJ Open. 2014;4(2):e004365.

38. Miní E, Varas R, Vicuña Y, Levano M, Rojas L, Medina J, et al. Self-medication behavior among pregnant women user of the Instituto Nacional Materno Perinatal, Peru 2011. Revista Peruana de Medicina Experimental Salud Publica. 2012;29(2):212–7.

39. Rocha R, Bezerra S, Lima J, Costa F. Consumption of medications, alcohol and smoking in pregnancy and assessment of teratogenic risks. Revista Gaúcha de Enfermagem. 2013;34(2):37–45.

40. Brum L, Pereira P, Felicetti L, da Silveira R. Utilização de medicamentos por gestantes usuárias do Sistema Único de Saúde no município de Santa Rosa (RS, Brasil). Revista Ciência & Saúde Coletiva. 2011;16:5.

41. Shamsi M, Bayati A. A survey of the prevalence of self-medication and the factors affecting it in pregnant mothers referring to health centers in Arak city, 2009. Paris Journal of Medical Sciences. 2010;7(3):34–42.

42. Abasiubong F, Bassey E, Udobang J, Akinbami O, Udoh S, Idung A. Self-medication: potential risks and hazards among pregnant women in Uyo, Nigeria. Pan African Medical Journal. 2012;13:1.

43. Gebremedhin G, Gomathi P. Assessment of drug use and effect in pregnant women attending antenatal care in hospitals of Mekelle, Tigray, Ethiopia. Journal of Drug Delivery and Therapeutics. 2014;4(6):75–82.

44. Ministry of Health. Health sector transformation plan 2015/16–2019/20. Addis Ababa; 2015. p. 23–31.

45. Addis Ababa City Council. [cited 2017 12 February]. Available from: http://www.ethioembassy.org.uk/about_us/regional_states/addis_ababa_city_council.htm.

46. Ministry of Health. Health and health related indictors. Policy planning directorate. Addis Ababa, Ethiopia, 2016.

47. Baraka M, Steurbaut S, Coomans D, Dupont A. Ethnic differences in drug utilization pattern during pregnancy: a cross-sectional study. J Matern Fetal Neonatal Med. 2013;26(9):900–7.

48. Ernst E. Herbal medicinal products during pregnancy: are they safe? BJOG: An International Journal of Obstetrics and Gynaecology. 2002;109(3):227–35.

49. Black R, Hill D. Over-the-counter medications in pregnancy. Am Fam Physician. 2003;67(12):2517–24.

50. Kebede B, Gedif T, Getachew A. Assessment of drug use among pregnant women in Addis Ababa, Ethiopia. Pharmacoepidemiol Drug Saf. 2009;18(6):462–8.

51. Abebe D, Debella A, Urga K. Medicinal plants and other useful plants of Ethiopia. 2003.

10

Epidemiology of bronchiolitis: a description of emergency department visits and hospitalizations in Puerto Rico, 2010–2014

Andrea Rivera-Sepulveda[1,2]* and Enid J. Garcia-Rivera[2,3]

Abstract

Background: Little is known about the epidemiology of bronchiolitis as a clinical diagnosis and its impact on emergency department visits and hospitalizations in tropical and semitropical regions. We described the epidemiology of bronchiolitis emergency visits and hospitalizations, its temporal trend and geographic distribution in Puerto Rico between 2010 and 2014.

Methods: We performed a retrospective descriptive analysis of a representative sample of privately insured children with bronchiolitis from January 2010 to December 2014. Data was provided by the largest private health insurer in Puerto Rico and identified children < 24 months of age with bronchiolitis by *International Classification of Diseases, Ninth Revision* code 466, 466.11, and 466.19. Chi-square and one-way ANOVA compared sex, age, diagnosis, and severity across the years. Joinpoint Poisson regression analysis evaluated the temporal trend distribution of bronchiolitis hospitalizations per calendar year. A *P* value less than 0.05 was statistically significant.

Results: During the study period, the annual proportion of emergency department visits and hospitalizations due to bronchiolitis increased from 3 to 5%, and 26 to 38%, respectively. The annual incidence rate of hospitalizations was 3.2 per 1000 privately insured children < 24 months. Non-RSV bronchiolitis was the most frequent diagnosis (51%). Hospitalizations occurred year-round, but increased significantly from August through December. Most children hospitalized resided in the metropolitan San Juan (35%) and surrounding urban areas. Total hospital charges decreased from $3.78 to $3.74 million, with an average cost per hospitalization of $4320.12 (11.3% increase; *P* = 0.0015).

Conclusions: This is the first study that evaluates the epidemiological characteristics of bronchiolitis in a primarily Hispanic population, living in a tropical country, and using data from a privately insured population. We found a small but significant increase in proportion of emergency visits and hospitalizations. Temporal trend shows year-round hospitalizations with an earlier seasonal peak and longer duration, consistent with Puerto Rico's seasonal rainfall throughout the study period. Further studies are needed to elucidate whether this epidemiologic pattern can also be seen in publicly insured children and whether Hispanic ethnicity is a risk factor for increased hospitalizations or is related to health disparities in the US healthcare system.

Keywords: Bronchiolitis, Pediatric, Children, Epidemiology, Hospitalization, Puerto Rico, Respiratory syncytial virus, Trend

* Correspondence: rivera.andreav@gmail.com
[1]Division of Pediatric Emergency Medicine, Department of Pediatrics, Saint Louis University School of Medicine, 1402 S. Grand Boulevard – Glennon Hall, Room 2717, 63104 Saint Louis, MO, USA
[2]School of Health Professions, University of Puerto Rico Medical Sciences Campus, and School of Medicine, San Juan, Puerto Rico
Full list of author information is available at the end of the article

Background

Bronchiolitis constitutes an important public health burden in the pediatric population worldwide [1–4], as the leading cause of emergency department visits and hospitalizations in infants younger than 2 years of age [5]. In the USA, emergency department visits and hospitalizations due to bronchiolitis have increased steadily over the last 30 years [6, 7], incurring in over 150,000 emergency visits and hospitalizations annually, and exceeding $1.7 billion in combined charges [1, 5, 7, 8]. Clinical manifestations associated with disease severity are influenced by sex, age, previous bronchiolitis, co-morbidities, environmental exposure, and the host's immune response to the infection [9]. About 1 in 9 infants develop bronchiolitis in the first year of life, classifying it as a major cause of clinical morbidity and rising inpatient healthcare costs [10, 11]. This is influenced by the significant variation in the frequency and type of intervention [12, 13], as well as healthcare resource utilization [14] and disparities in the healthcare system [15].

Past studies on bronchiolitis hospitalizations have focused on those caused by the respiratory syncytial virus (RSV), the most common etiologic agent [16]. In temperate climates, late fall and winter epidemics of bronchiolitis are usually linked to RSV, with slight variability in seasonal onset and duration [2, 16–19]. In tropical and semitropical climates with warm temperatures and seasonal rainfall like Puerto Rico, RSV occurs throughout the year [20], usually with outbreaks during the rainy season [9, 19–21]. This suggests that RSV bronchiolitis has unique epidemiologic characteristics depending on geographic region and climate [9, 21, 22].

Little is known about the epidemiology of bronchiolitis as a clinical diagnosis, with disregard as to the etiologic agent, and its impact on emergency visits and hospitalizations in tropical and semitropical regions like Puerto Rico. Therefore, the objectives of this study are to (1) describe demographic characteristics of emergency department visits due to bronchiolitis, (2) describe demographic and clinical characteristics of patients hospitalized with bronchiolitis, (3) examine temporal trend distribution of bronchiolitis hospitalizations, and (4) describe geographic distribution of bronchiolitis hospitalizations in Puerto Rico.

Methods
Study design

This retrospective descriptive study analyzed secondary data provided by the largest private health insurer in Puerto Rico. During the study period, two thirds of the population was covered under public health insurance; approximately one third under private health insurance. The insurer under study served an estimated average of 680,139 participants per year from 2010 to 2014, over 50% of privately insured Puerto Ricans on a yearly basis.

Data source

The insurer provided two aggregated and de-identified data sets: (1) children under 24 months of age who visited an emergency department in Puerto Rico from January 1, 2010, to December 31, 2014; and (2) children under 24 months of age with a primary or secondary diagnosis for acute bronchiolitis upon hospitalization in Puerto Rico from January 1, 2010, to December 31, 2014. Due to insurer data extraction procedures and codification, the databases for the emergency department visits and hospitalizations were mutually exclusive and independently analyzed.

Identification of sample

The diagnosis of bronchiolitis was defined using the *International Classification of Diseases, Ninth Revision, Clinical Modification* (ICD-9-CM) codes for acute bronchitis and bronchiolitis (ICD-9-CM: 466), acute bronchiolitis due to RSV (ICD-9-CM: 466.11), and acute bronchiolitis due to other infectious organism (ICD-9-CM: 466.19). An emergency visit due to bronchiolitis was defined as any patient < 24 months evaluated at the emergency department with a discharge diagnosis of bronchiolitis based on the ICD-9-CM code. A hospitalization due to bronchiolitis was defined as any patient < 24 months admitted with a primary or secondary diagnosis of bronchiolitis upon hospitalization based on the ICD-9-CM code. Severe bronchiolitis was defined as a hospitalization that required admission to the Pediatric Intensive Care unit (PICU).

Study variables

Emergency department data included (1) total visits per year by age group (months) and sex, and (2) total visits due to bronchiolitis per year by age group (months) and sex. Hospitalization data included (1) total number of patients hospitalized per year by age group (months) and sex, (2) number of hospitalizations due to bronchiolitis per year, (3) number of cases by diagnosis (ICD-9-CM code), (4) number of hospitalizations per month of admission, (5) number of hospitalizations per unit (general versus intensive care), (6) mean length of stay per month, (7) hospital charges per day based on number of patients hospitalized per year, and (8) number of hospitalizations per health insurance region based on municipality of residence.

Daily precipitation (inches) was monitored and provided by the National Oceanic and Atmospheric Administration from the primary weather station at the San Juan International Airport [23]. Total hospital charges reflected the total facility fees reported for the aggregated hospitalizations per year. Cost information was obtained from the insurer's billing reports. The geographical distribution of bronchiolitis hospitalizations were aggregated into seven health regions based on the categories used by the insurer and the Puerto Rico Department of Health.

Outcome measures

The primary outcome measures were (1) annual proportion of emergency department visits due to bronchiolitis, (2) annual proportion and annual incidence rate of bronchiolitis hospitalizations, and (3) temporal trend distribution of bronchiolitis hospitalizations per calendar year. Other outcomes of interest included disease severity, hospital charges, and proportion of bronchiolitis hospitalizations by geographic region.

Statistical analysis

Data was analyzed using descriptive statistics, including frequency distribution and measures of association. Categorical variables were analyzed using frequency and percentages; continuous variables were analyzed using means and standard deviation. To estimate the burden of bronchiolitis in this population, we calculated the annual proportion of bronchiolitis emergency visits among total emergency visits per year by age group, and the annual proportion of bronchiolitis hospitalizations among total hospitalizations per year by age group. The denominator of sex and age group distribution for bronchiolitis hospitalizations differed from ICD-9-CM codes and hospital unit due to post-adjustment measures provided by the insurer for billing purposes that included multiple admissions incurred by a single patient, coding, billing, and claim processing. To estimate the annual incidence rate of bronchiolitis hospitalizations per 1000 insured participants by age group, we used the insurer's enrollment data from June 2014; taking into consideration an adjustment for the annual fluctuation in health insurance enrollment with a stable descent of 13% since 2012 to estimate the insured population per year. To estimate the burden of economic inflation and facilitate direct comparisons between years for hospital charges in Puerto Rico and the USA, we used the medical care component of the Consumer Price Index [24]. Chi-square was used to evaluate if there were differences between sex, age, diagnosis, and severity distribution over time. One-way ANOVA was used to evaluate if there were differences between hospital charges and length of stay across the years. Temporal trend distribution of bronchiolitis hospitalizations per calendar year was evaluated by Joinpoint Regression Program, Version 4.2.0.2 June 2015 (Statistical Methodology and Applications Branch, Surveillance Research Program, National Cancer Institute) [25]. Joinpoint Poisson regression analysis consists of a series of permutation tests that define points in

time when the trend changed significantly. The estimated annual percentage change is represented by the magnitude of change in slopes within the accumulated monthly proportion of bronchiolitis hospitalizations per year in the time trend, alongside its 95% confidence intervals. We evaluated the total bronchiolitis hospitalizations by the month of diagnosis for the period of 5 years. A descriptive analysis was performed to evaluate the association between total precipitation (inches) and total bronchiolitis hospitalizations per month and year; and the geographic distribution of bronchiolitis hospitalizations per health region. A P value less than 0.05 was established as statistically significant. Analyses used STATA version 11 (Stata Corporation, College Station, TX, USA).

This study was approved by the University of Puerto Rico, Medical Sciences Campus (IORG000223) Institutional Review Board.

Results

Emergency department visits due to bronchiolitis

A total of 48,886 emergency department visits of children < 2 years were identified from 2010 to 2014, of which 2281 (4.7%; SD 1%) were due to bronchiolitis (Table 1). During the study period, there was a significant difference in the annual proportion of bronchiolitis emergency visits ($P < 0.001$). Infants < 12 months of age represented 68% of all bronchiolitis emergency visits. Subgroup analyses showed that the 3.1- to 6-month age group was most frequently diagnosed with acute bronchiolitis (12%; SD 1.6%) and represented 21% (SD 2.5%) of all bronchiolitis emergency visits. During the study period, the annual proportion of bronchiolitis emergency visits among sexes ($P = 0.15$), and age groups ($P = 0.116$) were relatively constant.

Demographics and selected characteristics of hospitalized children with bronchiolitis

A total of 13,833 hospitalizations were reported from 2010 to 2014, of which 4986 were due to bronchiolitis; corresponding to 37% (SD 6%) of all hospitalizations for children < 24 months (Table 1). Although the total number of bronchiolitis hospitalizations decreased from 941 in 2010 to 791 in 2014, the annual proportion of bronchiolitis hospitalizations showed a small but significant increase during the study period ($P < 0.001$). Bronchiolitis hospitalizations were most frequent in males (59 versus 41%, $P = 0.019$) and children < 1 year of age (62%; SD 13%) (Table 2). Subgroup analyses showed that the 3.1- to 6-month age group had the highest percentage of bronchiolitis hospitalizations (20%; SD 9%) during the study period, after which the hospitalization percentage declined steadily by age group ($P < 0.001$). We estimated the annual incidence rate of bronchiolitis

Table 1 Distribution of emergency department visits and hospitalizations due to bronchiolitis, 2010–2014

	Years, n (%)					
	2010	2011	2012	2013	2014	P value
Emergency department visits						
Total	12,515	10,609	10,403	8549	6810	
Due to bronchiolitis	434 (3)	553 (5)	525 (5)	423 (5)	346 (5)	< 0.001
Sex[a]						
Male	223 (3)	316 (6)	296 (5)	247 (5)	206 (6)	0.15
Female	211 (4)	237 (5)	229 (5)	176 (5)	140 (5)	
Age distribution[b]						
0 to 3 months	44 (6)	35 (7)	51 (11)	28 (8)	28 (9)	0.116
3.1 to 6 months	96 (10)	137 (14)	101 (12)	84 (13)	67 (11)	
6.1 to 9 months	94 (6)	119 (9)	121 (9)	89 (9)	74 (9)	
9.1 to 12 months	83 (5)	89 (6)	86 (6)	76 (6)	50 (6)	
12.1 to 24 months	117 (2)	173 (3)	166 (3)	146 (3)	127 (3)	
Hospitalizations						
Total	3624	3052	2604	2467	2086	
Due to bronchiolitis	941 (26)	1209 (40)	1076 (41)	969 (39)	791 (38)	< 0.001

[a]Percentage is based on annual proportion of bronchiolitis emergency visits among total emergency visits per sex
[b]Percentage is based on annual proportion of bronchiolitis emergency visits among total emergency visits per age group in months

hospitalizations as 3.2 per 1000 privately insured children < 24 months of age.

Bronchiolitis-related diagnoses

There were 5050 hospitalizations with a diagnosis of acute bronchiolitis upon hospitalization (Table 2). We found a significant change in the distribution of hospitalizations for acute bronchitis and bronchiolitis (5.3%; SD 1%), acute bronchiolitis due to RSV (43.8%; SD 10%) and acute bronchiolitis due to other infectious organism (50.9%; SD 9%) during the study period. The proportion of hospitalizations attributed to RSV bronchiolitis increased from 27% in 2010 to 45% in 2014, while the proportion of hospitalizations due to non-RSV bronchiolitis remained the most frequent diagnosis during the study period.

Temporal distribution of bronchiolitis hospitalizations

Joinpoint regression analysis showed a significant increase in bronchiolitis hospitalizations as of August, with an increasing trend until December in the years 2010, 2013, and 2014 (Fig. 1). The year 2011 did not show any discernible trend, while 2012 showed a significant early increase in trend from April to October. Bronchiolitis hospitalizations occurred throughout the year, increasing in September through December, with 44% (SD 7%) of bronchiolitis hospitalizations occurring during this 4-month period. The years 2011 and 2012 had an earlier increase in bronchiolitis hospitalizations above the yearly mean hospitalization percentage, starting in July and ending in October, for a cumulative hospitalization proportion of 37% (SD 1%) and 52% (SD 3%), respectively, (Fig. 2). Temporal analysis between bronchiolitis hospitalizations and amount of rainfall did not show any discernible distribution. However, a pattern of heavy cumulative rainfall representing over half (55%) the total amount of precipitation per year (1.4 inches; SD 0.54 inches) was seen during May through September, before each hospitalization surge, and 58% (SD 4.8%) of bronchiolitis hospitalizations occurred as of July through December, the start of the rainy season in Puerto Rico. Official data from a single weather station for the years 2010–2014 show a mean annual rainfall of 2.47 inches (SD 0.54 inches).

Bronchiolitis severity

Of the 4986 children, 91% had a single hospitalization, 8% had two hospitalizations, and 1% had three or more (P < 0.001). The proportion of severe bronchiolitis hospitalizations (3% PICU hospitalization rate, P = 0.54) and the mean length of stay (4.8 days, P = 0.42) remained stable throughout the study period.

Healthcare costs

Between 2010 and 2014, the mean cost per day increased 11.3% from $851.93 to $948.16, with an average cost of $4,320.12 per hospitalization, adjusted for inflation (1.7% mean yearly increase; P = 0.0015). Total hospital charges per year for bronchiolitis hospitalizations decreased from $3.78 to $3.74 million (Table 2).

Table 2 Demographics and characteristics of bronchiolitis hospitalizations, 2010–2014

Characteristics	Years, n (%)					P value
	2010	2011	2012	2013	2014	
Demographics	(n = 941)	(n = 1209)	(n = 1076)	(n = 969)	(n = 791)	
Sex[a]						
Male	565 (32)	705 (41)	586 (42)	582 (42)	485 (40)	0.019
Female	376 (20)	504 (37)	490 (41)	387 (36)	306 (35)	
Age distribution[b]						
0 to 3 months	124 (14)	176 (41)	134 (40)	88 (34)	91 (39)	< 0.001
3.1 to 6 months	190 (44)	289 (58)	233 (59)	120 (39)	169 (55)	
6.1 to 9 months	183 (43)	225 (54)	213 (56)	93 (30)	125 (45)	
9.1 to 12 months	137 (34)	153 (40)	158 (46)	80 (29)	116 (42)	
12.1 to 24 months	307 (21)	366 (28)	338 (29)	588 (44)	290 (29)	
Cost per hospitalization						
Mean	$4016	$4313	$4269	$4277	$4725	0.0015
Standard deviation	$3215	$2812	$3606	$3794	$3128	
Cost per day (mean)	$852	$865	$851	$910	$948	
Total charges per year	$3,779,161	$5,214,823	$4,593,615	$4,144,186	$3,737,647	
Hospitalizations	(n = 924)	(n = 1219)	(n = 1140)	(n = 969)	(n = 798)	
ICD-9-CM Code						
466	61 (7)	52 (4)	55 (5)	64 (7)	38 (5)	< 0.001
466.11	254 (27)	603 (50)	601 (53)	391 (40)	363 (45)	< 0.001
466.19	609 (66)	564 (46)	484 (42)	514 (53)	397 (50)	
Hospital unit						
General Ward	900 (97)	1183 (97)	1105 (97)	949 (98)	772 (97)	0.54
PICU	24 (3)	36 (3)	35 (3)	20 (2)	26 (3)	
Length of stay						
Total days	4436	6028	5396	4553	3942	
Mean (SD)	4.8 (3.2)	4.9 (2.8)	4.7 (3.2)	4.7 (3.6)	4.9 (3.6)	0.42

ICD-9-CM international classification of disease, 9th revision clinical modification, 466 acute bronchitis and bronchiolitis, 466.11 acute bronchiolitis due to Respiratory Syncytial Virus; 466.19 acute bronchiolitis due to other infectious organism, PICU Pediatric Intensive Care Unit, SD standard deviation
[a]Percentage is based on annual proportion of bronchiolitis hospitalizations among total hospitalizations per sex
[b]Percentage is based on annual proportion of bronchiolitis hospitalizations among total hospitalizations per age group in months

Geographical distribution of bronchiolitis hospitalizations
For the purpose of this analysis, Puerto Rico was divided into seven health regions based on municipality of residence. Hospitalizations were most frequent in the San Juan metropolitan area (35%; SD 1%), followed by the urban area of Bayamón (24%; SD 2%).

Discussion
We identified emergency department visits and hospitalizations due to bronchiolitis within a representative sample of privately insured children < 2 years between 2010 and 2014. Our study shows an annual proportion of emergency visits due to bronchiolitis of 5% (SD 1%) and an annual proportion of bronchiolitis hospitalizations of 37% (SD 6%). We estimated an annual incidence rate of 3.2 bronchiolitis hospitalizations per 1000 privately

insured children < 2 years of age within the general population. Bronchiolitis hospitalizations occurred year-round, increasing significantly as of August through December, and taking place more frequently in the main Metropolitan area of Puerto Rico.

During the study period, we identified more than 2200 emergency visits by children with bronchiolitis. Our data shows a similar annual proportion of bronchiolitis emergency visits to other studies in the USA. A study by Hasegawa et al. [26] based on a US nationally representative sample of 1,435,110 emergency visits with bronchiolitis had a similar (4.3%) annual proportion of bronchiolitis visits among total emergency visits. However, a study by Carroll et al. [27] based on a retrospective cohort of 103,670 infants enrolled in Tennessee Medicaid, reported that during the first year of life, 6.2%

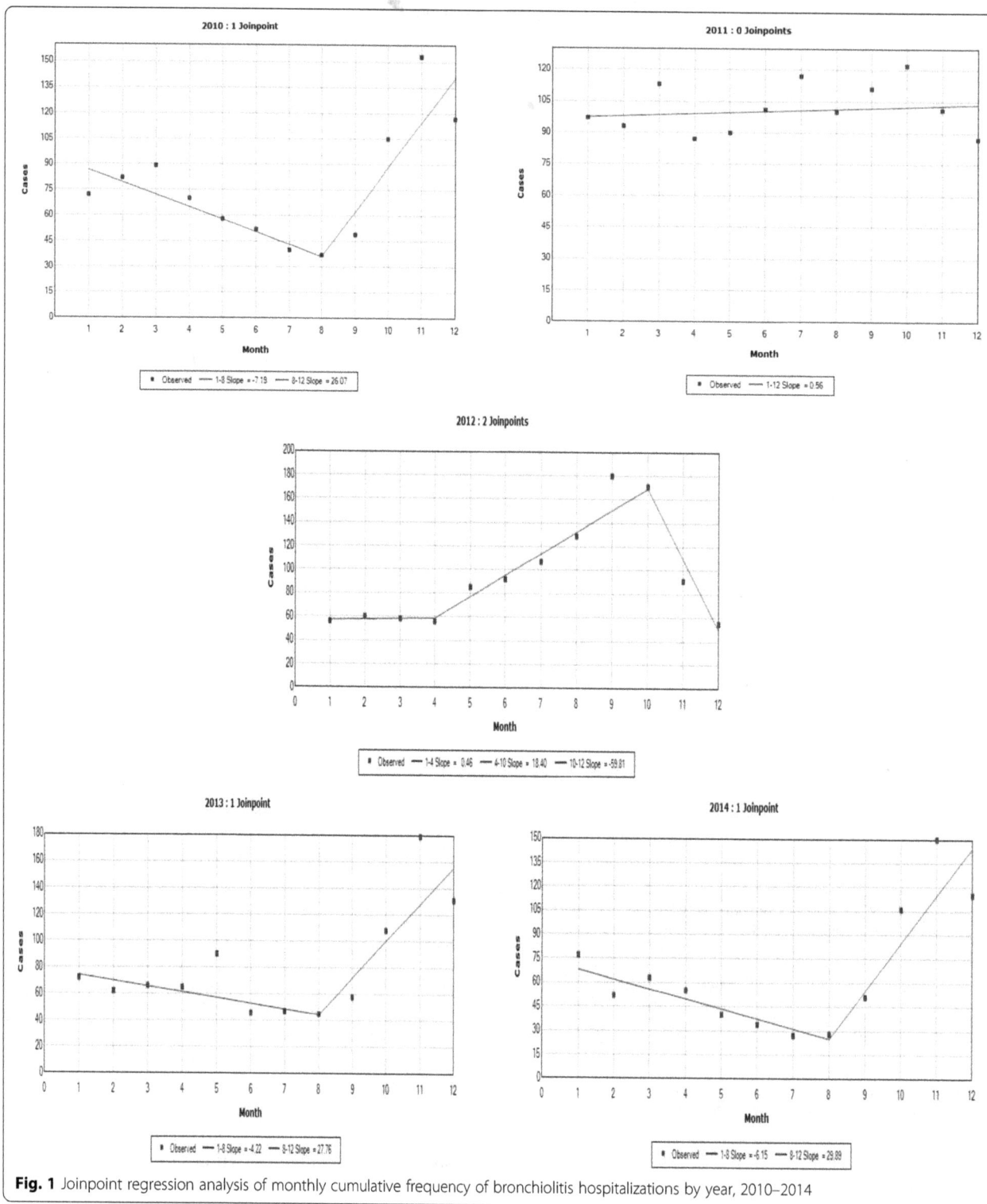

Fig. 1 Joinpoint regression analysis of monthly cumulative frequency of bronchiolitis hospitalizations by year, 2010–2014

of infants had an emergency visit due to bronchiolitis, with African-American and Latino infants being more likely to have such visits than white infants. The higher proportion of bronchiolitis emergency visits found in the Tennessee study may be explained by the inclusion of children under public insurance coverage, which is a risk

factor for increased bronchiolitis incidence and suggests a differential use of medical services [26, 27].

Previous studies have shown that in the USA, an increase in bronchiolitis hospitalizations was observed during the 1990s [6, 7] and early 2000s [2, 27], with a decrease in the mid-to-late 2000s in both the USA [1]

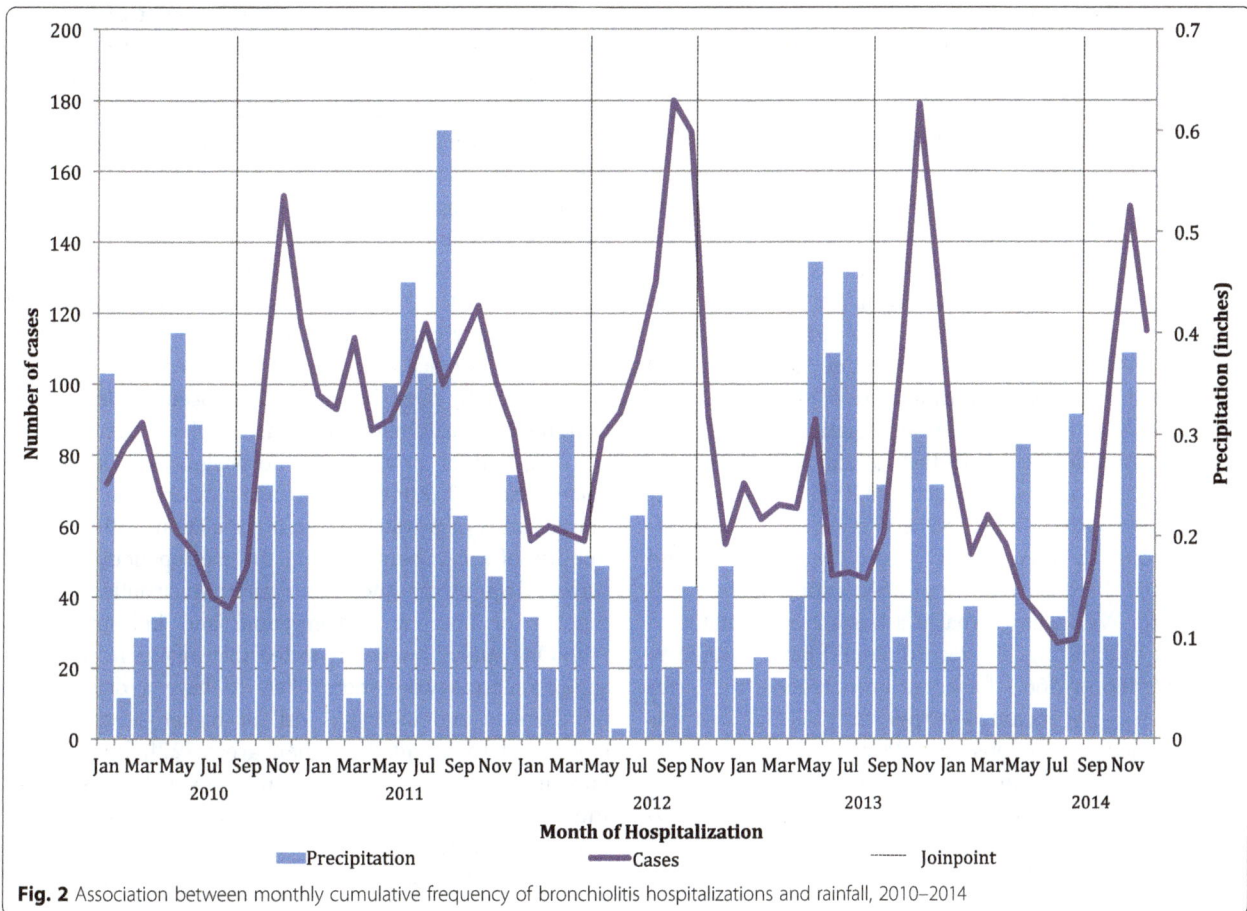

Fig. 2 Association between monthly cumulative frequency of bronchiolitis hospitalizations and rainfall, 2010–2014

and Spain [18]. Our study shows an annual proportion of bronchiolitis hospitalizations to be twice as high as that reported in a study by Hasegawa et al. (16%) [1]. Some studies, though not looking at incidence rate of hospitalizations due to bronchiolitis, have shown that Hispanic infants are twice as likely to be hospitalized for bronchiolitis than white infants [28, 29]. A study by Mansbach et al. [7], evaluating 1,868,000 emergency visits for children younger than 2 years of age, established that Hispanic ethnicity independently predicts both emergency visits and hospitalization. Another study of healthcare resource utilization among Latino infants in the USA showed that out of 674 previously healthy infants with acute respiratory illness, Latinos had lower thresholds for hospitalization than non-Hispanic whites and African Americans [14]. Authors suggested that this could be due to access to healthcare resources and language barriers. Our data shows that the annual proportion of bronchiolitis hospitalizations in Puerto Rico increased between 2010 and 2014, with a small but statistical significance. This however, does not equate to an increased incidence of bronchiolitis hospitalizations. This significant variation could be explained by a change seen from the year 2010 to 2011, when there was a 14% annual proportion increase

in bronchiolitis hospitalizations. Variations such as the one seen in our findings have been associated with changes in disease incidence and severity, as reported in a previous study [1]. Our study showed that the proportion of severe bronchiolitis remained constant throughout the study period and was similar to other studies [30–36]. Also, the highest annual proportion of bronchiolitis hospitalizations was consistent with the US peak bronchiolitis hospitalization, to be between 2 and 6 months of age [5, 6, 17, 32, 36–39]. This evidence suggests that age < 6 months may be a non-medical risk factor for bronchiolitis hospitalization in this population [9, 40].

During the study period, the proportion of RSV bronchiolitis hospitalizations varied significantly from 27 to 45%, with a 23% annual proportion increase from the year 2010 to 2011. One Canadian study reported the emergence of a new RSV variant, namely ON1 genotype (subgroup A), in late 2010 [41], associated with an altered immunogenicity and pathogenicity of the virus. Furthermore, after gradually spreading worldwide, one study described that the emergence of ON1 genotype was associated with an increased lower respiratory tract infection incidence and severity [42]. Although we lack information on the RSV genotype within our study population, the emergence of this new RSV variant in the current study site may also be important in the increase of RSV-attributed bronchiolitis hospitalizations. Overall, non-RSV bronchiolitis was more frequently diagnosed than RSV bronchiolitis, with the exception of 2011 and 2012. This finding is consistent with the RSV surveillance data provided by the Puerto Rico Department of Health [43], who reported that in 2011 and 2012, positive RSV tests doubled. This is different from studies in temperate areas, where it has been reported that RSV accounts for 50–80% of yearly bronchiolitis cases [39, 44, 45]. This may also be due to variations in codification processes and availability of diagnostic analyses such as antigen testing, virus isolation, and/or polymerase chain reaction (PCR) tests at admitting hospitals. Because laboratory confirmation for RSV is widely available in Puerto Rico, the ICD-9-CM code for acute bronchiolitis due to RSV (466.11) is only attributed and billed when there is evidence of RSV testing in the medical record. We assumed that if a hospital was unable to carry out this testing, the record should have an ICD-9-CM code 466 or 466.1 for acute bronchiolitis; the latter of which was not included in this study, as the data was not provided by the insurer. Because the ICD-9-CM code 466 represents an average of 5% of cases per year, we performed a secondary analysis between the ICD-9-CM codes 466.11 and 466.19, excluding 466, which did not change the significance of the distribution of diagnoses from 2010 to 2014.

Joinpoint regression analysis from 2010 to 2014 showed bronchiolitis hospitalizations year-round, with an increase during September through December. During the years 2011 and 2012, there was an increase in bronchiolitis hospitalizations from July through October, consistent with the reported RSV epidemic [43]. This was also consistent with the findings of the National Surveillance System that included the RSVAlert® program and the National Respiratory and Enteric Virus Surveillance System who determined that in Puerto Rico, RSV activity is perennial and lacks a discernible seasonal pattern [46], with an increased activity in RSV usually seen from September through December [47]. This seasonal trend is most closely related to the US Department of Health and Human Services (HHS) Region of Florida, which presents an earlier RSV season onset and longer duration than the rest of the USA [16]. The pattern of bronchiolitis hospitalizations suggests an association with Puerto Rico's seasonal rainfall (Fig. 2) [23], but we were not able to establish a statistical relationship. This may be because we are evaluating the relationship between a limited set of climate indicators and bronchiolitis as a clinical diagnosis and not as the result of an etiologic agent. Because a causative agent can be transmitted in different ways according to their atmospheric circumstance, thereby affecting the behavior of these infectious particles [48], it becomes important to elucidate the interaction between other environmental components and the transmission of the disease.

The decrease in total hospital charges during the study period is associated with a decrease in bronchiolitis hospitalizations and total hospital days. The cost of bronchiolitis hospitalizations were on average over 50% higher than the US $2815 geometric mean, reported by Hasegawa et al. [1] in 2009. The reason for this marked difference may be associated to hospital mean length of stay, which is twice as high in Puerto Rico.

In our study, most hospitalizations occurred in patients from the two main metropolitan areas, which together make up over half of bronchiolitis hospitalizations during the study period. This finding most likely reflects the socioeconomic status of privately insured population, with a higher number of subscribers living in the metropolitan area and surrounding urban and suburban municipalities, greater number of hospitals, urbanization, and industrialization [49]. One study however, reported that infants in rural and suburban areas were more likely to have a diagnosis of bronchiolitis and increased risk of higher severity when compared to infants in urban areas [27]. Because we lack information about the insurer's subscribers per municipality, month or year, we were unable to calculate the annual proportion of bronchiolitis hospitalizations by geographic region.

Limitations

There are several limitations of this study that should be considered. We used a database of admission-data level based on ICD-9-CM codification for which we might have overestimated bronchiolitis episodes by including early asthma and bronchitis or underestimated the frequency of bronchiolitis hospitalizations by not including misdiagnosed cases or those that developed bronchiolitis after hospitalization. This is an observational study based on aggregated and stratified data obtained for billing purposes. Changes in enrollment or discontinuation of private healthcare coverage by the insurer, as well as discrepancies in diagnostic-coding by physicians, hospitals, and post-adjustment measures for billing purposes could explain variations in bronchiolitis hospitalizations throughout the study period. The lack of individual patient characteristics and clinical information prevents us from determining and comparing annual incidence of bronchiolitis hospitalizations and its relationship with other risk factors and outcomes of interest, such as sociodemographic status, age-specific diagnosis, repeat hospitalization and PICU hospitalization, temporal distribution of bronchiolitis based on ICD-9-CM code, and presence of comorbidities. Furthermore, we lacked information about the ethnicity of children included in the study but note that the study is based in a tropical country with a primarily Hispanic population. However, a small portion of children of non-Hispanic ethnicity might have been included in the study. The codification of the etiology within this study did not specify the method by which RSV laboratory testing was confirmed. Because there are differences in sensitivity and specificity for RSV testing, we may have over- or under-reported RSV hospitalizations. However, increases seen in the proportion of RSV hospitalizations were consistent with RSV outbreaks reported by the Puerto Rico Department of Health. We also lack information about influenza outbreaks, which could have affected the proportion of non-RSV bronchiolitis cases that were hospitalized. Because the insurer's data on emergency visits and hospitalizations were mutually exclusive and analyzed separately, we cannot determine hospitalization rate after an emergency visit for bronchiolitis. Lastly, the study only included data from the private insurer. Procuring and including a representative sample that includes children covered by public health insurance or other insurance companies could strengthen future studies.

Strengths

This is the first study to evaluate the epidemiological features of bronchiolitis in Puerto Rico by using representative data of a privately insured population between 2010 and 2014 from the largest insurer in Puerto Rico. This allowed us to determine population-based emergency department visits and hospitalization distributions due to bronchiolitis with decreased health disparities in comparison to public health insurance holders. November and December 2014 were the only months to overlap with the publication of the updated bronchiolitis management guidelines by the American Academy of Pediatrics, which allowed us to evaluate epidemiologic distributions without influence to providers' decisions in hospitalizing children with bronchiolitis.

Conclusions

Between 2010 and 2014, we found that the proportion of emergency department visits due to bronchiolitis is similar to that reported in the USA, while bronchiolitis hospitalizations among children in Puerto Rico was found to be twice as high. Further studies are needed to elucidate whether Hispanic ethnicity is a risk factor for increased frequency of hospitalization or is related to health disparities in the US healthcare system. Temporal trend shows year-round hospitalizations with an earlier seasonal peak and longer duration, consistent with Puerto Rico's seasonal rainfall. This locally acquired data establishes the seasonality of bronchiolitis in Puerto Rico according to our epidemiology and helps us better define the pediatric population that has greater susceptibility so that interventions and prevention tools may be developed

to prevent and control transmission of this disease in the tropical environment of Puerto Rico. Further studies are needed to elucidate whether this epidemiologic pattern can also be seen in publicly insured children and whether Hispanic ethnicity is a risk factor for increased hospitalizations or is related to health disparities in the US healthcare system.

Abbreviations

RSV: Respiratory syncytial virus

Acknowledgements

Research reported is supported in part by the National Center on Minority Health and Health Disparities (NCMHD) of the National Institutes of Health (NIH) award number R25MD007607 and the University of Puerto Rico School of Medicine Endowed Health Services Research Center, award numbers 5S21MD000242 and 5S21MD000138. The content is solely the responsibility of the authors and does not necessarily represent the official views of the NCMHD or NIH.

Funding

The authors received no specific funding for this work.

Authors' contributions

Dr. RS conceptualized and designed the study, acquired, and interpreted data. Dr. GR made substantial contributions to conception and design, analysis, and interpretation of data. Both authors were involved in drafting, critically revising, and providing final approval of the manuscript.

Competing interests

The authors declare that they have no competing interests.

Author details

[1]Division of Pediatric Emergency Medicine, Department of Pediatrics, Saint Louis University School of Medicine, 1402 S. Grand Boulevard – Glennon Hall, Room 2717, 63104 Saint Louis, MO, USA. [2]School of Health Professions, University of Puerto Rico Medical Sciences Campus, and School of Medicine, San Juan, Puerto Rico. [3]Endowed Health Services, University of Puerto Rico School of Medicine, Medical Sciences Campus, San Juan, Puerto Rico.

References

1. Hasegawa K, Tsugawa Y, Brown D, Mansbach J, Camargo C. Trends in bronchiolitis hospitalizations in the United States, 2000–2009. Pediatrics. 2013;132(1):28–36.

2. Garcia C, Bhore R, Soriano-Fallas A, Trost M, Chason R, Ramilo O, et al. Risk factors in children hospitalized with RSV bronchiolitis versus non-RSV bronchiolitis. Pediatrics. 2010;126(6):e1453–60.

3. Stensballe L, Brunbjerg Simonsen J, Thomsen S, Hellesøe Larsen A, Hovmand Lysdal S, Aaby P, et al. The causal direction in the association between respiratory syncytial virus hospitalization and asthma. J Allergy Clin Immunol. 2009;123(1):131–7. e1

4. Hall C, Weinberg G, Iwane M, Blumkin A, Edwards K, Staat M, et al. The burden of respiratory syncytial virus infection in young children. N Engl J Med. 2009;360(6):588–98.

5. Corneli H, Zorc J, Holubkov R, Bregstein J, Brown K, Mahajan P, et al. Bronchiolitis. Pediatr Emerg Care. 2012;28(2):99–103.

6. Shay D. Bronchiolitis-associated hospitalizations among US children, 1980–1996. JAMA. 1999;282(15):1440–6.

7. Mansbach J, Emond J, Camargo C. Bronchiolitis in US emergency departments 1992 to 2000. Pediatr Emerg Care. 2005;21(4):242–7.

8. Pelletier A, Mansbach J, Camargo C. Direct medical costs of bronchiolitis hospitalizations in the United States. Pediatrics. 2006;118(6):2418–23.

9. Piedimonte G, Perez M. Respiratory syncytial virus infection and bronchiolitis. Pediatr Rev. 2014;35(12):519–30.

10. Viswanathan M, King V, Bordley C, Honeycutt A, Wittenborn J, Jackman A et al. Management of bronchiolitis in infants and children: summary. Rockville (MD): Agency for Healthcare Research and Quality (US); 2003 p. 1–5.

11. Joseph M. Evidence-based assessment and management of acute bronchiolitis in the emergency department. Pediatric Emerg Dep Pract. 2011;8(3):1–19.

12. Willson D, Horn S, Hendley J, Smout R, Gassaway J. Effect of practice variation on resource utilization in infants hospitalized for viral lower respiratory illness. Pediatrics. 2001;108(4):851–5.

13. Knapp J, Simon S, Sharma V. Variation and trends in ED use of radiographs for asthma, bronchiolitis, and croup in children. Pediatrics. 2013;132(2):245–52.

14. Valet R, Gebretsadik T, Carroll K, Minton P, Woodward K, Liu Z, et al. Increased healthcare resource utilization for acute respiratory illness among Latino infants. J Pediatr. 2013;163(4):1186–91.

15. Iwane M, Chaves S, Szilagyi P, Edwards K, Hall C, Staat M, et al. Disparities between black and white children in hospitalizations associated with acute respiratory illness and laboratory-confirmed influenza and respiratory syncytial virus in 3 US counties—2002–2009. Am J Epidemiol. 2013;177(7):656–65.

16. Center for Disease Control and Prevention. NREVSS|RSV National Trends|CDC[Internet]. Cdc.gov. 2015 [cited 17 May 2015]. Available from: http://www.cdc.gov/surveillance/nrevss/rsv/natl-trend.html

17. Ralston S, Lieberthal A, Meissner H, Alverson B, Baley J, Gadomski A, et al. Clinical practice guideline: the diagnosis, management, and prevention of bronchiolitis. Pediatrics. 2014;134(5):e1474–502.

18. Hervás D, Reina J, Yañez A, Valle J, Figuerola J, Hervás J. Epidemiology of hospitalization for acute bronchiolitis in children: differences between RSV and non-RSV bronchiolitis. Eur J Clin Microbiol Infect Dis. 2012;31(8):1975–81.

19. Weber M, Mulholland E, Greenwood B. Respiratory syncytial virus infection in tropical and developing countries. Tropical Med Int Health. 1998;3(4):268–80.

20. Molinari-Such M, García I, García L, Puig G, Pedraza L, Marín J, et al. Respiratory syncytial virus-related bronchiolitis in Puerto Rico. P R Health Sci J. 2009;24(2):137–40.

21. Rodríguez D, Rodríguez-Martínez C, Cárdenas A, Quilaguy I, Mayorga L, Falla L, et al. Predictors of severity and mortality in children hospitalized with respiratory syncytial virus infection in a tropical region. Pediatr Pulmonol. 2013;49(3):269–76.

22. Mullins J, Lamonte A, Bresee J, Anderson L. Substantial variability in community respiratory syncytial virus season timing. Pediatr Infect Dis J. 2003;22(10):857–63.

23. National Oceanic and Atmospheric Administration. Datasets|Climate Data Online (CDO)|National Climatic Data Center (NCDC) [Internet]. Ncdc.noaa. gov. 2015 [cited 15 March 2015]. Available from: http://www.ncdc.noaa.gov/cdo-web/datasets.

24. US Department of Labor, Bureau of Labor Statistics. Consumer Price Index (CPI) [Internet]. Bls.gov. 2015 [cited 10 June 2015]. Available from: http://www.bls.gov/cpi/home.htm

25. Kim H, Fay M, Feuer E, Midthune D. Permutation tests for joinpoint regression with applications to cancer rates. Stat Med. 2000;19(3):335–51. correction: 2001;20:655

26. Hasegawa K, Tsugawa Y, Brown D, Mansbach J, Camargo C. Temporal trends in emergency department visits for bronchiolitis in the United States, 2006 to 2010. Pediatr Infect Dis J. 2014;33(1):11–8.

27. Carroll K, Gebretsadik T, Griffin M, Wu P, Dupont W, Mitchel E, et al. Increasing burden and risk factors for bronchiolitis-related medical visits in infants enrolled in a state health care insurance plan. Pediatrics. 2008;122(1):58–64.

28. McConnochie K. Parental smoking, presence of older siblings, and family history of asthma increase risk of bronchiolitis. Arch Pediatr Adolesc Med. 1986;140(8):806–12.

29. Simoes E, King S, Lehr M, Groothuis J. Preterm twins and triplets: a high-risk group for severe respiratory syncytial virus infection. Am J Dis Child. 1993; 147(3):303–6.

30. Tsolia M, Kafetzis D, Danelatou K, Astra H, Kallergi K, Spyridis P, et al. Epidemiology of respiratory syncytial virus bronchiolitis in hospitalized infants in Greece. Eur J Epidemiol. 2002;18(1):55–61.

31. Díez-Domingo J, Pérez-Yarza E, Melero J, Sánchez-Luna M, Aguilar M, Blasco A, et al. Social, economic, and health impact of the respiratory syncytial virus: a systematic search. BMC Infect Dis. 2014;14(1):544.

32. Green C, Yeates D, Goldacre A, Sande C, Parslow R, McShane P et al. Admission to hospital for bronchiolitis in England: trends over five decades, geographical variation and association with perinatal characteristics and subsequent asthma. Arch Dis Child. 2015;: archdischild-2015-308723.

33. Mansbach J, Piedra P, Teach S, Sullivan A, Forgey T, Clark S, et al. Prospective multicenter study of viral etiology and hospital length of stay in children with severe bronchiolitis. Arch Pediatr Adolesc Med. 2012;166(8):700–6.

34. Zamora-Flores D, Busen N, Smout R, Velasquez O. Implementing a clinical practice guideline for the treatment of bronchiolitis in a high-risk Hispanic pediatric population. J Pediatr Health Care. 2015;29(2):169–80.

35. Calvo C, Pozo F, García-García M, Sanchez M, Lopez-Valero M, Pérez-Breña P, et al. Detection of new respiratory viruses in hospitalized infants with bronchiolitis: a three-year prospective study. Acta Paediatr. 2010;99(6):883–7.

36. Gil-Prieto R, Gonzalez-Escalada A, Marín-García P, Gallardo-Pino C, Gil-de-Miguel A. Respiratory syncytial virus bronchiolitis in children up to 5 years of age in Spain. Medicine. 2015;94(21):e831.

37. Colón Blanco Z, Colón Rivera C, Matos González M, Pérez Valentín B, Rivera Fernández R, Santiago Méndez I, et al. Epidemiologic descriptive study of the clinical characteristics of acute bronchiolitis in patients hospitalized at the pediatric unit of the Manatí Medical Center Hospital. Bol Asoc Med PR. 2014;106(2):4–8.

38. Johnson L, Robles J, Hudgins A, Osburn S, Martin D, Thompson A. Management of bronchiolitis in the emergency department: impact of evidence-based guidelines? Pediatrics. 2013;131(Supplement):S103–9.

39. Zorc J, Hall C. Bronchiolitis: recent evidence on diagnosis and management. Pediatrics. 2010;125(2):342–9.

40. Simoes E. Environmental and demographic risk factors for respiratory syncytial virus lower respiratory tract disease. J Pediatr. 2003;143(5):118–26.

41. Eshaghi A, Duvvuri V, Lai R, Nadarajah J, Li A, Patel S, et al. Genetic variability of human respiratory syncytial virus a strains circulating in Ontario: a novel genotype with a 72 nucleotide G gene duplication. PLoS One. 2012;7(3):e32807.

42. Yoshihara K, Le M, Okamoto M, Wadagni A, Nguyen H, Toizumi M, et al. Association of RSV-A ON1 genotype with increased pediatric acute lower respiratory tract infection in Vietnam. Sci Rep. 2016;6(1):27856.

43. Puerto Rico Department of Health. Estadísticas Virus Respiratorio Sincitial (RSV). Período 2003–2012; 2016 p. 1.

44. Miller E, Gebretsadik T, Carroll K, Dupont W, Mohamed Y, Morin L, et al. Viral etiologies of infant bronchiolitis, croup and upper respiratory illness during 4 consecutive years. Pediatr Infect Dis J. 2013;32(9):950–5.

45. Omer S, Sutanto A, Sarwo H, Linehan M, Djelantik I, Mercer D, et al. Climatic, temporal, and geographic characteristics of respiratory syncytial virus disease in a tropical island population. Epidemiol Infect. 2008;136(10):1319–27.

46. McGuiness C, Boron M, Saunders B, Edelman L, Kumar V, Rabon-Stith K. Respiratory syncytial virus surveillance in the United States, 2007–2012. Pediatr Infect Dis J. 2014;33(6):589–94.

47. Matías I, García I, García-Fragoso L, Puig G, Pedraza L, Rodríguez L, et al. Trends of respiratory syncytial virus infections in children under 2 years of age in Puerto Rico. P R Health Sci J. 2016;34(2):98–101.

48. Fernstrom A, Goldblatt M. Aerobiology and its role in the transmission of infectious diseases. J Pathogens. 2013;2013:1–13.

49. Simoes E, Carbonell-Estrany X. Impact of severe disease caused by respiratory syncytial virus in children living in developed countries. Pediatr Infect Dis J. 2003;22(Supplement):S13–20.

11

Malaria impact of large dams at different eco-epidemiological settings in Ethiopia

Solomon Kibret[1,4]* , G. Glenn Wilson[1], Darren Ryder[1], Habte Tekie[2] and Beyene Petros[3]

Abstract

Background: Dams are important to ensure food security and promote economic development in sub-Saharan Africa. However, a poor understanding of the negative public health consequences from issues such as malaria could affect their intended advantages. This study aims to compare the malaria situation across elevation and proximity to dams. Such information may contribute to better understand how dams affect malaria in different eco-epidemiological settings.

Methods: Larval and adult mosquitoes were collected from dam and non-dam villages around the Kesem (lowland), Koka (midland), and Koga (highland) dams in Ethiopia between October 2013 and July 2014. Determination of blood meal sources and detection of *Plasmodium falciparum* sporozoites was done using enzyme-linked immunosorbent assay (ELISA). Five years of monthly malaria case data (2010–2014) were also collected from health centers in the study villages.

Results: Mean monthly malaria incidence was two- and ten-fold higher in the lowland dam village than in midland and highland dam villages, respectively. The total surface area of anopheline breeding habitats and the mean larval density was significantly higher in the lowland dam village compared with the midland and highland dam villages. Similarly, the mean monthly malaria incidence and anopheline larval density was generally higher in the dam villages than in the non-dam villages in all the three dam settings. *Anopheles arabiensis*, *Anopheles pharoensis*, and *Anopheles funestus s.l.* were the most common species, largely collected from lowland and midland dam villages. Larvae of these species were mainly found in reservoir shoreline puddles and irrigation canals. The mean adult anopheline density was significantly higher in the lowland dam village than in the midland and highland dam villages. The annual entomological inoculation rate (EIR) of *An. arabiensis*, *An. funestus s.l.*, and *An. pharoensis* in the lowland dam village was 129.8, 47.8, and 33.3 infective bites per person per annum, respectively. The annual EIR of *An. arabiensis* and *An. pharoensis* was 6.3 and 3.2 times higher in the lowland dam village than in the midland dam village.

Conclusions: This study found that the presence of dams intensifies malaria transmission in lowland and midland ecological settings. Dam and irrigation management practices that could reduce vector abundance and malaria transmission need to be developed for these regions.

Keywords: Malaria, Mosquito breeding, *An. arabiensis*, *An. pharoensis*, *An. funestus*, Water management, Dams, Irrigation, Africa

* Correspondence: s.kibret@gmail.com
[1]Ecosystem Management, School of Environmental and Rural Science, University of New England, Armidale, NSW 2351, Australia
[4]Present address: Program in Public Health, University of California, Irvine, CA 92697, USA
Full list of author information is available at the end of the article

Background

The sub-Saharan Africa region is ranked lowest in the world for average water withdrawal [1], suggesting the pressing need for targeted development of water resource infrastructure. New water storages are currently being extensively developed to help improve the region's food security and promote sustainable economic development [2, 3]. However, the link between dams and malaria has been widely recognized as a public health challenge [4–6] which could hamper the intended advantages provided by these water infrastructures.

Ninety percent of the global malaria burden occurs in sub-Saharan Africa, resulting in transmission and disease management being a leading public health challenge [7]. With the current high level of dam construction in the region [8], links between the spatial distribution of dams in the landscape and malaria outcomes must be better understood for an assessment of any potential negative public health outcomes from dam development. Previous studies have indicated that dams increase malaria by providing breeding sites for malaria-transmitting mosquitoes in areas with unstable/seasonal malaria [9–19]. For example, a study around the Akosombo Dam in Ghana documented a 20% increase in malaria incidence in populations within a 3-km radius of the reservoir compared with those residing more than 7 km from the reservoir [17]. The occurrence and persistence of shallow shoreline puddles around the edge of the reservoir providing breeding habitats for the primary malaria vector species, *Anopheles gambiae*, were indicated to underpin the increased malaria incidence [20].

A number of environmental factors determine the degree of intensity of malaria transmission in Africa. Elevation has long been known for its effect on malaria transmission, mainly due to its influence on ecological and climatic drivers. A study in Tanzania found that malaria prevalence decreases by 21% in every 100 m increase in elevation [21]. Higher temperatures and other ecological characteristics associated with lower altitudes have been indicated to support higher rates of malaria transmission in the lowlands than in the highlands, which are considered as epidemic-prone.

Although dams can increase malaria in unstable areas (i.e., areas with seasonal malaria), it is not clear whether the impact of dams on malaria varies in different ecological settings. As Africa is experiencing a new era of dam building, with numerous dams planned or currently under construction [5], understanding the link between dams and malaria transmission across different eco-epidemiological settings is crucial in order to devise malaria control strategies and enable appropriate allocation of limited resources for intervention around water resources development schemes.

The present study assessed the link between three dams and malaria at different eco-epidemiological settings in Ethiopia. The objective of this study was to identify mosquito breeding sites and compare adult and larval abundances around three dams in highland, midland, and lowland settings of Ethiopia. This study aims to compare the malaria situation across elevations and proximity to dams. Such information may contribute to better understand how dams affect malaria in different eco-epidemiological settings.

Methods
Study area

This study was carried out around three dams in Ethiopia (Fig. 1): Kessem Dam (912 m above sea level (asl)), Koka Dam (1551 m asl), and Koga Dam (1,950 m asl). One village located within 5 km from the reservoir shorelines and another located farther away (>5 km) but not in downstream direction were selected for this study at each dam site. Generally, villages >5 km downstream of the dam were excluded as they are affected by water releases from the dam.

Kesem Dam (9°13′60′′ N, 40°6′0′′ E), hereafter referred to as the lowland dam, is located on the Awash River in the Ethiopian Rift Valley in east-central Ethiopia, 220 km from Addis Ababa. Its capacity is 500 million m^3, and the primary use of its water is for irrigation of sugarcane crops that cover 20,000 hectares of floodplain downstream of the dam. The region is classified as arid with long-term average rainfall between 500 and 600 mm per year and a mean annual temperature of 26 °C (National Meteorological Agency, unpublished report). Sabure (932 m asl), hereafter referred as the lowland dam village, is the nearest settlement (<1 km) to the dam with a population of 3608 in 2012 (Sabure Health Center, unpublished report). Inhabitants live close to their irrigated fields. Meli (936 m asl), hereafter referred as lowland non-dam village, is located 15 km from the Kesem reservoir shoreline and was selected as a control village (beyond the vector impact range of the reservoir). Most of the inhabitants of both villages were agrarians, but only dam villages practiced irrigation. According to the local health center, malaria is a serious health problem in this region with intensive seasonal malaria transmission (Oromia Health Bureau, unpublished report).

Koka Dam (8°28′ N, 39°9′ E), hereafter referred as the midland dam, is located 100 km south-east of Addis Ababa, in the midland region of Central Ethiopia. The area is classified as semi-arid with 600 to 800 mm of annual rainfall, a mean annual temperature of 20 °C, and unstable/seasonal malaria transmission (National Meteorology Agency, unpublished report). Commissioned in 1969, Koka Dam was constructed to provide 46 MW of

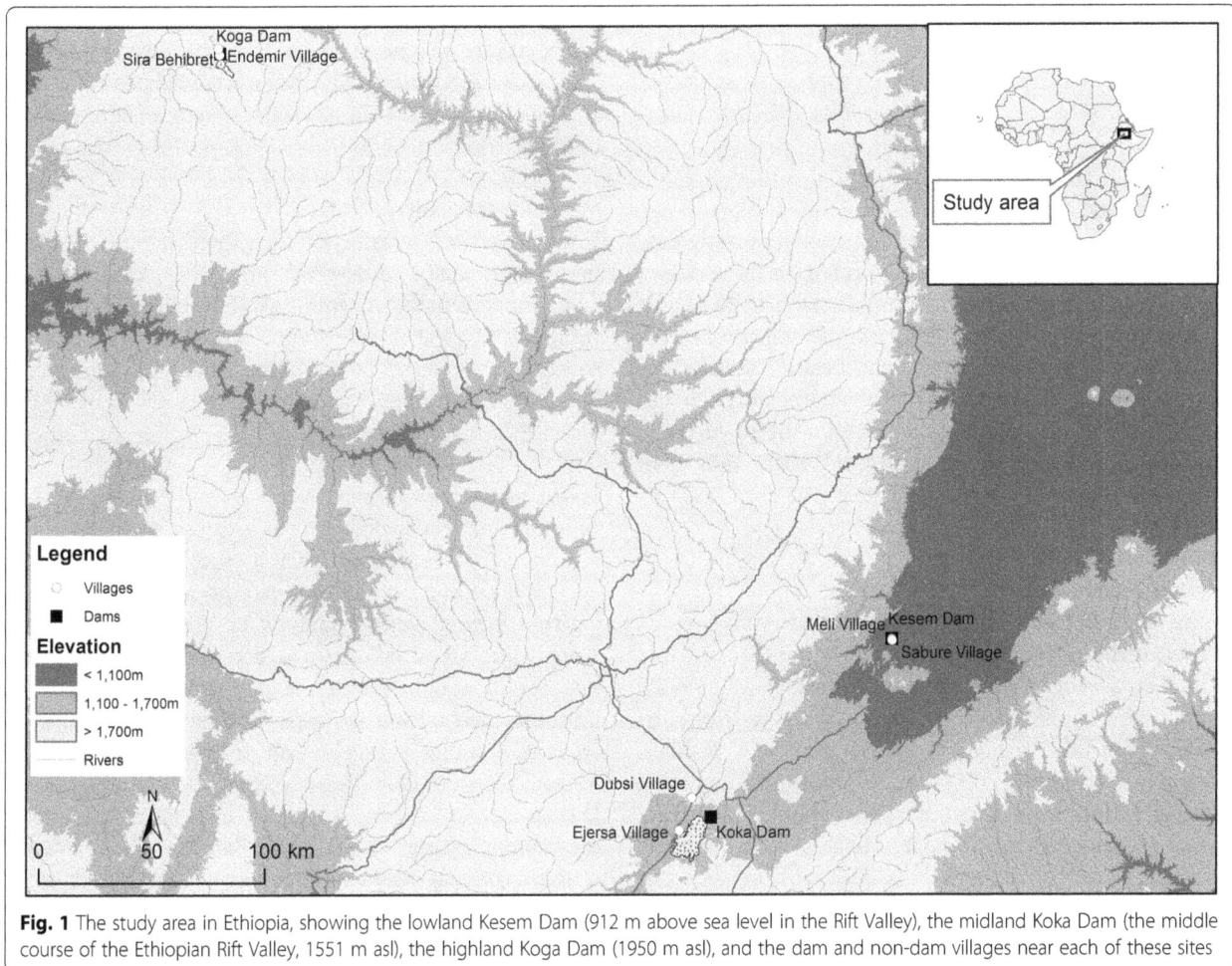

Fig. 1 The study area in Ethiopia, showing the lowland Kesem Dam (912 m above sea level in the Rift Valley), the midland Koka Dam (the middle course of the Ethiopian Rift Valley, 1551 m asl), the highland Koga Dam (1950 m asl), and the dam and non-dam villages near each of these sites

hydro-electricity to Addis Ababa and has a capacity of 1850 million m^3. Ejersa (1564 m asl; population 4236), hereafter referred to as the midland dam village, is a rural village located adjacent (<1 km) to the Koka Reservoir shoreline. No irrigation was practiced around Koka. Dubsi (1566 m asl; population 3,421; Adama Health Center, unpublished report), hereafter referred as the midland non-dam village, is located about 10 km from Koka Reservoir, and was used as a control village. The inhabitants of both villages are largely agrarians. Malaria is common in both villages, with the main transmission season occurring from September to November, immediately following the long rainy season (June–August).

Koka Dam (11°25′ N, 37°09′ E), hereafter referred as the highland dam, is located on the Koga River, one of the major tributaries of the Blue Nile River in northwest Ethiopia, 556 km from Addis Ababa. The area is classified as a highland with an average annual rainfall of 1500 mm and has a mean annual temperature of 18 °C (National Meteorological Agency, unpublished report). Koga Dam has a storage capacity of 83.1 million m^3 with the reservoir inundating an area of 17.5 km^2.

Commissioned in 2009, Koga Dam was constructed to provide water security for 7000 ha of irrigated land growing wheat, corn, and teff downstream of the dam. Endemir (1955 m asl), hereafter referred as the highland dam village, is located adjacent (<1 km) to the reservoir shoreline and had a population of 2907 in 2013 (Merawi Health Center, unpublished report). Sira Behibret (1942 m asl), hereafter referred as the highland non-dam village, is located 12 km from the reservoir shoreline and had a population of 3241 in 2013 (Merawi Health Center, unpublished report). The inhabitants of both villages are agrarians, and cattle herding is also common. Only dam villages use irrigation.

Vector control that involves use of bed nets and indoor residual spraying is commonly practiced in all study villages. No socioeconomic or intervention differences was observed among study villages. *Plasmodium falciparum* is the most common malaria parasite species, causing between 60 and 80% of malaria cases in the study area, with *Plasmodium vivax* causing the remaining malaria illnesses [12]. *Anopheles arabiensis* (the most widely distributed *An. gambiae sensu lato* species in Ethiopia) is the major malaria vector species, while *An. pharoensis* plays a secondary role [16]. In this study, it was assumed that all *An. gambiae s.l.* collected were *An. arabiensis* based on previous PCR identifications [22, 23].

Clinical malaria data collection

To assess the risk of malaria around dams, monthly data of retrospective microscope-confirmed malaria cases were obtained from health centers in each of the three dam sites (2010–2014). Inhabitants of the study area commonly visit these government health facilities for medical consultation since they provide medical services free of charge. The malaria dataset was sorted for each of the six villages (three dam and three non-dam villages) and species of malaria parasite as confirmed by microscopy.

Mosquito sampling

Larval and adult mosquitoes were sampled every 3 weeks in each of the study villages from October 2013 to July 2014. Larval stages were sampled from any water body such as rain pools, man-made pools, reservoir shoreline puddles, irrigation canals, and irrigated field paddies. During each survey, all potential mosquito breeding habitats within a 1-km radius of the study village were sampled using 350 mL standard dippers [24]. First, the surface area of the each potential mosquito breeding site was estimated in square meters (m^2), and sampling was undertaken at a rate of six dips per m^2 [24]. At least one dip was taken when the breeding habitat was too small (<0.2 m^2). Larval anopheline samples were then counted and stored in vials by direct pipetting, killed by gentle heating, and preserved in 70% alcohol for later taxonomic identification. Larval samples from each mosquito habitat were placed in separate vials. Preserved larval anophelines were identified to species by microscope in the laboratory using morphological characteristics [25].

Adult mosquitoes were collected using CDC light traps (Model 512; J W Hock Co, Atlanta, USA). In each study village, a total of ten light traps were deployed for overnight mosquito collection from 1800 to 0630 h. Five of the light traps were deployed inside human homesteads and the other five were installed outdoors. Houses for light trap mosquito collection were randomly selected, and sampling was conducted in the same houses throughout the period of the study. Each indoor light trap was placed in a bedroom, near a wall, with the bulb about 50 cm above a person sleeping under an untreated bed net [15]. The outdoor light traps were installed on trees nearby open cattle enclosures where some of the villagers spent the evening. The following morning, light traps were collected and emptied into paper boxes containing a silica gel desiccant. Anophelines

were later sorted out from other mosquito taxa, counted, and identified to species in the laboratory using morphological characteristics [26]. Female anophelines were kept at room temperature (22–25 °C) with silica gel desiccator until processed.

Mosquito processing

The head-thorax portion of each dried female anopheline was processed to detect *P. falciparum* circumsporozoite antigens using enzyme-linked imminosorbent assay (ELISA) [27]. To determine mosquito blood meal sources (human vs bovine), the abdomen portion of blood-engorged female anophelines was tested using the direct ELISA technique [28].

Statistical analysis

Monthly malaria incidence was express as the number of microscope-confirmed malaria cases in a given month per 1000 population [29]. Larval and adult counts were log-transformed before analysis to normalize the data. Anopheline larval density was determined as the mean number of anopheline larvae per square meter. Adult mosquito density was expressed as the mean number of adult mosquitoes per light trap per night, separated for indoor and outdoor traps within each study village. Differences in malaria incidence and larval and adult mosquito densities were tested among the elevation settings (pairing reservoir and non-reservoir villages at each site) using one-way analysis of variance (ANOVA) with post hoc HSD Tukey's test applied to test differences between villages within each dam site [30].

The sporozoite rate was expressed as the proportion of mosquitoes positive for *Plasmodium* sporozoites from the total number of mosquitoes of a species tested by ELISA. Human biting rates were derived from light trap catches by dividing adult anopheline density by a factor of 1.5 to match light trap catches with human landing catches, as determined by Yohannes et al. [15]. The human biting rate was then multiplied by the sporozoite rate to estimate the entomological inoculation rate (EIR). For each *Anopheles* species, the human blood index (HBI) was determined as the proportion of samples positive for human blood from the total samples tested by blood meal ELISA. All analyses were done using Microsoft Excel 2010 and SPSS statistical software version 22 (SPSS Inc, Chicago, IL, USA). The level of significance used for all tests was 0.05.

Results

Malaria incidence

The mean monthly malaria incidence was generally higher in the dam villages than in the non-dam villages in all three study dam sites (degree of freedom (df) = 2; $P < 0.05$) (Fig. 2). The mean monthly malaria incidence

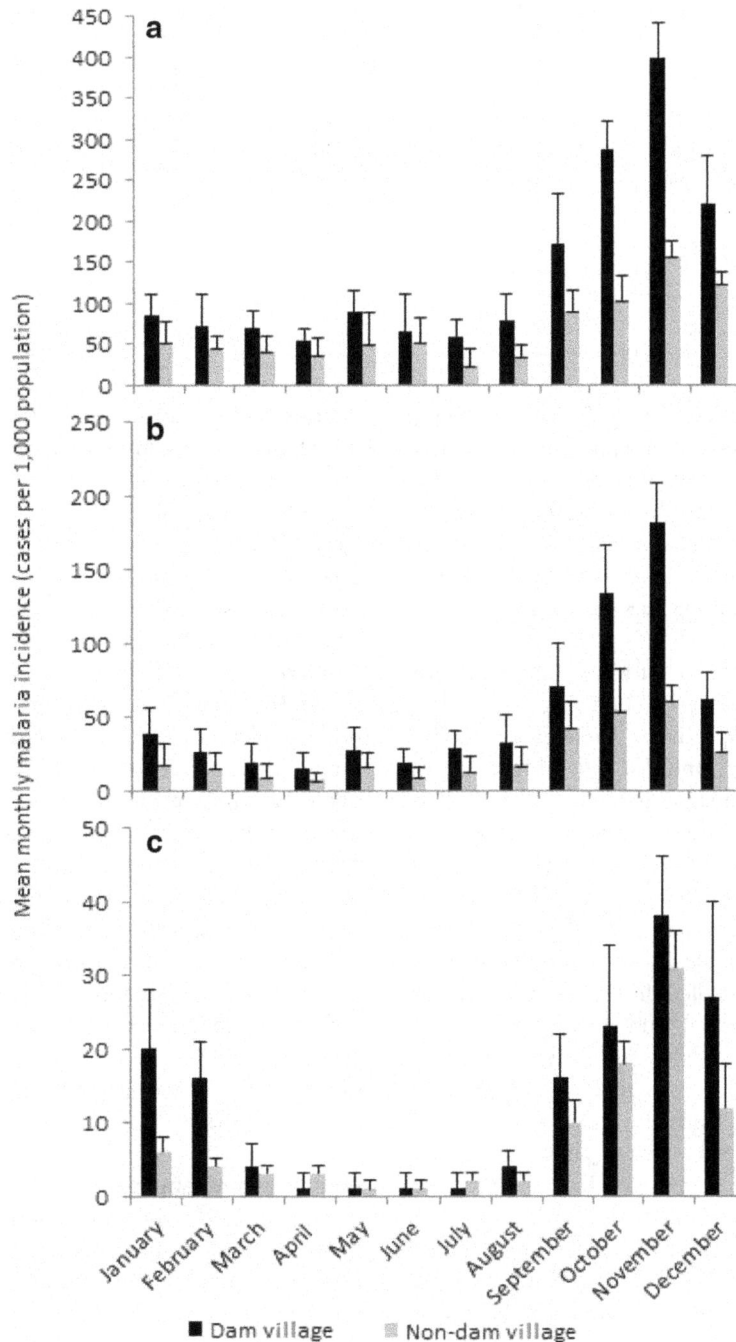

Fig. 2 Mean monthly malaria incidence (cases per 1000 population) in the **a** lowland, **b** midland, and **c** highland dam and non-dam villages in Ethiopia, 2010–2014. Note the different scales on the Y-axes. Error bars are the standard error

at the lowland dam village (mean = 137.4; 95% CI = 86.3–188.5) was twofold higher than at the midland dam village (54.4; 95% CI = 38.2–70.6) and over tenfold higher than at the highland dam village (12.7; 95% CI = 10.2–15.2). A significant difference in malaria incidence among the three dam sites was found (ANOVA df = 2; F = 5.673; $P < 0.05$). The peak period of malaria incidence at all study sites was between September and November.

Mosquito breeding sites and larval density

A total of 1838 potential mosquito larval sites were surveyed during the study period (Table 1). Of these, 1556 (84.7%) were encountered in the dam villages, while only 282 (15.3%) were from non-dam villages. Anopheline larvae were detected at 454 (29.2%) and 43 (15.2%) of these sites at dam and non-dam villages, respectively. At the lowland, the number of positive

Table 1 Summary of anopheline larval surveys conducted in the lowland (Kesem), midland (Koka) and highland (Koga) dam and non-dam villages in Ethiopia between October 2013 and July 2014

	Village	No. of potential anopheline breeding sites	No. of positive anopheline breeding sites	Total area of potential mosquito breeding sites (m^2)	Total area of positive anopheline breeding sites (m^2)	Total no. of anopheline larvae sampled	Mean larval density (no. of larvae per m^2)
Lowland dam	Dam village	712	271	202.1	153.4	793	10.8
	Non-dam village	148	22	71.6	56.3	398	3.7
Midland dam	Dam village	508	115	164.2	116.5	308	5.1
	Non-dam village	83	16	64.1	48.1	122	1.4
Highland dam	Dam village	336	68	121.5	84.2	165	0.5
	Non-dam village	51	11	39.8	18.5	74	0.2

anopheline breeding sites was over 12 times higher in the dam village ($n = 271$) than in the non-dam village ($n = 22$). At the midland, the number of positive anopheline breeding sites was nearly nine times higher in the dam village ($n = 115$) than in the non-dam village ($n = 16$). Similarly, the number of anopheline breeding sites was six times higher in the dam village ($n = 68$) than in the non-dam village ($n = 11$).

A total of 354.1 and 122.7 m^2 of water body was found supporting anopheline mosquito breeding in the dam and non-dam villages, respectively. The area of anopheline breeding sites was 1.3 and 1.8 times higher in the lowland dam village compared to that in the midland and highland dam villages, respectively. The surface area of anopheline larval sites in the dam villages was generally 3–5 times higher than in the non-dam villages.

A total of 1860 anopheline larvae were sampled during the period of the study (Table 1). Of which, the majority (64%; $n = 1,191$) were sampled from the lowland dam while the rest 23% ($n = 430$) and 13% ($n = 239$) were from the midland and highland dam sites, respectively. Anopheline larval abundance was generally higher in the dam villages than in the non-dam villages at all study dam sites. The mean larval density (larvae per square meter) was significantly higher in the lowland dam village (ANOVA mean = 10.8; 95% CI = 7.9–13.7; $F = 31.413$; $P < 0.01$) than in the midland (mean = 5.1; 95% CI = 4.0–6.2) and highland (mean = 0.5; 95% CI = 0.3–0.7) dam villages. Overall, controlling for elevation differences, the variation in mean larval density among the three dam sites was significant (ANOVA $F = 8.453$; $P < 0.01$).

Five *Anopheles* species were identified as larvae across the study area: *An. gambiae s.l.* (hereafter referred as *An. arabiensis*), *An. pharoensis*, *An. funestus s.l.*, *An. coustani s.l.*, and *An. cinereus* (Table 2). Among these, larvae of *An. arabiensis* was predominant in all study villages, accounting for 58% ($n = 1083$) of total larval collections, followed by *An. pharoensis* (24%; $n = 453$), *An. coustani s.l.* (10%; $n = 189$), and *An. funestus s.l.* (7%; $n = 131$). Larvae of *An. funestus s.l.* were found only in the lowland dam village, predominantly in the shoreline

puddles and irrigation canals. In the lowland setting, *An. arabiensis* was predominantly found in irrigation canals and shoreline puddles, contributing to 56 and 37% of the total larval collection from these habitats, respectively. Shoreline puddles accounted for 70.1% of this species' larvae in the midland dam village, while irrigation canals and shoreline puddles accounted for 49.5 and 12.6% in the highland dam village, respectively. Similarly, *An. pharoensis* larvae were primarily found within irrigation canals and/or shoreline puddles at each of the dam villages. In control villages, larval *An. arebiensis* was predominant, commonly found in rain pools and man-made pools. Overall, while anopheline larvae at the midland dam village were collected mainly from shoreline puddles, both shoreline puddles and irrigation canals were the dominant larval habitats at the lowland and highland dam villages.

Anopheline larval density peaked between October and November, dropping during the dry season, and building up to the wet season in all study villages (Fig. 3). However, overall mean larval density was generally higher in the dam villages than in the non-dam villages at all three study areas.

Adult mosquito abundance

A total of 5140 adult anopheline mosquitoes were collected during the study period. Of these, 68% ($n = 3503$), 29% ($n = 1506$), and 3% ($n = 131$) were from lowland, midland, and highland study sites, respectively (Table 3). *Anopheles arabiensis* was the predominant species in all villages, accounting for 53% of the total adult anopheline collections. *Anopheles pharoensis* was the next most abundant species (31%), followed by *An. funestus s.l.* (9.4%), *An. coustani s.l.* (6.4%), and *An. cinereus* (0.2%).

Similar to larvae, anopheline adult density peaked between October and November, fell during the dry season, and increased again in June with the commencement of the wet season in all study villages (Fig. 4). Overall mean adult anopheline density varied significantly across villages (ANOVA $F = 23.89$; $P < 0.001$) and was generally higher at the dam villages than at the non-

Table 2 Distribution of *Anopheles* species across different types of larval breeding habitats in the lowland (Kesem), midland (Koka), and highland (Koga) dam and non-dam villages in Ethiopia, between October 2013 and July 2014

Site	Village	Type of breeding habitat	Number of positive mosquito breeding sites	Area of positive mosquito breeding sites sampled (m²)	An. arabiensis	An. pharoensis	An. coustani	An. funestus	An. cinereus	Total no. of Anopheles larvae found
Lowland dam	Dam village	Shoreline puddle	188	77.3	164	75	10	61	0	310
		Rain pools	12	15.2	26	6	5	0	2	39
		Man-made pools	8	4.9	8	0	9	0	1	18
		Irrigation canals	63	56	248	89	26	63	0	426
		Total	271	153.4	446	170	50	124	3	793
	Non-dam village	Shoreline puddle	−a	−	−	−	−	−	−	−
		Rain pools	18	49	177	110	51	0	0	338
		Man-made pools	4	7.3	31	17	12	0	0	60
		Irrigation canals	−	−	−	−	−	−	−	−
		Total	22	56.3	208	127	63	0	0	398
Midland dam	Dam village	Shoreline puddle	90	84.8	129	84	19	4	0	236
		Rain pools	10	17.2	18	2	3	0	0	23
		Man-made pools	15	14.5	37	3	8	0	1	49
		Irrigation canals	−	−	−	−	−	−	−	−
		Total	115	116.5	184	89	30	4	1	308
	Non-dam village	Shoreline puddle	−	−	−	−	−	−	−	−
		Rain pools	12	37.1	47	27	9	0	0	83
		Man-made pools	4	11	32	5	2	0	0	39
		Irrigation canals	−	−	−	−	−	−	−	−
		Total	16	48.1	79	32	11	0	0	122
Highland dam	Dam village	Shoreline puddle	10	12.1	14	2	6	1	0	23
		Rain pools	17	15.8	28	0	10	0	0	38
		Man-made pools	2	1.5	4	0	2	0	0	6
		Irrigation canals	28	54.8	65	17	14	2	0	98
		Total	57	84.2	111	19	32	3	0	165
	Non-dam village	Shoreline puddle	−	−	−	−	−	−	−	−
		Rain pools	8	12.4	47	11	3	0	0	61
		Man-made pools	3	6.1	8	5	0	0	0	13
		Irrigation canals	0	0	0	0	0	0	0	0
		Total	11	18.5	55	16	3	0	0	74

a - indicates that this type of breeding habitat did not exist

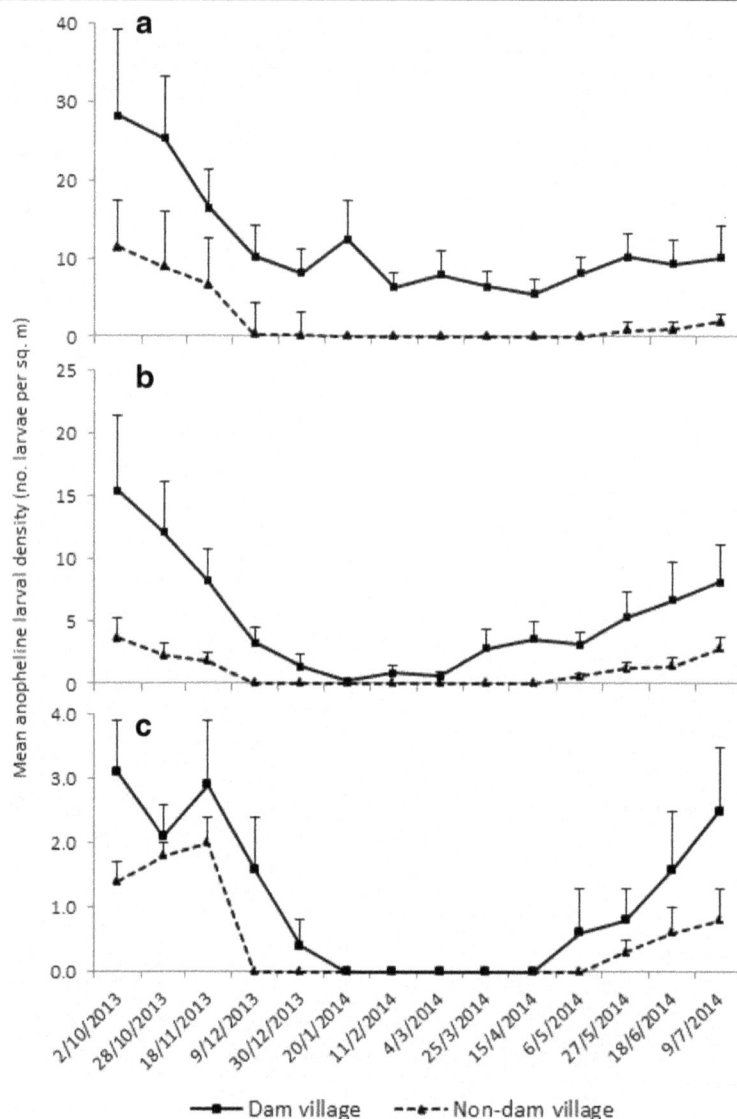

Fig. 3 Mean anopheline larval density (no. larvae per m²) in the **a** lowland, **b** midland, and **c** highland dam and non-dam villages in Ethiopia, between October 2013 and July 2014. Note the different scales on the Y-axes. Error bars are the standard error

dam villages in all three study areas. The highest density was recorded at the lowland dam village (mean = 10.8 anopheline per trap per night; 95% CI = 6.2–15.4) and the lowest at the highland non-dam village (mean = 0.2; 95% CI = 0.1 – 0.4). Similarly, the overall mean adult anopheline density at the lowland dam village was 2.2 times higher than at the midland dam village and 22 times higher than at the highland dam village.

Indoor and outdoor adult mosquito sampling detected *An. arabiensis* predominantly indoors in all study villages (Table 4). The density of *An. pharoensis* was also higher indoors than outdoors at the lowland dam site but not at the midland and highland dam sites. In contrast, *An. coustani s.l.* and *An. funestus s.l.* were predominantly sampled from outdoor traps in all study sites.

Blood meal sources and entomological inoculation rate

ELISA results indicated that *An. funestus s.l.* (human blood index (HBI) = 87.2%) and *An. arabiensis* (HBI = 82.4%) were the most anthropophagic species in the lowland dam village (Table 5). Slightly lower HBI values (70.7–72.7%) were recorded for *An. arabiensis* in the other dam villages. In contrast, the proportion of blood meals of *An. arabiensis* originating from bovine sources appeared to increase from lowland (22%) to midland (34%) and highland (36%). *An. pharoensis* preferred human blood meals over bovine sources, while *An. coustani s.l.* preferred bovine over human blood in all study villages.

A total of 4848 female anophelines were tested for *P. falciparum* sporozoite infections (Table 6). The highest

Table 3 Number and mean density of adult anophelines and collected in the lowland (Kesem), midland (Koka), and highland (Koga) dam and non-dam villages in Ethiopia, between October 2013 and July 2014

		An. arabiensis		An. pharoensis		An. coustani		An. funestus		An. cinereus		Total Anophelines	
		No. (%)	Mean density[a]	No. (%)	Mean density	No. (%)	Mean density	No. (%)	Mean density	No. (%)	Mean density	No. (%)	Mean density
Lowland dam	Dam village	1423	15.81	782	8.69	99	1.10	449	4.99	2	0.02	2755	30.61
	Non-dam village	466	5.18	251	2.79	31	0.34	0	0.00	0	0.00	748	8.31
Midland dam	Dam village	541	6.01	421	4.68	103	1.14	36	0.40	8	0.09	1109	12.32
	Non-dam village	205	2.28	126	1.40	66	0.73	0	0.00	0	0.00	397	4.41
Highland dam	Dam village	64	0.71	16	0.18	12	0.13	0	0.00	0	0.00	92	1.02
	Non-dam village	23	0.26	0	0.00	16	0.18	0	0.00	0	0.00	39	0.43
Total	Dam village	2028	7.51	1219	4.51	214	0.79	485	1.80	10	0.04	3.956	14.65
	Non-dam village	694	2.57	377	1.40	113	0.42	–	–	0	0.00	1.184	4.39

[a]Mean density refers to the mean number of adult anophelines per trap per night during the sampling period

sporozoite infection rate was detected in the lowland dam village where 4.5% (20/449), 4.1% (59/1423), and 2.3% (18/782) of *An. funestus s.l.*, *An. arabiensis*, and *An. pharoensis*, respectively, were found to be positive. In the lowland non-dam village, 1.7% (8/466) of *An. arabiensis* and 1.2% (3/251) of *An. pharoensis* tested positive for *P. falciparum* sporozoites. In the midland dam village, the sporozoite rate of *An. arabiensis* and *An. pharoensis* was 2% (11/541) and 1.4% (6/421), respectively, while only a single female *An. arabiensis* (0.5%, 1/205) tested positive for *P. falciparum* sporozoite in the midland non-dam village. All sporozoite-infected anophelines were collected during the main transmission season. None of the samples from the highland dam villages tested positive for *P. falciparum* sporozoites.

The annual entomological inoculation rate (EIR) for *An. arabiensis*, *An. funestus s.l.*, and *An. pharoensis* at the lowland dam village was found to be 129.8, 47.8, and 33.3 infective bites per person per year (ib/p/y), respectively (Table 6). In contrast, the annual EIR of *An. arabiensis* and *An. pharoensis* at the lowland non-dam village was 15.6 and 5.0 ib/p/y, respectively. At the midland dam village, the annual EIR was found to be 20.7 and 10.2 ib/p/y by *An. arabiensis* and *An. pharoensis*, respectively, while the annual EIR in the midland non-dam village was 2.0 ib/p/y by *An. arabiensis*. Overall, the data revealed that dams resulted in 10 and 15-fold increases in EIR in the lowland and midland areas, respectively, compared to that in the non-dam villages in the same settings.

Discussion

The present study indicates the link between dams and malaria in different eco-epidemiological settings in Ethiopia. At the lowland and midland settings, reservoir shoreline puddles and irrigation canals were the major malaria vector breeding habitats, contributing to 70–80% of the anopheline larval breeding sites. *Anopheles arabiensis* and *An. pharoensis* were the major malaria vectors, occurring in higher abundance at lowland and midland dam villages than at the highland dam villages.

Anopheles arabiensis and *An. pharoensis* were primarily breeding in shoreline puddles and irrigation canals in the lowland, midland, and highland dam villages, although their abundance differed among villages. The abundance of these vector species peaked between October and November when the water level started receding following peak water level between July and August: this creates breeding sites at the shorelines. A previous study around the Koka Dam indicated that while *An. arabiensis* prefers shallow sunlit shoreline puddles, *An. pharoensis* breeds in semi-permanent and partly covered large water pools [16]. A preference for similar breeding habitats was documented for these species in the neighboring Ziway area [31], around microdams in northern Ethiopia [15] and elsewhere in Ethiopia [11, 32].

Larval and adult vector densities decreased from the lowland to midland to highland dam villages. Climate variables such as temperature are the major factors that determine rates of mosquito breeding, adult longevity, and malaria parasite development at different elevation settings [33]. Dams in lowland areas create ideal breeding sites for mosquitoes where rainfall is the limiting factor underpinning the availability of mosquito breeding habitats. Moreover, irrigation activities increase vector breeding habitats by creating waterlogged sites in the irrigated fields as well as irrigation canals. A previous study in central Ethiopia where irrigation is commonly practiced indicated that poor irrigation water management led to increased mosquito breeding habitats with a

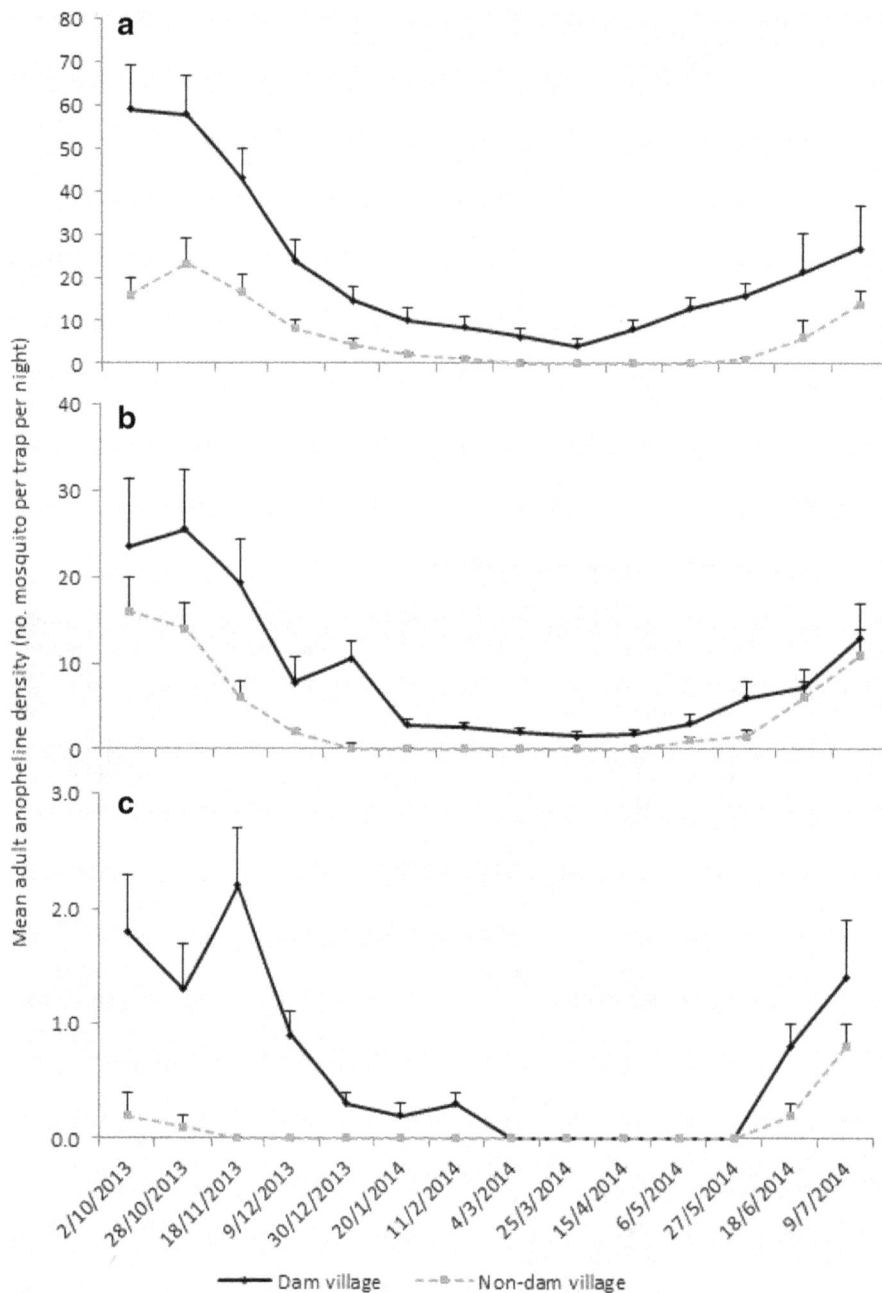

Fig. 4 Mean adult anopheline density (number of mosquitoes per trap per night) in the **a** lowland, **b** midland, and **c** highland dam villages and non-dam villages in Ethiopia, between October 2013 and July 2014. Note the different scales on the Y-axes. Error bars are the standard error

high risk of malaria transmission [34]. A number of studies in sub-Saharan Africa have also revealed the link between irrigation and malaria and the need for targeted planning and implementation of mosquito control measures in order to reduce mosquito breeding [35–40]. Similarly, the present study identified that the lowland irrigation dam had increased mosquito vector abundance and malaria transmission.

A higher vector density along with a high HBI and EIR in the lowland dam village revealed the serious potential

negative impact of dams on malaria in lowland Ethiopia. Moreover, the presence of three vector species (*An. arabiensis*, *An. pharoensis*, and *An. funestus s.l.*) with a combined annual EIR of 210 per person per year around the Kesem Dam highlights the pressing need to devise vector control strategies around lowland dams. Nevertheless, the annual EIR of *An. arabiensis* (129.8) and *An. funestus s.l.* (47.4) in the lowland dam village was lower than those reported (314 and 88, respectively) from the Lower Moshi irrigation area of northern Tanzania for

Table 4 Indoor and outdoor mean adult anopheline density (no. of mosquitoes per trap per night) in the lowland (Kesem), midland (Koka), and highland (Koga) dam and non-dam villages in Ethiopia, between October 2013 and July 2014

Study site		An. arabiensis		An. pharoensis		An. coustani		An. funestus		An. cinereus		Total	
		Indoor	Outdoor	Indoor	Outdoor	Indoor	Outdoor	Indoor	Outdoor	Indoor	Outdoor	Indoor	Outdoor
Lowland	Dam village	20.87	10.76	10.13	7.24	0.71	1.49	0.91	9.07	0.00	0.04	32.62	28.60
	Non-dam village	6.89	3.47	4.18	1.40	0.22	0.47	0.00	0.00	0.00	0.00	11.29	5.33
Midland	Dam village	7.20	4.82	2.51	6.84	0.47	1.82	0.16	0.64	0.00	0.18	10.33	14.31
	Non-dam village	3.11	1.44	1.04	1.76	0.53	0.93	0.00	0.00	0.00	0.00	4.69	4.13
Highland	Dam village	1.13	0.29	0.13	0.22	0.07	0.20	0.00	0.00	0.00	0.00	1.33	0.71
	Non-dam village	0.31	0.20	0.00	0.00	0.09	0.27	0.00	0.00	0.00	0.00	0.40	0.47
Total	Dam village	29.20	15.87	12.78	14.31	1.24	3.51	1.07	9.71	0.00	0.22	44.29	43.62
	Non-dam village	10.31	5.11	5.22	3.16	0.84	1.67	0.00	0.00	0.00	0.00	16.38	9.93

Table 5 Blood meal sources of female anophelines in the lowland (Kesem), midland (Koka), and highland (Koga) dam and non-dam villages in Ethiopia, between October 2013 and July 2014

Site	Village	An. arabiensis	An. pharoensis	An. funestus	An. coustani
Lowland dam	Dam village				
	No. tested	924	508	311	47
	Positive for human blood (%)	761 (82.4)	348 (68.5)	272 (87.5)	18 (38.3)
	Positive for bovine blood (%)	203 (22.0)	209 (41.1)	40 (12.9)	32 (68.1)
	Unidentified (%)	9 (1.0)	5 (1.0)	2 (0.6)	3 (6.4)
	Non-dam village				
	No. tested	278	199	0	20
	Positive for human blood (%)	202 (72.7)	122 (61.3)	0	6 (30.0)
	Positive for bovine blood (%)	88 (31.7)	72 (36.2)	0	15 (75.0)
	Unidentified (%)	4 (1.4)	7 (3.5)	0	1 (5.0)
Midland dam	Dam village				
	No. tested	392	314	18	73
	Positive for human blood (%)	277 (70.7)	201 (64.0)	11 (61.1)	28 (38.4)
	Positive for bovine blood (%)	135 (34.4)	123 (39.2)	7 (38.9)	54 (74.0)
	Unidentified (%)	14 (3.6)	17 (5.4)	0 (0)	3 (4.1)
	Non-dam village				
	No. tested	168	91	0	44
	Positive for human blood (%)	118 (70.2)	61 (67.0)	0	18 (40.9)
	Positive for bovine blood (%)	62 (36.9)	32 (35.2)	0	34 (77.3)
	Unidentified (%)	7 (4.2)	3 (3.3)	0	2 (4.5)
Highland dam	Dam village				
	No. tested	45	9	0	5
	Positive for human blood (%)	32 (71.1)	6 (66.7)	0	2 (40.0)
	Positive for bovine blood (%)	16 (35.6)	4 (44.4)	0	3 (60.0)
	Unidentified (%)	0 (0.0)	1 (11.1)	0	0 (0.0)
	Non-dam village				
	No. tested	11	0	0	16
	Positive for human blood (%)	8 (72.7)	0	0	7 (43.8)
	Positive for bovine blood (%)	4 (36.4)	0	0	9 (56.3)
	Unidentified (%)	1 (9.1)	0	0	1 (6.3)

Table 6 *Plasmodium falciparum* sporozoite rate and annual entomological inoculation rate (EIR) of *Anopheles* mosquitoes in the lowland (Kesem), midland (Koka), and highland (Koga) dam and non-dam villages in Ethiopia, between October 2013 and July 2014

Site	Village		An. arabiensis	An. pharoensis	An. funestus	An. coustani
Lowland dam	Dam village					
		No. tested	1423	782	449	99
		No. positive (%)	59 (4.1)	18 (2.3)	20 (4.5)	0 (0.0)
		Annual EIR	129.8	33.3	47.8	0
	Non-dam village					
		No. tested	466	251	36	103
		No. positive (%)	8 (1.7)	3 (1.2)	0 (0.0)	0 (0.0)
		Annual EIR	15.6	5.0	0	0
Midland dam	Dam village					
		No. tested	541	421	36	103
		No. positive (%)	11 (2.0)	6 (1.4)	0 (0.0)	0 (0.0)
		Annual EIR	20.7	10.2	0	0
	Non-dam village					
		No. tested	205	126	−[a]	66
		No. positive (%)	1 (0.5)	0 (0.0)	−	0 (0.0)
		Annual EIR	2.0	0	−	0
Highland dam	Dam village					
		No. tested	64	16	−	12
		No. positive (%)	0 (0.0)	0 (0.0)	−	0 (0.0)
		Annual EIR	0	0	−	0
	Non-dam village					
		No. tested	23	0	0	16
		No. positive	0 (0.0)	−	−	0 (0.0)
		Annual EIR	0	0	0	0

EIR refers to the number of infective bites per person per year
[a]− (minus) refers to absence of the species in that area

the same species [41]. The annual EIR in the midland dam village was comparable to previously documented EIR in the same study area [16] and in western [32] and southwestern Ethiopia [42]. The higher EIR and malaria incidence in the lowland dam village is likely to have been driven by the greater climatic suitability of lowland areas for malaria transmission. Moreover, due to high humidity in the lowland dam area, people often sleep outside under trees (personal observation), which increases the chance of mosquito bites as bed nets are not suitable for outdoor use. Additional malaria intervention measures are thus required particularly for outdoor-dominant *An. funestus s.l.* in the lowland dam village and *An. pharoensis* in the midland dam village since the current malaria intervention strategies entirely target indoor mosquitoes.

The present study has documented for the first time in four decades the role of *An. funestus s.l.* in malaria transmission in the lowland regions of Ethiopia. This species disappeared from several wetland areas of

Ethiopia in the 1970s due to land use changes [32]. The presence of *P. falciparum* sporozoite-infected *An. funestus s.l.* along with a high HBI confirms the role of this species in malaria transmission in the lowland dam area. The reported high sporozoite rate of *An. funestus s.l.* (4.5%) in the lowland dam village was comparable to that reported from Uganda (5.3%) [43] but lower than that documented in Eritrea (9.5%) [44]. Krafsur [45] reported a lower sporozoite rate (1.1%) for this species in the wetlands of the Gambella Region in western Ethiopia. Erlanger et al. [46] reported that the density of *An. funestus s.l.* was 25-fold higher in the irrigated sites as compared to that in non-irrigated sites in the sub-Saharan Africa. The present study documented the link between *An. funestus s.l.* and irrigation dams in the lowland areas of Ethiopia which otherwise would not have been identified.

Malaria incidence and vector density peaked in all study villages between October and November immediately after the main wet season. The impact of the dams was to intensify the malaria transmission instead of extending the period of transmission. Similar findings were documented in the Gilgel-gibe Dam in south Ethiopia [13], the Bemendjin Dam of Cameroon [9], the Kamburu Dam of Kenya [10], the Mthera Dam of Tanzania [47], and the Usuma Reservoir of Nigeria [48]. A recent review work reported that dams intensify malaria transmission in seasonally unstable areas since they provide breeding habitats for mosquito vectors [5]. Reservoir shoreline puddles and irrigation canals provide suitable breeding habitats for malaria vector mosquitoes around dam sites. A previous study around Koka Dam indicated that lower water level drawdown rates between September and November led to increased formation of reservoir shoreline puddles [12]. Reservoir water management is thus crucial to minimize the presence and persistence of reservoir shoreline puddles. In addition, irrigation canals do not operate during the wet season as farmers use rainfed agriculture during this period, leaving irrigation canals waterlogged from rainfall and thus providing ideal breeding grounds for malaria vector mosquitoes (personal observation). Draining irrigation canals and reducing water logging in agricultural fields were previously shown to be effective in reducing larval breeding habitats around microdams in northern Ethiopia [15]. Reservoirs need to be operated in such a way to suppress mosquito breeding as previously done in Tennessee Valley of the USA where faster drawdown of reservoir water levels were associated with lower larval mosquito abundance at the shoreline of the reservoir [49].

This study did not include data for all months of a year. For instance, September lies in the peak malaria transmission season and its inclusion would improve the seasonality of malaria transmission in each eco-epidemiological settings. Future longitudinal research is required to verify the results of this study and assess interannual water level variations on malaria transmission across dams in different ecological settings. Similarly, molecular work is needed to provide the taxonomic resolution for the species of the *An. funestus* complex in the lowland regions of Ethiopia.

Conclusions

The link between dams and malaria must be considered while planning, designing, and operating large dams in sub-Saharan Africa where malaria is a primary public health challenge. The present study confirmed that dams in semi-arid lowland and midland areas intensify malaria transmission due to mosquito vector breeding in associated shoreline and irrigation habitats. However, such an effect was not detected at the highland dam area. Proper management of dams and associated shallow shoreline and canal habitats is thus essential to reduce malaria vector breeding around these economically important water infrastructures. Such environmental management techniques along with conventional vector interventions should be targeted to reduce malaria transmission around these critical infrastructures.

Abbreviations
ANOVA: Analysis of variance; ASL: Above sea level; DF: Degree of freedom; EIR: Entomological inoculation rate; ELISA: Enzyme-linked immunosorbent assay; ib/p/y: Infective bites per person per year

Acknowledgements
The authors wish to thank the Addis Ababa University for the laboratory space; Mr. Tesfaye Abebe for the field assistance; and the inhabitants of the study villages for allowing mosquito collections in their homesteads. Koka, Kesem, and Koga area health centers are also acknowledged for the provision of malaria data.

Funding
This study was financially supported by the University of New England and the International Foundation for Science (IFS, grant no. W/4752-2).

Authors' contributions
SK, GGW, and DR contributed to the conception and design of the study and interpretation of the data. SK conducted the fieldwork and laboratory analysis, performed the statistical analysis, and drafted the manuscript. BP and HT supervised the field data collection and laboratory analysis. All authors critically revised the draft manuscript and approved the final manuscript. SK takes the first authorship responsibility.

Competing interests
The authors declare that they have no competing interests.

Author details
[1]Ecosystem Management, School of Environmental and Rural Science, University of New England, Armidale, NSW 2351, Australia. [2]Department of Zoological Sciences, Addis Ababa University, PO Box 1176, Addis Ababa, Ethiopia. [3]Department of Microbial, Cellular and Molecular Biology, Addis Ababa University, PO Box 1176, Addis Ababa, Ethiopia. [4]Present address: Program in Public Health, University of California, Irvine, CA 92697, USA.

References
1. World Bank. The water resources sector strategy: an overview. Washington DC: The World Bank; 2004.
2. International Commission on Large Dams (ICOLD). World Register of Dams. Paris: ICOLD; 2003.
3. Rosegrant MW, Perez ND. Water resources development in Africa: a review and synthesis of issues, potentials, and strategies for the future. EPTD Discussion Paper No. 28. Washington DC: International Food Policy Research Institute; 1997.
4. Keiser J, Castro MC, Maltese MF, et al. Effect of irrigation and large dams on the burden of malaria on a global and regional scale. Am J Trop Med Hyg. 2005;72:392–406.
5. Kibret S, Wilson GG, Ryder D, et al. The influence of dams on malaria transmission in sub-Saharan Africa. EcoHealth. 2015. doi:10.1007/210393-015-1029-0.

6. Kibret S, Lautze J, McCartney M, et al. Malaria impact of large dams in sub-Saharan Africa: maps, estimates and predictions. Malar J. 2015;14:339.

7. World Health Organization (WHO). World malaria report 2012. Geneva: WHO; 2013.

8. Cole MA, Elliott RJR. Climate change, hydro-dependency, and the African Dam boom. World Dev. 2014;60:84–98.

9. Atangana S, Foumbi J, Charlois M, et al. Epidemiological study of onchocerciasis and malaria in Bamendjin dam area (Cameroon). Medecine tropicale. 1979;39:537–43.

10. Oomen J. Monitoring health in African dams: The Kamburu dam as a test case. PhD thesis. The Netherlands: Rotterdam University; 1981.

11. Lautze J, McCartney M, Kirshen P, et al. Effect of a large dam on malaria risk: the Koka Reservoir in Ethiopia. Trop Med Int Health. 2007;12:982–9.

12. Kibret S, McCartney M, Lautze J, et al. Malaria transmission in the vicinity of impounded water: evidence from the Koka Reservoir, Ethiopia. Colombo: International Water Management Institute (IWMI Research Report 132); 2009.

13. Yewhalaw D, Legesse W, van Bortel W, et al. Malaria and water resource development: the case of Gilgel-Gibe hydroelectric dam in Ethiopia. Malar J. 2009;8:21.

14. Ghebreyesus TA, Haile M, Witten KH, Getachew A, Yohannes AM, Yohannes M, Teklehaimanot HD, Lindsay SW, Byss P. Incidence of malaria among children living near dams in northern Ethiopia: community based incidence survey. BMJ. 1999;319:663–6.

15. Yohannes M, Mituku H, Ghebreyesus TA, et al. Can source reduction of mosquito larval habitat reduce transmission of malaria in Tigray, Ethiopia? Trop Med Int Health. 2005;10:1274–85.

16. Kibret S, Lautze J, Boelee E, et al. How does an Ethiopian dam increase malaria? Entomological determinants around the Koka Reservoir. Trop Med Int Health. 2012;11:1320–8.

17. Mba CJ, Aboh IK. Prevalence and management of malaria in Ghana: a case study of Volta region. Afri Pop Stud. 2007;22:137–71.

18. Baudon D, Robert V, Darriet F, et al. Impact of building a dam on the transmission of malaria: malaria survey conducted in southeast Mauritania. Bull Soc Pathol Exot. 1986;79:123–9.

19. Ndiath MO, Sarr JB, Gaayeb L, et al. Low and seasonal malaria transmission in the middle Senegal River basin: identification and characteristics of Anopheles vectors. Parasit Vectors. 2012;5:12.

20. Badu K, Brenya RC, Timmann C, et al. Malaria transmission intensity and dynamics of clinical malaria incidence in a mountainous forest region of Ghana. MWJ. 2013;4:14.

21. Drakeley CJ, Carneiro I, Reyburn H, et al. Altitude-dependent and-independent variations in Plasmodium falciparum prevalence in northeastern Tanzania. J Infect Dis. 2005;15:1589–98.

22. Balkew M, Ibrahim M, Koekemoer LL, et al. Insecticide resistance in Anopheles arabiensis (Diptera: Culicidae) from villages in central, northern and south west Ethiopia and detection of kdr mutation. Parasite Vector. 2010;3:1.

23. Fettene M, Olana D, Christian RN, et al. Insecticide resistance in Anopheles arabiensis from Ethiopia. African Entomol. 2013;21:89–94.

24. Silver JB. Mosquito ecology: field sampling methods. Springer Science & Business Media: The Netherlands; 2007.

25. Verrone G. Outline for the determination of malarial mosquitoes in Ethiopia. Part II. Anopheline larvae. Mosq News. 1962;22:394–401.

26. Verrone G. Outline for the determination of malarial mosquitoes in Ethiopia. Part I. Adult female anophelines. Mosq News. 1962;22:37–49.

27. Wirtz RA, Zavala F, Charoenvit Y, et al. Comparative testing of monoclonal antibodies against Plasmodium falciparum sporozoites for ELISA development. Bull World Health Organ. 1987;65:39–45.

28. Beier JC, Perkins PV, Wirtz RA, et al. Blood meal identification by enzyme-linked immunosorbent assay (ELISA), tested on Anopheles (Diptera: Culicidae) in Kenya. J Med Entomol. 1988;25:9–16.

29. World Health Organization (WHO). Disease surveillance for malaria control: an operational manual. Genève: WHO; 2012.

30. Ott RL, Longnecker M. Statistical methods and data analysis. Duxbury: California; 2001.

31. Kibret S, Alemu Y, Boelee E, et al. The impact of a small-scale irrigation scheme on malaria transmission in Ziway area, Central Ethiopia. Trop Med Intl Health. 2010;15(1):41–50.

32. Woube M. Geographical distribution and dramatic increases in incidences of malaria: consequences of the resettlement scheme in Gambella, SW Ethiopia. Indian J Malariol. 1997;34:140–63.

33. Zhou G, Minakawa N, Githeko AK, et al. Association between climate variability and malaria epidemics in the East African highlands. Proc Natl Acad Sci. 2004;101:2375–80.

34. Kibret S, Wilson GG, Tekie H, et al. Increased malaria transmission around irrigation schemes in Ethiopia and potential of water management to mitigate malaria. Malar J. 2014;13:360.

35. Ijumba JN, Lindsay SW. Impact of irrigation on malaria in Africa: paddies paradox. Med Vet Entomol. 2001;15:1–11.

36. Muturi E, Shililu J, Jacob B, et al. Mosquito species diversity and abundance in relation to land use in riceland agro-ecosystem in Mwea, Kenya. J Vector Biol. 2006;31:129–37.

37. Mwangangi MJ, Shililu J, Muturi EJ, et al. Anopheles larval abundance and diversity in three rice agro-village complexes Mwea irrigation scheme, central Kenya. Malar J. 2010;9:228.

38. Dolo G, Briet OJT, Dao A, et al. Malaria transmission in relation to rice cultivation in the irrigated Sahel of Mali. Acta Trop. 2004;89:147–59.

39. Robert V, van de Broek A, Stevens P, et al. Mosquitoes and malaria transmission in irrigated rice-fields in the Benoue Valley of northern Cameroon. Acta Trop. 1992;52:201–4.

40. Mutero CM, Kabutha C, Kimani V, et al. A transdisciplinary perspective on the links between malaria and agroecosystems in Kenya. Acta Trop. 2004;89:171–86.

41. Ijumba JN, Mosha FW, Lindsay SW. Malaria transmission risk variations derived from different agricultural practices in an irrigated area of northern Tanzania. Med Vet Entomol. 2002;16:28–38.

42. Massebo F, Balkew M, Gebre-Michael T, et al. Blood meal origins and insecticide susceptibility of Anopheles arabiensis from Chano in South-West Ethiopia. Parasit Vector. 2013;6:44.

43. Mulamba C, Irving H, Riveron JM, et al. Contrasting Plasmodium infection rates and insecticide susceptibility profiles between the sympatric sibling species Anopheles parensis and Anopheles funestus s.s: a potential challenge for malaria vector control in Uganda. Parasit Vectors. 2014;7:71.

44. Shililu JI, Maier WA, Seitz HM, et al. Seasonal density, sporozoite rates and entomological inoculation rates of Anopheles gambiae and Anopheles funestus in a high-altitude sugarcane-growing zone in Western Kenya. Trop Med Int Health. 1998;3:706–10.

45. Krafsur ES. Malaria transmission in Gambella, Illubabor Province. Ethiop Med J. 1971;9:75–94.

46. Erlanger TE, Keiser J, De Castro MC, et al. Effect of water resource development and management on lymphatic filariasis, and estimates of populations at risk. Am J Trop Med Hyg. 2005;73:523–33.

47. Njunwa KJ. Intense malaria transmission in Mtera dam area: need for promoting insecticide treated nets among fishermen, Tanesco staff, and villagers living around the dam. Tanzan Health Res Bull. 2000;2:2.

48. Ujoh F, Ikyernum J, Ifatimehin OO. Socio-environmental considerations at the Usuma Reservoir in Abuja, Nigeria. Frontiers in Science. 2012;2(6):169–74.

49. Kitron U, Spielman A. Suppression of transmission of malaria through source reduction: antianopheline measures applied in Israel, the United States, and Italy. Rev Inf Dis. 1989;11(3):391–406.

12

"Alert-Audit-Act": assessment of surveillance and response strategy for malaria elimination in three low-endemic settings of Myanmar in 2016

Aye Mon Mon Kyaw[1*], Soundappan Kathirvel[2,3], Mrinalini Das[4], Badri Thapa[5], Nay Yi Yi Linn[1], Thae Maung Maung[6], Zaw Lin[1] and Aung Thi[1]

Abstract

Background: Myanmar, a malaria endemic country of Southeast Asia, adopted surveillance and response strategy similar to "1-3-7" Chinese strategy to achieve sub-national elimination in six low-endemic region/states of the country. Among these, Yangon, Bago-East, and Mon region/states have implemented this malaria surveillance and response strategy with modification in 2016. The current study was conducted to assess the case notification, investigation, classification, and response strategy (NICR) in these three states.

Methods: This was a retrospective cohort study using routine program data of all patients with malaria diagnosed and reported under the National Malaria Control Programme in 2016 from the above three states. As per the program, all malaria cases need to be notified within 1 day and investigated within 3 days of diagnosis and response to control (active case detection and control) should be taken for all indigenous malaria cases within 7 days of diagnosis.

Results: A total of 959 malaria cases were diagnosed from the study area in 2016. Of these, the case NICR details were available only for 312 (32.5%) malaria cases. Of 312 cases, the case notification, investigation, and classification were carried out within 3 days of malaria diagnosis in 95.5% cases (298/312). Of 208 indigenous malaria cases (66.7%, 208/312), response to control was taken in 96.6% (201/208) within 7 days of diagnosis.

Conclusion: The timeline at each stage of the strategy namely case notification, investigation, classification, and response to control was followed, and response action was taken in nearly all indigenous malaria cases for the available case information. Strengthening of health information and monitoring system is needed to avoid missing information. Future research on feasibility of mobile/tablet-based surveillance system and providing response to all cases including imported malaria can be further studied.

Keywords: Reactive case detection, Low endemicity, Indigenous malaria, Case notification, Case investigation, Operational research

* Correspondence: dramkyaw@gmail.com
[1]National Malaria Control Programme/Vector Borne Disease Control, Department of Public Health, Ministry of Health and Sports, Nay Pyi Taw, Myanmar
Full list of author information is available at the end of the article

Background

Malaria is still among the top 10 causes of mortality despite reduction by 48% of malaria incidence rate and 44% of mortality between 2010 and 2016 in the Southeast Asian region (SEAR) [1]. The Global Technical Strategy for Malaria 2016–2030 (GTS) calls for elimination of malaria in 10 countries by 2020 and 35 countries by 2030 [2].

Robust surveillance and response mechanism is necessary to accelerate and ensure malaria elimination which is identified as one of the three pillars under GTS framework [2, 3]. Surveillance assists the healthcare system to actively identify the unreported cases and also to identify the hidden infection source for further control of malaria [4]. Among the 14 countries of Asia Pacific Malaria Elimination Network (APMEN), 13 countries reported the availability of such surveillance system in place. Similarly, the member countries have reported about the malaria case investigations to all or part of cases notified depending on the burden and type of malaria cases (indigenous or imported malaria) [5].

China is one of the member countries of APMEN who successfully established a good surveillance and response system called as "1-3-7" strategy (case notification within 1 day, case investigation and classification within 3 days, and focus investigation and response within 7 days of malaria diagnosis) under its national program [6, 7]. The performance of 1-3-7 strategy in China was encouraging but suggested the need for proactive malaria hotspot mapping, assessment of genetic diversity, and population dynamics to eliminate malaria [6–9].

Myanmar, a malaria endemic SEAR country, has made significant progress in reducing malaria morbidity and mortality in 2016 compared to 2012 [4]. Despite these advancements, malaria remains to be the country's major public health problem with annual parasite incidence of 3.5 per 1000 population and 21 deaths in 2016 [1]. The country has adopted similar malaria surveillance and response strategy like China with modifications to achieve sub-national elimination as per Myanmar National Plan for Malaria Elimination (NPME) 2016–2030 of National Malaria Control Programme (NMCP) [10]. It has been proposed to eliminate falciparum malaria from six low-endemic states and regions namely Yangon, Bago, Mon, Mandalay, Magway, and Nay Pyi Taw regions/states of Myanmar by 2020 and in the remaining nine regions/states by 2030. Among these, Yangon, Bago-East, and Mon regions/states have implemented this strategy in 2016, and the remaining states started implementing from 2017 [11].

Though the malaria surveillance and response strategy has been rolled out, assessment of this strategy has not yet been studied systematically. Assessment is needed to further review and strengthen the existing surveillance

and response mechanism to accelerate the malaria elimination. Thus, this study was conducted to assess the malaria case notification, investigation, and response strategy in three low-endemic settings (Yangon, Bago-East, and Mon region/states) of Myanmar. The specific objectives were to assess the (a) number and proportion of patients diagnosed with malaria (stratified for socio-demographic and clinical characteristics), (b) number and proportion of patients with malaria notified within 1 day of diagnosis, (c) number and proportion of patients with malaria investigated and classified within 3 days of diagnosis, and (d) number and proportion of indigenous malaria cases for which the response to control action has been taken within 7 days of diagnosis.

Methods

Study design

This was a retrospective cohort study using electronic record review of routine program data collected under NMCP.

General setting

The Republic of the Union of Myanmar, a WHO SEAR country, is administratively divided into 14 regions/states and Nay Pyi Taw Council Territory. Malaria is endemic in 291 out of 330 townships in Myanmar [12]. NMCP is carrying out malaria control and elimination activities, and the services are provided free of charge to the population. Basic health staff (BHS; health assistant, lady health visitor, midwives, and public health supervisors) of the formal public health system provides malaria diagnostic and treatment services at a facility level, and village health volunteers (VHV) provide the malaria control services at a community level with the special focus on rural, hard to reach areas.

Specific setting

Yangon (45 townships), Bago-East (14 townships), and Mon (10 townships) region/states (Fig. 1) of Myanmar have a population of 7.5, 2.95, and 2.1 million, respectively [10, 12]. The annual parasite index (API) of Yangon, Bago-East, and Mon region/states was 0.07, 0. 86, and 2.25 in respectively in 2015 [13]. In total, all townships of Bago-East and Mon and 11/45 townships of Yangon are malaria endemic.

Case notification, investigation, classification (NIC), and response (NICR) strategy

Malaria NICR strategy in Yangon, Bago-East, and Mon region/states has been implemented since January 2016. As per the strategy, all malaria-positive cases must be notified within 24 h. Case investigation and classification of notified cases should be carried out using the standard investigation form within 3 days of diagnosis, and

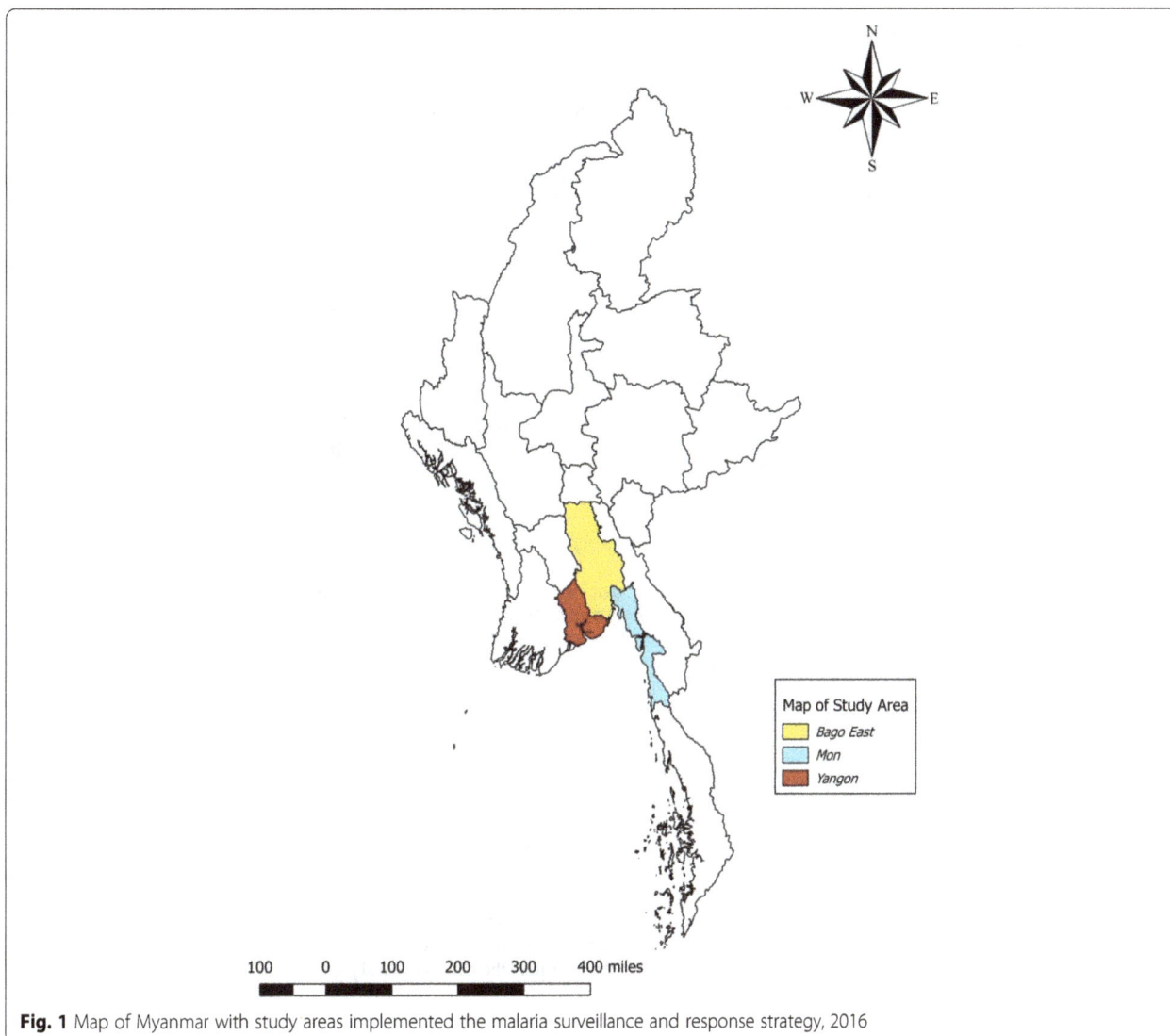

Fig. 1 Map of Myanmar with study areas implemented the malaria surveillance and response strategy, 2016

response to control should be taken within 7 days of malaria diagnosis. The foci investigation and response has not been started by the program which also needs to be carried out within 7 days.

Patients with undifferentiated fever are tested using a malaria dual antigen (both *Plasmodium vivax* and *Plasmodium falciparum*) rapid diagnostic test by VHV at the village level and BHS at facility/outreach. Once a malaria case is diagnosed by a VHV, it is informed to BHS by phone call. BHS further informs the township/regional vector borne disease control (VBDC) office again by phone call. Similarly, cases diagnosed by BHS are notified to VBDC office directly over phone. The township VBDC staff and health assistant at the township health department are informed further to carry out the case NIC. Once the case investigation and classification is done, the township VBDC team sends the filled form to regional/state VBDC officials. The regional/state VBDC

team is asked to verify the case investigation and classification and suggests the appropriate response to be carried out in case of indigenous malaria. The case was classified as "indigenous" or "imported" or "introduced" based on the travel history and the link with imported malaria case. The process of case NICR is described in Fig. 2, and operational definitions NICR and malaria case classification are detailed in Table 1 [3, 11, 14].

Study population and period
All patients with malaria diagnosed and reported under NMCP between January and December 2016 in Yangon, Bago-East, and Mon region/states were included in the study.

Data variables and source of data
Details of all patients with undifferentiated fever screened for malaria by BHS and VHV are routinely

Screening and diagnosis

Patients with undifferentiated fever attended by health staff are tested using rapid diagnostic test/ microscopic examination

Treatment

Patients with malaria are provided treatment according to type of malaria within 24 hours, or referred to other health centers if required

Notification

The health staff notifies about each patient diagnosed with malaria to the township Vector Borne Disease control (VBDC) office within 24 hours

Case investigation and classification

The VBDC officials visit each malaria cases who were notified and interviews the case using standard case investigation form about date of onset of fever, age, sex, occupation, residential and workplace malaria stratum, travel history, date of examination, type of test and species, treatment provision, time of treatment within 3 days.

b) Case classification: Township/Regional/State officials would classify and confirm the patients as 'indigenous' or 'imported' or 'introduced' case

Response

Case investigation and appropriate response
- Complete treatment of index case, Indoor residual sparying
- Active case detection around the index case and prevention and control within seven days

Fig. 2 Case notification, investigation, classification, and response strategy in Yangon, Bago-East, and Mon region/states of Myanmar, 2016

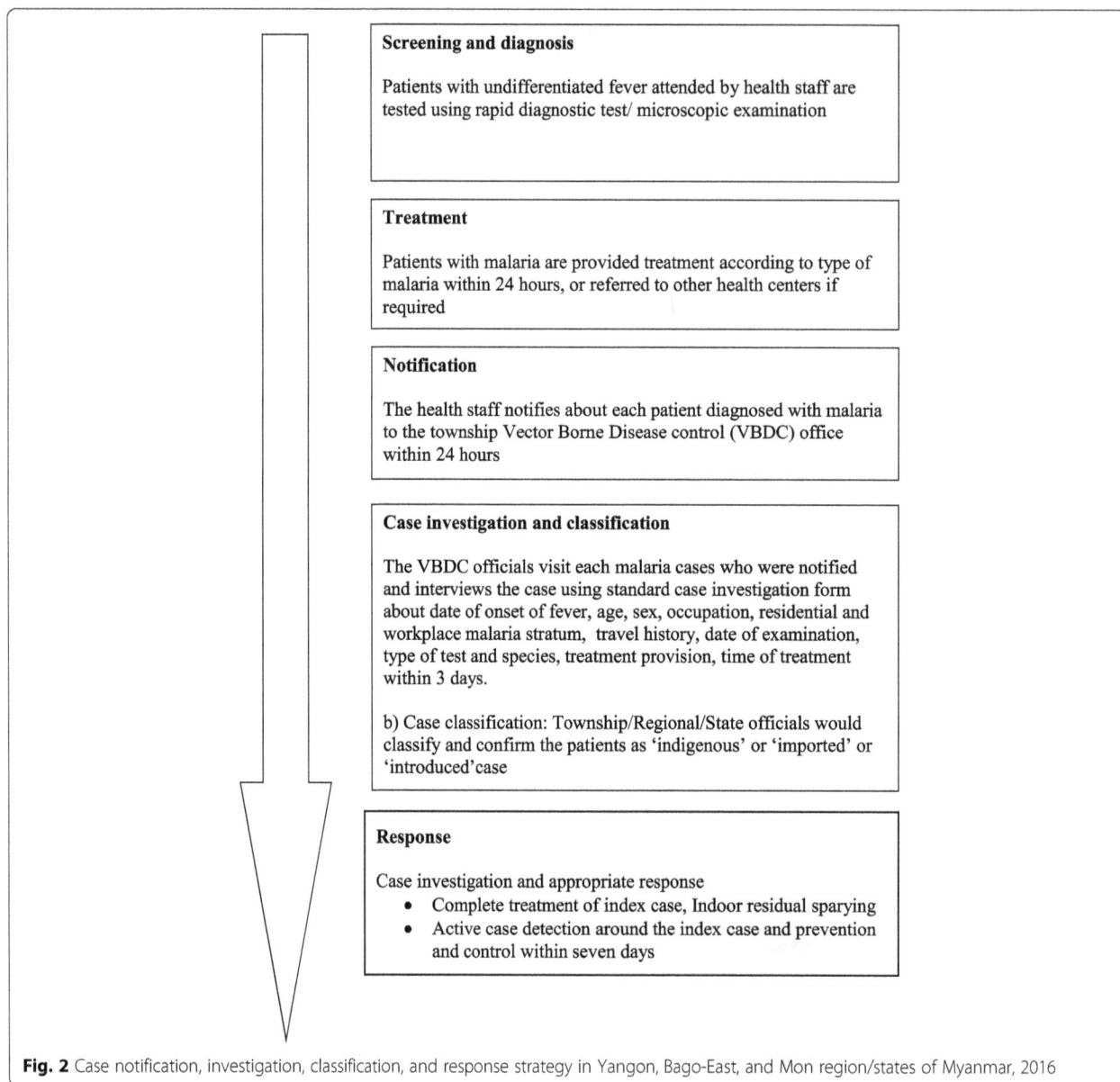

collected in carbonless registers and sent to township VBDC office every month. The same is further sent to regional/state-level VBDC office. The data are entered in a national malaria compile database (Microsoft Office Excel) at the township/regional level by a data assistant. The socio-demographic (age, sex, region/state, type of healthcare provider) and clinical (type of test, malaria species, severity, and treatment status) characteristics of malaria cases diagnosed were obtained from the national malaria compile database.

There is no formal mechanism of maintaining the notified malaria cases, as all new cases are informed over phone with township VBDC staff. The filled case investigation forms submitted at the regional/state level are routinely entered into the case investigation database (Microsoft Office Excel) by the data assistant. There is no specific identifier (name or other unique identifier) available to match the data between the national malaria compile database and case investigation form. The day of case notification, case investigation, and classification from the day of diagnosis (categorized as first, third, or seventh day), and time of response to control (categorized as third or seventh day from diagnosis) and the type of response to control were collected.

Analysis and statistics

The electronic data entered in the national malaria compile database and case investigation database are separately exported to Statistical Package for Social Science (IBM Corp. Version 18) for analysis. Numbers and

Table 1 Operational definitions for malaria case notification, investigation, classification, and response strategy implemented in low-endemic settings of Myanmar, 2016 [3, 10, 11, 14]

Malaria stratum	The malaria stratum are classified as high (> 5/1000 population), moderate (1–5 case per 1000 population), low (< 1 case per 1000 population), and potential transmission and malaria free areas based on the annual parasite incidence, presence, or absence of indigenous cases, presence or absence of main vectors of malaria, and ecology. Each village is classified as malarious (stratum 3), potentially malarious (stratum 2), or malaria-free area (stratum 1). The malarious villages are further stratified into high risk (3a), moderate risk (3b), and low risk (3c).
Case notification	Compulsory reporting of detected cases of malaria by all medical units and medical practitioners, to either the health department or the malaria elimination service.
Case investigation	Collection of information to allow classification of a malaria case by origin of infection, i.e., whether it was imported, introduced, indigenous, or induced. Case investigation includes administration of a standardized questionnaire to a person in whom a malaria infection is diagnosed.
Response to control	Response to control refers to the response following the case investigation which consists of (a) active case detection through blood examination/symptom screening of the febrile cases in and around 10 households of the index cases and (b) vector control measures are IRS, distribution of LLINs (for positive cases), larval source management, and IEC/BCC activities.
Malaria case classification	
Indigenous case	A case contracted locally with no evidence of importation and no direct link to transmission from an imported case.
Imported case	Malaria case or infection in which the infection was acquired outside the area (outside region or state or country) in which it is diagnosed.
Introduced case	A case contracted locally, with strong epidemiological evidence linking it directly to a known imported case (first-generation local transmission).

proportions of patients diagnosed with malaria, notified, and case-investigated within 1, 3, or 7 days of diagnosis, type of malaria classified (indigenous, imported, or introduced), and response to control carried out in indigenous malaria were calculated. Similarly, number and proportions are calculated for socio-demographic and clinical characteristics of patients diagnosed with malaria and case-investigated. Chi-square tests were performed to compare the proportions of the categorical variables. The p value < 0.05 was taken as statistically significant.

Results

Burden of malaria

A total of 959 (0.4%) of patients with undifferentiated fever were found malaria positive among 231,098 patients with fever, screened from Yangon, Bago-East, and Mon region/states. The annual parasite index (number of new parasitologically confirmed malaria cases per 1000 population at risk per year) of malaria cases detected under NMCP in 2016 for Yangon, Bago-East, and Mon was 0.01 (52/7,510,139), 0.14 (414/2,952,897), and 0.24 (493/2,096,099), respectively (data not tabulated).

Characteristics of patients with malaria

Of 959 patients with malaria, 83.6% (802/959) were aged ≥ 15 years and 75.4% (723/959) were males. BHS diagnosed 77.7% (745/959) of malaria cases. *Plasmodium vivax* was the most common (55%, 436/793) species identified in these cases. The socio-demographic and clinical characteristics of patients diagnosed

with malaria in these three areas are described in Table 2.

NICR information availability

NICR details were available only for 312 (32.5%) malaria cases. For the remaining cases (67.5%, 647/959), neither electronic data from case investigation database nor hard copy of the case investigation form was available. The socio-demographic and clinical characteristics of the patients with malaria for whom NICR information is available are given in Table 2. Compared to the malaria cases for which the information is not available, the study did not miss cases systematically in any particular age group, sex, or malaria species ($p > 0.05$). However, the information of VHV-treated cases (80.8%, 173/2/214) were significantly missing ($p < 0.001$) compared to BHS-treated cases (63.6%, 474/745). The proportion of availability of NICR information in Yangon, Bago-East, and Mon region/states was 100% (52/52), 18.1% (75/414), and 37.5% (185/493), respectively. Among the NIC information available cases, 40.1% (125/312), 12.2% (38/312), 21.2% (66/312), and 13.1% (41/312) were forest goers, farmers, construction workers, and others (student/housewife/retired), respectively (data not tabulated).

Case notification, investigation, classification (NIC), and response strategy (NICR)

The flow of patients with malaria under NICR strategy in Yangon, Bago-East, and Mon state/regions is given in Fig. 3. The number of proportion of malaria cases notified with 24 h of diagnosis was not calculated since no

Table 2 Socio-demographic, clinical characteristics of patients with malaria in three low-endemic settings of Myanmar, 2016

Characteristics		All malaria		Malaria NIC information available		Malaria NIC information not available		p value
		n	(%)[a]	n	(%)[b]	n	(%)[b]	
Total		959		312		647		
State/region	Yangon	52	(5.4)	52	(100)	0	(0)	
	Bago-East	414	(43.2)	75	(18.1)	339	(81.9)	
	Mon	493	(51.4)	185	(37.5)	308	(62.5)	
Age (years)	0–14	157	(16.4)	59	(37.6)	98	(62.4)	0.17
	≥ 15	802	(83.6)	253	(31.5)	549	(68.5)	
Sex	Male	723	(75.4)	238	(32.9)	485	(67.1)	0.72
	Female	236	(24.6)	74	(31.4)	162	(68.6)	
	Pregnant[c]	5	(2.1)	na				
Type of healthcare provider	Basic health staff	745	(77.7)	271	(36.4)	474	(63.6)	< 0.001
	Village health volunteer	214	(22.3)	41	(19.2)	173	(80.8)	
Malaria species[d]	Plasmodium vivax	436	(55.0)	171	(39.2)	265	(60.8)	0.99
	Plasmodium falciparum	321	(40.5)	126	(39.3)	195	(60.7)	
	Mixed	35	(4.4)	15	(42.9)	20	(57.1)	
	Plasmodium ovale	1	(0.1)	–				
Severity	Uncomplicated	927	(96.7)	na		na		
	Complicated	32	(3.3)	na		na		

NIC case notification, investigation, and investigation; Mixed both Plasmodium falciparum and Plasmodium vivax positive; na information not available
[a]Column percentage
[b]Row percentage
[c]Percentage among total female
[d]Data for 166 patients among all malaria is not available

such data on case notification was separately maintained. As the exact date/day of notification was not available, it was combined with case investigation and classification details and reported. For the available case information, the malaria case NIC were carried out within 3 days in 95.5% cases. For the remaining 4.5% of cases, NIC was carried out within 7 days (fourth to seventh day) of malaria diagnosis.

Among the total 312 cases, 66.7% (208/312), 31.7% (99/312), and 1.6% (5/312) cases were classified as indigenous, imported, and introduced malaria, respectively, as per operational definition. The response to control was taken in 96.6% (201/208) of cases within 7 days of malaria diagnosis of all indigenous malaria cases. In 34.8% (70/201) of cases, the response action was taken within 3 days of malaria diagnosis. During response to control, 1185 undifferentiated febrile patients were identified, and all were tested negative for malaria.

Discussion
Summary
The current study assessed the malaria NICR implemented for malaria elimination in Yangon, Bago-East, and Mon region/states of Myanmar in 2016. The NICR

details were not available for nearly two thirds of cases. Among the malaria cases for which the information was available, case NIC were done within 3 days of malaria diagnosis in 95.5% of cases. Nearly two thirds of the investigated malaria cases were classified as indigenous and warranted response action. The response to control like mass symptom/blood screening, treatment of cases detected, and distribution of the insecticide impregnated bed nets was taken within 7 days in 96.6% of indigenous malaria cases. The results positively indicate that case NICR is being implemented as planned in Myanmar.

Strengths
This is the first study conducted to assess the case NICR strategy under NMCP in Myanmar after the implementation. This could guide the program further to place standard operating procedures, build capacity of the health workers, improve the data quality, and strengthen the existing health system to prevent and control malaria. The study included all malaria cases diagnosed in Yangon, Bago-East, and Mon region/states from January 2016 to December 2016. The use of routinely collected programmatic data is one of the strengths of this study which reflects the field reality.

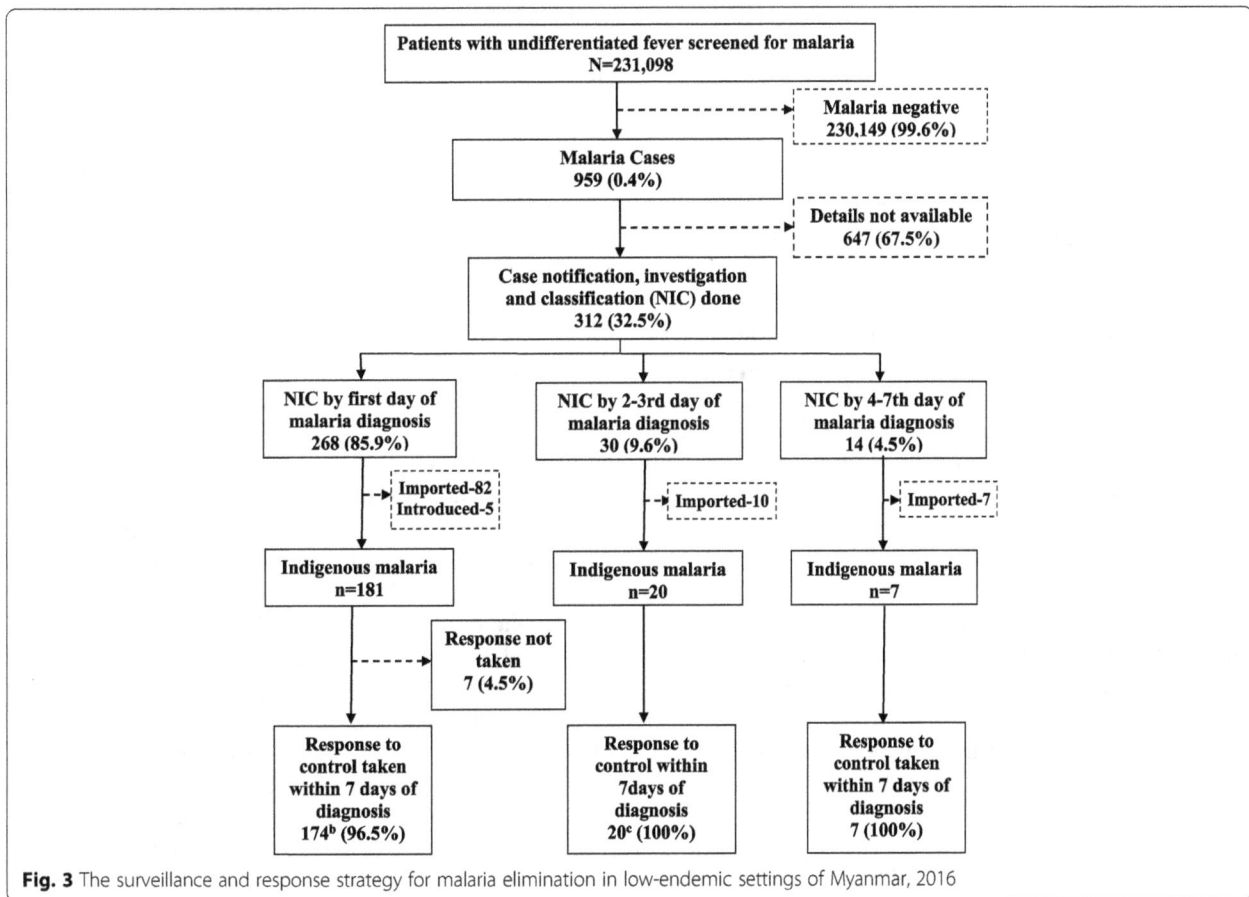

Fig. 3 The surveillance and response strategy for malaria elimination in low-endemic settings of Myanmar, 2016

Case notification within 1 day

The day/date of case notification is not maintained as it happens over phone. The date of diagnosis and notification should be collected to assess the timeliness of the surveillance system and to initiate the investigation of index malaria case for further response and control. Similarly, the BHS or VHV have to report the malaria cases twice first for the surveillance system over phone immediately after diagnosis of a malaria case and monthly by carbonless registers (paper based) to township VBDC office. It is to be noted that nearly two thirds of malaria cases are diagnosed at the community level in Myanmar which necessitates the strengthening surveillance at the community level using information and communication technology interventions [1, 7–9]. Establishment of real-time web-based health information system (HIS) in Myanmar will ensure the immediate availability of notification data and may reduce the workload and double reporting by BHS and VHV. NMCP has recently piloted mobile or tablet-based case NICR, and the results of the same are awaited.

Case investigation and classification within 3 days

The proportion of malaria cases investigated and classified within in 3 days was 95.5% in Myanmar which

aligns well with other countries in APMEN, such as China (85–100%), Indonesia (90.8%), and Thailand (86. 7%) [7–9, 15]. This is a remarkable achievement for the Myanmar NMCP which has just started its sub-national elimination activities in 2016. Though case investigation and classification is possible within 1 day of diagnosis, the 86% achievement questions the adherence by VBDC staff to comprehensive steps involved in case investigation and classification as these are done by different teams. This can be due to case investigation of index case over telephone or at health facility immediately after the diagnosis.

As Myanmar is aiming for malaria (sub-national) elimination, classification of the cases needs careful attention. Misclassification of indigenous case as imported is possible as there is huge population mobility between borders of states/regions with heterogeneous malaria transmission in the country [9, 16, 17]. Similarly, case NICR for mobile, migrant population is one of the key challenges in effective implementation of surveillance strategy and in achieving elimination. This warrants mapping of the mobile and migrant clusters, target profiling, and strengthening the existing mobile, migrant follow-up units of the country to conduct active surveillance and response. It is also important to document previous episodes of malaria infection and necessary post-treatment follow-up to classify cases correctly for appropriate action [3].

Response to control malaria by seventh day

The response to control like complete treatment of index case, indoor residual spray, reactive case detection (RACD) in family and neighborhood is well placed within the surveillance system. However, the foci investigation (identification, characterization, classification, and follow-up) and response are yet to be implemented in the study area which is one of the important components for sustained elimination. There is also a need to specify who should be tested during foci investigation in standard operating procedure (it is under development by the country), e.g., only symptomatic cases or all asymptomatic cases [3, 7, 9, 16].

High burden (67%) of indigenous malaria indicates the existing active transmission. As the elimination effort gains momentum, the regions/states tend to get more imported cases rather than indigenous cases and this is likely to flip in few years of time in these three regions/ states. The imported malaria also warrants action in future following detailed investigation and classification if sustainable elimination is needed.

Limitations

The findings of this study should be interpreted with caution in view of the following limitations. The case NIC details were not available for nearly two thirds of malaria cases diagnosed during the study period. The investigators made all their efforts to trace the forms (either in hard or soft copy) to extract the data but failed. However, except for cases diagnosed and treated by VHV, the study did not systematically miss cases with regard to age, sex, and malaria species compared to cases for which the information is missing. The high proportion of missing information of patients treated by VHV may be due to delayed involvement of VHV in surveillance, delayed reporting of cases, failure of reporting by VHV to BHS or BHS to township VBDC staff, or could be due to non-traceable cases especially in rural and remote areas.

The BHS and VHV primarily use rapid diagnostic test (RDT) kits rather than microscopic examination for diagnosis of cases in Myanmar. The primary and sole use of RDT for diagnosis may miss the low-density malaria infections and the elimination target [7, 9, 16]. Identification and notification of all malaria case is one of the rate limiting factors for malaria elimination; a dual diagnostic method, i.e., use of highly sensitive RDT and quality control mechanism, is needed. Simultaneous collection of blood smear in a sample/all patients tested with RDT and reconfirmation at township health facility

could validate the findings. Similarly, review meetings at regular intervals to discuss sample of cases at the township or higher level could also validate the findings; in addition, it could improve the capacity of health workers.

Complete tracking of patients from fever to diagnosis, case notification, investigation, or response was not carried out as the national malaria compile database and case investigation databases could not be linked due to non-availability of a specific identifier. The RACD monitoring and evaluation tool is tested in China, Indonesia, and Thailand which can be adopted by Myanmar with modifications for the local needs.

Recommendations

Malaria case notification should be made mandatory at least in these three study regions/states by all healthcare providers namely private healthcare providers, informal health providers, military, and health departments other than public health departments. Uptake of RACD monitoring and evaluation tool and developing/adopting clear SOP specifying the responsibilities of health workforce at each level along with timeline is needed. Adequate capacity building of the staff is necessary based on the SOP. Development of web-based HIS linked with mobile phones may potentially improve the availability of information and coverage and speed up the response to control. At different levels, the reporting system should be linked by a unique identification number to get the complete details of a case and validation of the obtained data. Quality assurance strategies like reconfirmation of diagnosis using blood microscopy or other advanced diagnostic methods may be included in the SOP and implemented. Similarly, regular review meeting to discuss the cases at the township or higher level should be established. Gradually, the townships of neighbor regions/states should also be included for reporting to understand about the imported malaria. Myanmar should adopt best malaria elimination standard practices from other malaria-eliminated countries and neighboring countries which are in the verge of elimination and tailor to the existing program infrastructure and needs.

Conclusion

The timeline at each stage of the strategy namely case notification, investigation, classification, and response to control was followed, and response action was taken in nearly all indigenous malaria cases for the available case information. Strengthening of health information and monitoring system is needed to avoid missing information. Future research on feasibility of mobile/tablet-based surveillance system and providing response to all cases including imported malaria can be further studied.

Abbreviations

API: Annual parasite index; APMEN: Asia Pacific Malaria Elimination Network; BHS: Basic health staffs; CISDCP: China Information System for Disease Control and Prevention; GTS: Global Technical Strategy for Malaria 2016–2030; HIS: Health information system; NIC: Notification, investigation, and classification; NICR: Notification, investigation, classification and response strategy; NMCP: National Malaria Control Programme; NPME: Myanmar National Plan for Malaria Elimination 2016–2030; RACD: Reactive case detection; RDT: Rapid diagnostic test; SEAR: Southeast Asian region; SOP: Standard operating procedures; VBDC: Vector borne disease control; VHV: Village health volunteers; WHO: World Health Organization

Acknowledgements

This research was conducted through the Structured Operational Research and Training Initiative (SORT IT). The model is based on a course developed jointly by the International Union Against Tuberculosis and Lung Disease (The Union) and Medécins sans Frontières (MSF/Doctors Without Borders). The specific SORT IT program which resulted in this publication was jointly organized and implemented by the following: The Centre for Operational Research, The Union, Paris, France; The Union Country Office, Mandalay, Myanmar; The Union South-East Asia Office, New Delhi, India; and MSF Brussels Operational Center.

Funding

The training program in which this paper was developed was funded by the Department for International Development (DFID), UK. The funders had no role in study design, data collection and analysis, decision to publish, or preparation of the manuscript.

Authors' contributions

The work was designed by AMMK, SK, MD, BT and NYYL. The data analysis was performed by AMMK, SK, BT. AMMK, SK, MD, BT, NYYL, TMM, ZL, and AT contributed to writing the paper. All authors read and approved the final manuscript.

Competing interests

The authors declare that they have no competing interests.

Author details

[1]National Malaria Control Programme/Vector Borne Disease Control, Department of Public Health, Ministry of Health and Sports, Nay Pyi Taw, Myanmar. [2]International Union Against Tuberculosis and Lung Disease, Southeast Asia, New Delhi, India. [3]Department of Community Medicine, School of Public Health, Postgraduate Institute of Medical Education and Research, Chandigarh, India. [4]Médecins Sans Frontières (MSF) OCB, New Delhi, India. [5]World Health Organization Country Office for Myanmar, Yangon, Myanmar. [6]Department of Medical Research, Ministry of Health and Sports, Nay Pyi Taw, Myanmar.

References

1. World Health Organization. World Malaria Report 2017 [Internet]. Geneva; 2017 [cited 2017 Dec 15]. p. 160. Available from: http://apps.who.int/iris/bitstream/10665/259492/1/9789241565523-eng.pdf?ua=1.
2. World Health Organization. Global Technical Strategy for Malaria 2016-2030 [Internet]. Geneva; 2015 [cited 2017 Mar 9]. p. 29. Available from: http://apps.who.int/iris/bitstream/10665/176712/1/9789241564991_eng.pdf?ua=1.
3. World Health Organization. A framework for malaria elimination [Internet]. Geneva; 2017 [cited 2018 Jan 11]. p. 100. Available from: http://apps.who.int/iris/bitstream/10665/254761/1/9789241511988-eng.pdf?ua=1.
4. 1. Ministry of Health and Sports. National Strategic Plan for Intensifying Malaria Control and Accelerating Progress towards Malaria Elimination (2016-2020) [Internet]. Myanmar; 2016 [cited 2017 Mar 9]. p. 47. Available from: http://www.searo.who.int/myanmar/documents/malarianationalstrategicplan2016-2020.pdf?ua=1.
5. Smith Gueye C, Sanders KC, Galappaththy GN, Rundi C, Tobgay T, Sovannaroth S, et al. Active case detection for malaria elimination: a survey among Asia Pacific countries. Malar J. 2013;12(1):358.
6. Cao J, Sturrock HJW, Cotter C, Zhou S, Zhou H, Liu Y, et al. Communicating and monitoring surveillance and response activities for malaria elimination: China's '1-3-7' strategy. PLoS Med. 2014;11(5):1–6.
7. Zhou S-S, Zhang S-S, Zhang L, Rietveld AEC, Ramsay AR, Zachariah R, et al. China's 1-3-7 surveillance and response strategy for malaria elimination: is case reporting, investigation and foci response happening according to plan? Infectious Diseases of Poverty. 2015;4(1):55.
8. Wang D, Cotter C, Sun X, Bennett A, Gosling RD, Xiao N. Adapting the local response for malaria elimination through evaluation of the 1–3–7 system performance in the China–Myanmar border region. Malar J. 2017;16(1):54.
9. Feng J, Liu J, Feng X, Zhang L, Xiao H, Xia Z. Towards malaria elimination: monitoring and evaluation of the "1-3-7" approach at the China-Myanmar border. Am J Trop Med Hyg. 2016 Oct 5;95(4):806–10.
10. 1. Ministry of Health and Sports. National Plan for Malaria Elimination in Myanmar 2016-2030 [Internet]. Nay Pyi Taw; 2016 [cited 2017 Mar 9]. p. 72. Available from: http://www.searo.who.int/myanmar/documents/nationalplanformalariaeliminationinmyanmar2016-2030.pdf?ua=1.
11. Ministry of Health and Sports. Standard Operating Procedure for Malaria Interventions in RAI Project Areas. Nay Pyi Taw; 2017 [unpublished].
12. Ministry of Health and Sports. Health in Myanmar 2014 [Internet]. Ministry of Health. 2014 [cited 2018 Jan 14]. p. 1–142. Available from: http://mohs.gov.mm/Main/content/publication/health-in-myanmar-2014.
13. Minsitry of Health and Sports. National malaria control programme-Annual report 2015. Nay Pyi Taw; 2016 [unpublished].
14. World Health Organisation. WHO malaria terminology [Internet]. Geneva; 2017 [cited 2017 Mar 30]. p. 38. Available from: http://apps.who.int/iris/bitstream/handle/10665/208815/WHO_HTM_GMP_2016.6_eng.pdf?sequence=1 .
15. Cotter C, Sudathip P, Herdiana H, Cao Y, Liu Y, Luo A, et al. Piloting a programme tool to evaluate malaria case investigation and reactive case detection activities: results from 3 settings in the Asia Pacific. Malar J. 2017; 16(1):347.
16. Lu G, Liu Y, Beiersmann C, Feng Y, Cao J, Müller O. Challenges in and lessons learned during the implementation of the 1-3-7 malaria surveillance and response strategy in China: a qualitative study. Infectious Diseases of Poverty. 2016;5(1):94.
17. Canavati SE, Quintero CE, Lawford HLS, Yok S, Lek D, Richards JS, et al. High mobility, low access thwarts interventions among seasonal workers in the Greater Mekong Sub-region: lessons from the malaria containment project. Malar J. 2016;15(1):434.

13

Awareness of malaria and treatment-seeking behaviour among persons with acute undifferentiated fever in the endemic regions of Myanmar

Phyo Aung Naing[1*], Thae Maung Maung[1], Jaya Prasad Tripathy[2], Tin Oo[1], Khin Thet Wai[1] and Aung Thi[3]

Abstract

Background: Myanmar has a high burden of malaria with two-third of the population at risk of malaria. One of the basic elements of the Roll Back Malaria Initiative to fight against malaria is early diagnosis and treatment within 24 h of fever. Public awareness about malaria is a key factor in malaria prevention and control and in improving treatment-seeking behaviour.

Methods: A large community-based survey was carried out in 27 townships of malaria endemic regions in Myanmar in 2015 which reported on the knowledge, behaviour and practices around malaria in the general population. We used the data already collected in this survey to assess (i) general public awareness of malaria and (ii) treatment-seeking behaviour and associated factors among persons with acute undifferentiated fever.

Results: A total of 6597 respondents from 6625 households were interviewed (response rate of 99.5%). About 85% of the respondents were aware that mosquito bite was the mode of transmission of malaria and 90% mentioned that malaria was preventable. However, only 16% of the respondents knew about anti-malaria drug resistance. There were certain misconceptions about the transmission of malaria such as dirty water, same blood group, sharing shelter, sleeping/eating together and poor hygiene. Health facility staff were the most common source of information about malaria (80%). Nearly one-fourth (23%) of the respondents with fever resorted to self-medication. Around 28% of the respondents with fever underwent blood testing, less than half of whom (44%) were tested within 24 h. Elderly age group, females, those with poor knowledge about malaria and those residing in non-Regional Artemisinin Resistance Initiative townships were associated with poor treatment-seeking behaviour in case of fever.

Conclusion: Although there is fair knowledge on mosquito bite as a mode of transmission and prevention of malaria, there are some misconceptions about transmission of malaria. Those having poor knowledge about malaria have poor treatment-seeking behaviour. A considerable number of respondents seek care from informal care providers and seek care late. Thus, there is a need to promote awareness about the role of early diagnosis and appropriate treatment and address misconceptions about transmission of malaria.

Keywords: Treatment-seeking behaviour, Myanmar, Malaria/diagnosis, Health knowledge, Attitudes, Practice, Plasmodium infections

* Correspondence: phyoaungnaing84@gmail.com
[1]Department of Medical Research, Ministry of Health and Sports, No. 5, Ziwaka Road Dagon Township, Yangon 11191, Myanmar
Full list of author information is available at the end of the article

Background

Malaria is an acute febrile illness caused by *Plasmodium* parasite. It is considered a serious public health threat because of its severity and often fatal outcome. Over half of the population is known to be at risk of malaria globally; and most of them are children under-5 years of age [1]. World Health Organization (WHO) reports that in the Asia and Pacific region, which covers 22 countries, about 2.1 billion people (80% of the total population) are at risk of getting malaria. A total of 212 million cases and an estimated 429,000 deaths were reported in 2015 globally [1].

Myanmar has a high burden of malaria with more than two-third of the population at risk of malaria. Myanmar has the greatest malaria incidence in the Greater Mekong Sub-region (GMS) with 253 cases per 100,000 population [2]. A total of 183,000 confirmed cases were reported in the country in 2015 against an estimated number of 240,000 [3]. Myanmar, located in the tropical zone, provides a favourable wet and moist climate for breeding of *Anopheles* mosquito. Nearly three-fourth of the cases of malaria are caused by *Plasmodium falciparum*. Myanmar is at the third position among the countries in the South East Asian Region (SEAR) with contribution of malaria cases, and at top among the countries in GMS which is known for artemisinin resistance [4].WHO has emphasised early diagnosis and prompt treatment within 24 h of onset of symptoms to decrease the risk of severe complications and onward transmission [5]. One of the basic elements of the Roll Back Malaria Initiative to fight against malaria is early diagnosis and treatment of malaria (EDTM). It is thus recommended that patients should seek early medical advice following the onset of fever, a common symptom of malaria [5].

Studies in the SEAR such as Bangladesh, India, Nepal and Bhutan have found that public awareness about malaria is a key factor in malaria prevention and control. It also plays a key role in improving treatment-seeking behaviour [6–9]. Earlier studies in this region have reported that poor treatment-seeking behaviour was associated with poor socio-economic status, rural residence, proximity to health facilities, accessibility to trained providers, availability of transportation and knowledge of malaria [10–13]. However the studies in Myanmar were done in a selected sample and thus did not represent the whole country [11, 12, 14, 15].

A large community-based survey was carried out in the endemic regions of Myanmar in 2015 which reported on the knowledge, behaviour and practices around malaria in the general population. We used the data already collected in this survey to assess (i) general public awareness of malaria and source of information about malaria and (ii) treatment-seeking behaviour and associated factors among persons with acute undifferentiated fever in the previous 2 weeks. This information would be useful in designing appropriate health education content and in formulating effective interventions to improve health-seeking behaviour in the event of fever in the endemic regions.

Methods

Study design

It was a cross-sectional analytical study involving analysis of secondary data from a community-based survey conducted by the National Malaria Control Program (NMCP) in Myanmar in 2015. The key outcome variables are knowledge about cause, transmission and prevention of malaria and drug resistance. Other outcome variables are the proportion of respondents with undifferentiated fever who had poor treatment-seeking behaviour, got their blood tested for malaria and timing of test done.

General setting

The Republic of the Union of Myanmar is one of the South East Asian countries neighboured by countries like Bangladesh, India, China, Laos and Thailand in the North and East [16]. It is divided administratively, into the capital territory (Nay Pyi Taw Council Territory), seven states and seven regions. There are 74 districts with 330 townships. According to the last census, Myanmar has an estimated population of 51.5 million with nearly 70% residing in rural areas [17]. Ministry of Health and Sports (MOHS) provides health care services to the whole population through hospitals by Department of Medical Services (DMS). Primary health care services are provided by the Department of Public Health especially in the rural areas [3].

Specific setting: epidemiological profile, intervention policies and strategies for malaria in Myanmar

Malaria is endemic in 284 out of 330 townships in Myanmar. The country constitutes of high transmission (> 1 case per 1000 population), low transmission (0–1 case per 1000 population) and malaria-free areas (zero cases) represented by 16, 44 and 40% of the total population, respectively [2]. It remains a public health problem due to climatic and ecological changes, population migration and ecological development activities such as mining, forestry and development of drug resistant *Plasmodium falciparum* parasite.

In Myanmar, National Malaria Control Programme (NMCP) is carrying out malaria control activities in line with the Global and National Malaria Control Strategies in collaboration with national and international partners. The key programme interventions include information, education and communication; free distribution of insecticide-treated nets in areas of high malaria transmission; indoor residual spraying; diagnostic testing for suspected malaria cases; and artemisinin-based combination therapy (ACT), all of which are provided free-of-cost. According to the anti-malarial treatment policy, case management with ACT was initiated in all endemic townships in 2009 [18].

Community-based survey

A nationwide community-based survey was conducted jointly by the Department of Medical Research (DMR) and NMCP in 2015 to understand the knowledge, attitude and health-seeking behaviour towards malaria in the general population in all endemic States and Regions of Myanmar except Mandalay Region and Chin State. A multistage sampling procedure was used in this survey. Firstly, 27 townships were selected using the probability proportionate to size (PPS) method. At the township level, 8 villages were randomly selected from each township. In each village, 25–30 households were systematically selected by using a predefined list of village households. Figure 1 shows a map depicting the malaria endemic townships where the community-based survey was carried out. In the selected households, face to face interview was conducted with preferably the female adult respondent or any other adult using a semi-structured questionnaire by trained interviewers. Questionnaires were pre-tested and all interviewers were well trained in each State/Region by NMCP and DMR.

A total of 6625 households in 216 villages located in 27 townships were covered out of which 6597 respondents completed the interview. Survey data was double entered and validated using EpiData Entry software (version 3.1, EpiData Association, Odense, Denmark). This community-based malaria survey database is available with the NMCP, Ministry of Health and Sports, Myanmar.

Study population

For the first objective, the study population comprises of the general population in endemic regions of Myanmar covered under the survey. Persons with acute undifferentiated fever in the last 2 weeks in endemic regions of Myanmar constitute the study population for the second objective.

Operational definition

Poor treatment-seeking behaviour is defined as no medication or self-medication or seeking treatment from traditional healer.

Knowledge score

Questions related to knowledge about malaria—its transmission, prevention, anti-malarial drug resistance and management were scored as 1 (yes) and 0 (no). A total of 14 questions on the abovementioned questions were included in the scoring with a Cronbach's score of

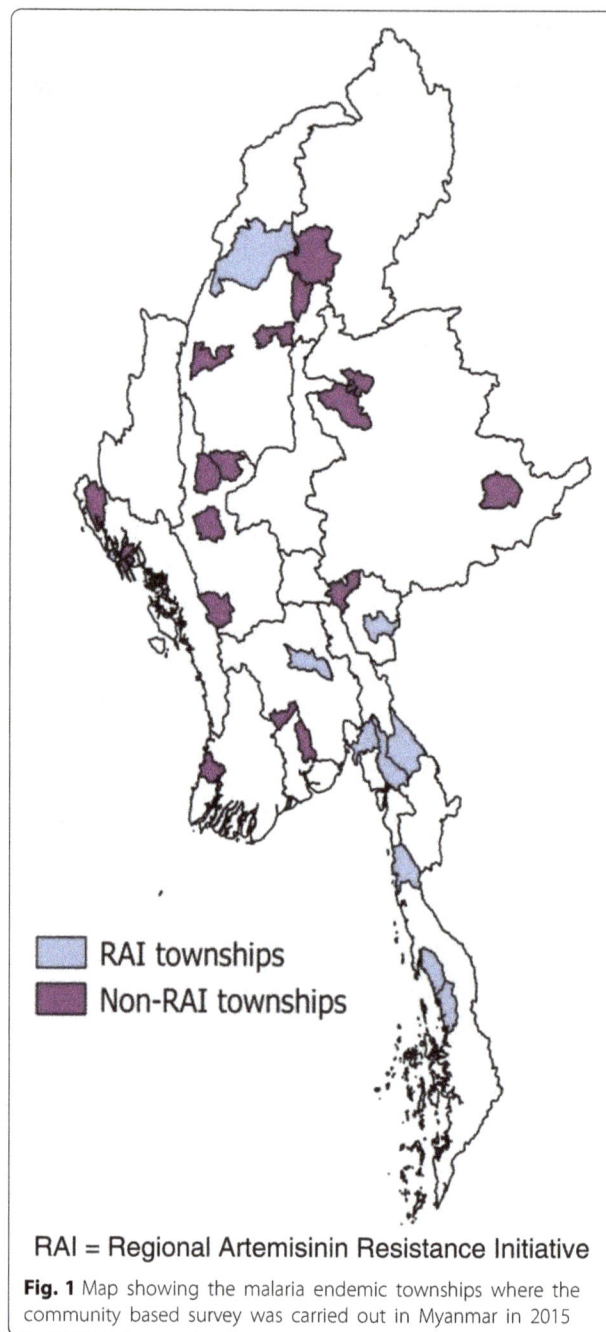

Fig. 1 Map showing the malaria endemic townships where the community based survey was carried out in Myanmar in 2015

0.76 (measure of internal reliability). The maximum and minimum scores were 0 and 14. The median (IQR) of the scores was 7 (3–10). The scores were then added up to get a knowledge score for each individual in the survey. The score was then categorised into high and low based on the median cut-off value.

Regional Artemisinin Resistance Initiative (RAI) townships

In 2009–2010, Myanmar reported suspected artemisinin resistance. Myanmar Artemisinin Resistance Containment (MARC) Framework was developed and endorsed

Awareness of malaria and treatment-seeking behaviour among persons with acute undifferentiated fever...

141

in April 2011 to control the emergence of artemisinin resistance. Areas of artemisinin resistance are stratified into three Tiers. *Tier 1* are areas where there is credible evidence of artemisinin resistance; *tier 2* includes areas with significant inflow of people from tier 1, including those immediately bordering Tier 1; *tier 3* are areas with no evidence of artemisinin resistance and limited contact with Tier 1 areas. There are 31 townships in tier 1, 21 in tier 2 and 258 in tier 3. In 2013, the project was transferred to the Three Millennium Development Goal (3MDG) and renamed as Regional Artemisinin Initiative (RAI) in March, 2014. The RAI project area includes 52 townships in tiers 1 and 2. In 2015, the RAI area was expanded to 72 townships, and in 2016, the RAI area was further extended up to 76 townships [19]

Data analysis

Data were extracted from EpiData database and imported into STATA (version 11, StataCorp, TX, USA) for analysis. Measures of descriptive statistics, i.e. proportions were used to summarise categorical variables related to knowledge about malaria-its transmission, prevention, drug resistance and management and source of information. These are presented in the form of bar diagrams. Incidence of fever was reported by different socio-demographic characteristics in the form of proportions. Chi-square test was used to study the association between socio-demographic variables and poor treatment-seeking behaviour. Multivariable logistic analysis (enter method) was performed to find out the factors associated with poor treatment-seeking behaviour in the event of fever. Due to the clustered sample design and non-response in the survey, weights were calculated where each participant was given a value/weight. Sampling and non-response weights were used to calculate the final weight which is a product of the two weights. This study reports weighted estimates.

Results

Community awareness about malaria

Out of 6625 households, 6597 respondents, i.e. one respondent from each household (response rate of 99.5%), completed the interview. There were 31,165 members in these households.

Of all the household respondents interviewed, 5771 (87.5%) had heard of malaria, among whom 5004 (87%) knew mosquito bites as the mode of transmission of malaria. Besides, other common misconceptions around transmission of malaria included drinking dirty water (13%), poor hygiene (6.4%), same blood group (5.3%), sharing shelter (4%), bad food (3.8%) and sleeping together (3%). Figure 2 Nearly 90% of respondents were of the view that malaria is preventable. The common methods of preventing malaria as reported by the respondents were mosquito nets (76%) followed by ITNs (28.9%) Fig. 3.

Again, 90% of the respondents said that malaria can be treated, and among whom, 85% believed that modern medicine could treat malaria. Around 16.3% of the respondents were aware of anti-malarial drug resistance. The common methods for preventing drug resistance as reported are sleeping under ITN (49%) and protection from mosquito bite in the forest (21%) (Fig. 4). Figure 5 shows that health facility staff (80%) was the most common source of information about malaria followed by Village Health Volunteer (VHV)/Village MidWife (VMW) (28%) and family/friends/neighbours (16%).

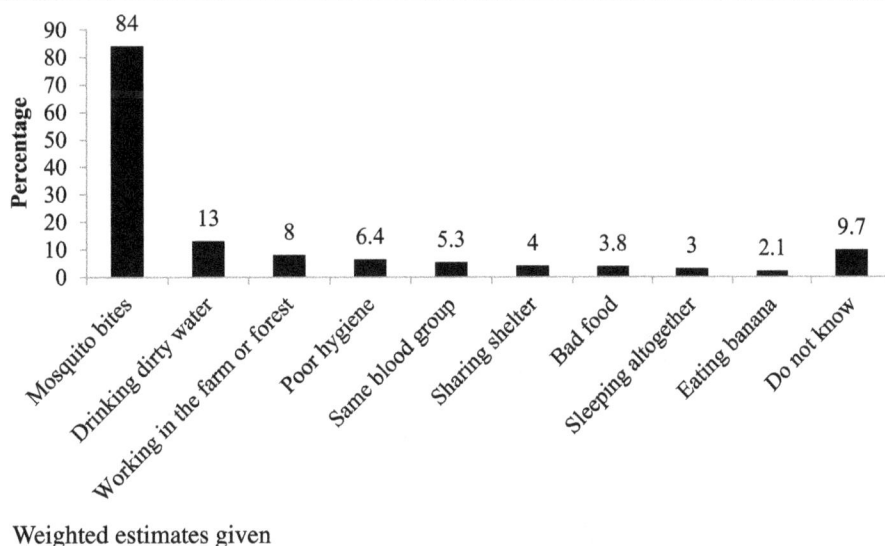

Weighted estimates given

Fig. 2 Awareness about cause and transmission of malaria among the general population in the endemic regions of Myanmar in 2015

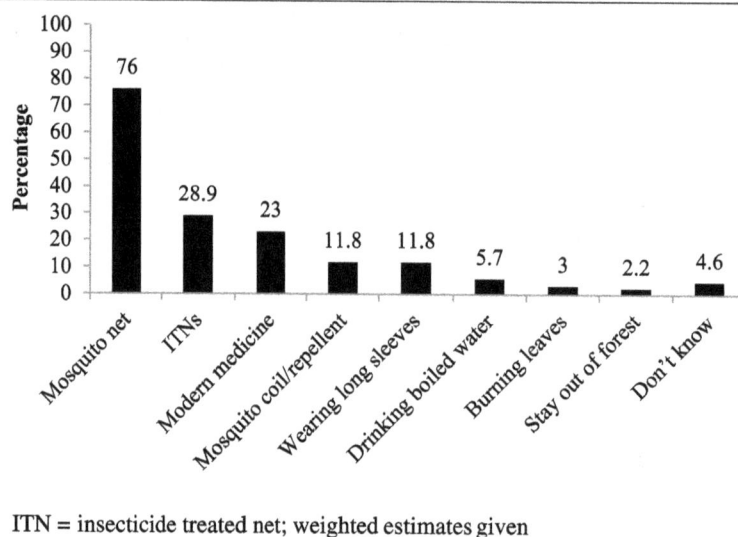

ITN = insecticide treated net; weighted estimates given

Fig. 3 Awareness about prevention of malaria among the general population in the endemic regions of Myanmar in 2015

Treatment-seeking behaviour for acute undifferentiated fever

Of 6597 households, 938 (14.2%) households had any family member contracting fever within the last 2 weeks. Among 31,165 household members contacted, 1180 (3.8%) had fever within the last 2 weeks. The incidence of fever was significantly higher among children < 5 years ($p < 0.001$, 9.4%), certain occupation groups and manual labourers (4.8–5.0%) and those who had high knowledge scores ($p = 0.04$, 4.8%). Table 1.

Among persons with undifferentiated fever, only 28.2% underwent a blood test for confirmation of diagnosis.

Less than half (~ 44%) of the blood tests were done within 24 h of fever. Nearly half of the respondents with fever approached a government health facility (48.4%) for treatment followed by self-medication (22.8%) and private clinic (22.1%) Table 2.

Elderly age group 60 years and above (9.0, 95% CI = 6.0–17.2, $p = 0.01$), female sex (1.5, 95% CI = 1.0–1.9, $p = 0.03$), illiteracy (3.5, 95% CI = 2.0–7.8, $p = 0.0018$), poor knowledge about malaria (2.9, 95% CI = 1.6–6.2, $p < 0.001$) and non-RAI townships (2.0, 95% CI = 1.4–2.6, $p < 0.001$) are associated with poor treatment behaviour in case of fever Table 3.

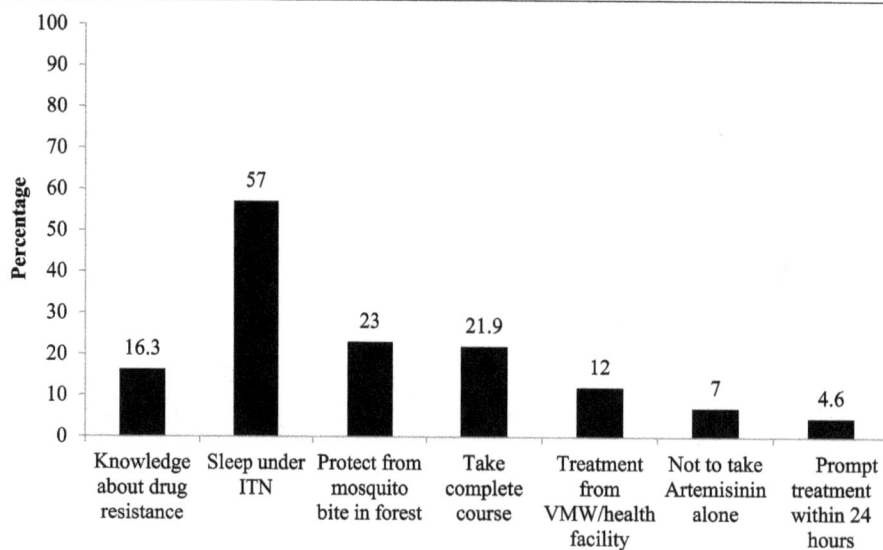

ITN = insecticide treated net, VMW = village Midwife, weighted estimates given

Fig. 4 Awareness about anti-malarial drug resistance and its prevention among the general population in the endemic regions of Myanmar in 2015

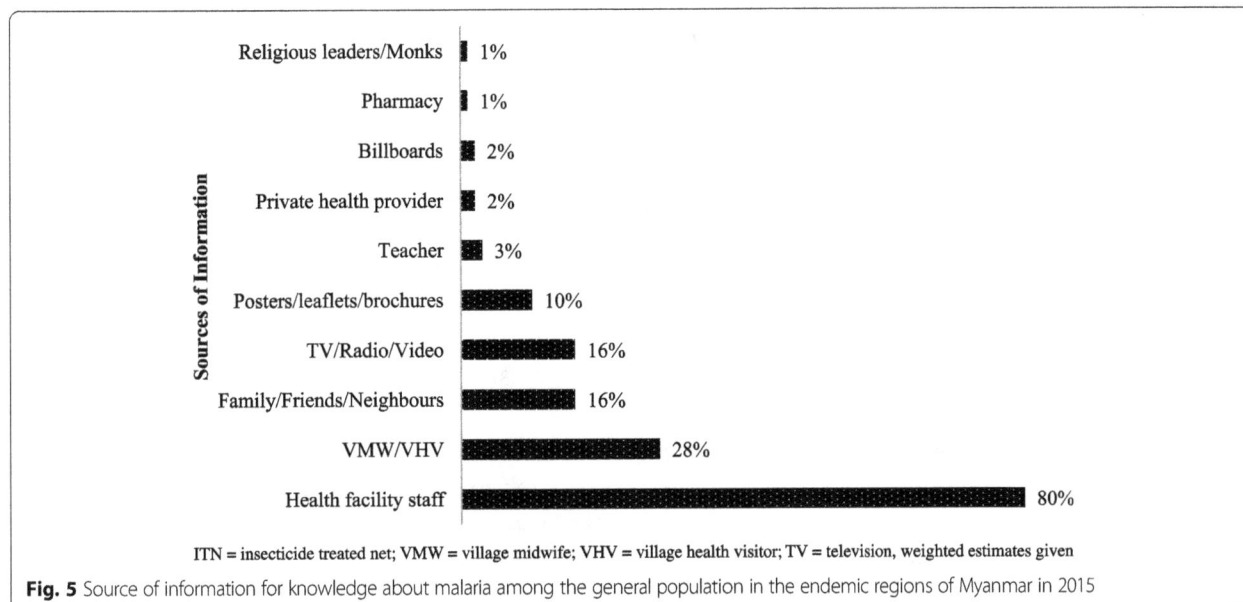

ITN = insecticide treated net; VMW = village midwife; VHV = village health visitor; TV = television, weighted estimates given

Fig. 5 Source of information for knowledge about malaria among the general population in the endemic regions of Myanmar in 2015

Discussion

The key highlights of the study are (a) although there is fair knowledge about transmission and prevention of malaria, there is poor awareness about anti-malarial drug resistance and certain misconceptions about the transmission of malaria, (b) health facility staff and VHV/ VMW are the most common source of information about malaria, (c) nearly one-fourth of the respondents with fever resorted to self-medication, (d) less than one-third of the respondents with fever underwent blood testing; less than half of whom were tested within 24 h, and (e) elderly, females, those with poor knowledge about malaria and those residing in non-RAI townships were associated with poor treatment-seeking behaviour in case of fever.

Overall, there was fair knowledge about mosquito bites as a mode of transmission and prevention of malaria. The majority of the respondents reported that malaria could be transmitted from person-to-person through mosquito bites and could be prevented by the use of mosquito net. On the other hand, many misconceptions emerged around transmission of malaria, such as drinking dirty water, same blood group, sharing shelter, sleeping/eating together and poor hygiene. There was poor knowledge about drug resistance, its cause and prevention. These findings were consistent with other studies from Myanmar [20, 21]. The participants related malaria to water, food, hygiene and proximity which indicates poor awareness in the community. Although many people knew about the correct mode of transmission of malaria, i.e. mosquito bite, people who knew that also had some misconceptions as they cited multiple modes of transmission. Thus, a clear simple message that mosquito bite is the only mode of transmission of malaria

should be disseminated. Also, health facility staff and others such as VMW/VHV, being the most common source of information about malaria, should be mobilised for disseminating the health education content. Other channels of dissemination such as television/ radio/print media/village meetings should also be utilised in health education campaigns depending on the local context. Health education campaign should be designed to address the knowledge gaps identified in this study such as anti-malarial drug resistance, prevention of drug resistance through early diagnosis and treatment and misconceptions around the transmission of malaria.

Anti-malarial drug resistance is a major threat in this region with the emergence of artemisinin drug resistance. Prevention of drug resistance requires improving the way drugs are used through rational prescribing, better follow-up practices and patient compliance and discouraging self-medication or medication from informal providers [22]. The present study showed poor public awareness about drug resistance and its prevention and also reported substantial proportion of self-medication. Improving general awareness about drug resistance and its prevention might lead to improved compliance to therapy [23]. Thus, health education campaigns must be tailored to plug the gaps around causes and prevention of drug resistance in order to prevent the emergence and spread of resistance.

Nearly one-fourth of the respondents with fever resorted to self-medication. Available published literature shows that self-medication and seeking assistance from drug vendors were the most common practices in certain regions of Myanmar [12]. With 80% target of providing appropriate treatment within 24 h, WHO advocates strategies to improve home-based management

Table 1 Socio-demographic characteristics of the respondents who reported fever within 2 weeks in the endemic regions of Myanmar, 2015

Characteristics		Total	Reported fever within 2 weeks n (%, 95% CI)	p value
Age group				p < 0.001
	Under 5	2673	250 (9.4, 7.2–12.0)	
	5–14	6638	337 (5.1, 3.3–7.3)	
	15–59	18,989	510 (2.7, 1.3–5.4)	
	60 and above	2793	83 (3.0, 1.2–4.8)	
Sex				p = 0.09
	Male	15,069	599 (4.0, 3.0–6.1)	
	Female	16,096	581 (3.6, 2.4–5.0)	
Occupation				p < 0.001
	Agriculture	18,950	625(3.4, 2.0–5.0)	
	Seller	2316	73(3.2, 1.4–5.5)	
	Casual labour	6719	325(4.8, 2.9–7.0)	
	Others	2785	138(5.0, 3.0–6.9)	
Education				p = 0.088
	Illiterate	4429	182(4.1, 3.0–5.0)	
	Up to primary	17,234	660(3.8, 2.3–5.5)	
	High school	8191	310(4.0, 2.8–5.4)	
	Higher education	805	18(2.2, 1.6–3.0)	
Townships				p = 0.18
	RAI	11,775	471(4.0, 3.1–5.0)	
	Non-RAI Townships	18,995	702(3.7, 2.8–4.8)	
Knowledge about malaria				p = 0.04
	High	1432	69(4.8, 3.0–6.8)	
	Low	29,733	1111(3.7, 2.6–5.0)	

Weighted estimates given
RAI Regional Artemisinin Resistance Initiative

Table 2 Source of treatment and timing of blood test by age group among persons with undifferentiated fever within 2 weeks in the endemic regions of Myanmar in 2015

Age group (in years)		Under 5 (n = 246)	5–15 (n = 336)	15–59 (n = 504)	60 and above (n = 81)	Total (n = 1167)
Source of treatment		n (%)	n (%)	n (%)	n (%)	n (%)
	No medication taken	3 (1.2)	11 (3.3)	9 (1.8)	3 (3.7)	26 (2.2)
	Self-medication	42 (17.1)	78 (23.2)	128 (25.4)	18 (22.2)	266 (22.8)
	Traditional healer	8 (3.3)	10 (3.0)	17 (3.4)	5 (6.2)	40 (3.4)
	Government's Health Centre	135(54.9)	155(46.2)	240(47.7)	34(41.9)	564(48.4)
	Private Health Centre	58(23.5)	78(23.2)	102(20.2)	19(23.5)	257(22.1)
	Others/DNK	0 (0)	4 (1.2)	8 (1.6)	2(2.5)	14 (1.2)
Blood test done		55 (22.5)	88 (26.2)	162 (32.1)	20 (24.7)	325 (27.8)
Timing of blood test		(N = 55)	(N = 88)	(N = 162)	(N = 20)	(N = 325)
	Within 24 h	26 (47.3)	35 (39.8)	75 (46.3)	8 (40.0)	144 (44.3)
	24–48 h	19 (34.6)	29 (33.0)	49 (30.3)	7 (35.0)	104 (32.0)
	More than 48 h	7 (12.7)	21 (23.9)	25 (15.4)	3 (15.0)	56 (17.2)
	Not sure	3 (5.5)	3 (3.4)	13 (8.0)	2 (10.0)	21 (6.5)

Weighted estimates given
DNK do not know

Table 3 Association of socio-demographic characteristics of respondents with poor treatment-seeking behaviour of those who reported fever within the last 2 weeks in the endemic regions of Myanmar, 2015

Characteristics		Total N	Poor treatment seeking behaviour (N)	Crude OR (95% CI)	p value	Adjusted OR (95% CI)	p value
Age group					0.008		
	Under 5	246	53	1.0		1.0	
	5–14	334	99	1.5 (1.1–2.3)		1.3 (0.8–2.5)	0.3
	15–59	500	154	1.6 (1.1–2.3)		1.4 (0.8–2.3)	0.2
	60 and above	81	64	10.7 (7.4–19.4)		9.0 (6.0–7.2)	0.01
Sex					0.008		
	Male	594	152	1.0		1.0	
	Female	567	181	1.4 (1.1–1-8)		1.5 (1.0–1.9)	0.03
Occupation					0.9		
	Agriculture	625	178	1.0		–	
	Seller	73	21	1.0 (0.6–1.7)		–	
	Casual labourer	319	94	1.1 (0.8–1.4)		–	
	Others	137	38	0.9 (0.6–1.5)		–	
Education level					< 0.001		
	Illiterate	177	88	3.4 (1.8–8.7)		3.3 (1.8–7.9)	0.0018
	Up to primary	656	172	1.2 (0.4–3.8)		1.0 (0.5–3.2)	0.3
	Middle and High school	307	68	1.0 (0.3–3.1)		0.8 (0.3–2.9)	0.5
	Higher education	18	04	1.0		1.0	
Knowledge score about malaria					< 0.001		
	Low	1092	329	3.8 (1.7–8.4)		2.9 (1.6–6.2)	<0.001
	High	69	07	1.0		1.0	
Type of townships							
	RAI townships	466	102	1.0	< 0.001	1.0	
	Non-RAI townships	695	231	1.8 (1.4–2.3)		2.0 (1.4–2.6)	<0.001

OR odds ratio, RAI Regional Artemisinin Resistance Initiative

Poor treatment-seeking behaviour is defined as no medication or self-medication or seeking treatment from traditional healer; weighted estimates given

of malaria, with drug retailers being seen as one possible channel [24, 25]. This could be one of strategies addressing timely and appropriate treatment of malaria in Myanmar.

A majority of respondents did not seek appropriate care within 24 h of fever. Delays of more than 24 h in care seeking has also been reported in other settings as well [12, 26]. More efforts are needed to ensure prompt malaria diagnosis and treatment since case fatality rises if treatment is delayed beyond 24 h after the onset of clinical symptoms [1]. The study reports that among those with undifferentiated fever, less than one-third get their blood tests done for malaria despite the fact that most of them seek care. This calls for intervention at the level of the health care provider including the drug retailers in terms of educating them on the need for testing for malaria in any case of fever before starting antimalarial medications. Those who get their blood tested for malaria, less than half get it done within 24 h which

requires a wider engagement of the community and rapid access to RDTs [27].

The study showed that families were more likely to seek appropriate care if patients were male or children under 15 years old similar to another cross-sectional study in Myanmar [12]. Women are dependent on family members for seeking care and thus, usually start with home remedies at the onset of symptoms which partly explains their poor treatment-seeking behaviour. On the other hand, there is more emphasis on children in a family and they are likely to be assisted by a caregiver in seeking treatment. Thus, programme interventions to improve treatment-seeking behaviour should prioritise these vulnerable groups.

It was also found that those who had greater knowledge score about malaria were over two times more likely to seek care from trained providers than those without sufficient knowledge which is supported by other studies in the literature [11, 28]. This also supports another finding in this study which reports significantly higher incidence of fever in respondents who had a higher knowledge score. This might be due to the fact that awareness about the condition leads to timely and appropriate decision making about seeking care. Future efforts should focus on improving knowledge for malaria treatment and prevention, particularly in endemic regions.

Strengths and limitations

The major strengths of the study were that the data were obtained from a large national representative survey covering all the endemic regions of Myanmar; the response rate was high; the interviewers were well trained and supervised; and the subject is an identified national operational research priority. Data quality was ensured though double data entry and validation using EpiData entry software. We also adhered to The Strengthening the Reporting of Observational Studies in Epidemiology (STROBE) guidelines for the reporting of observational studies [29].

The study had some limitations as well. The study could not provide detailed information on early diagnosis and appropriate treatment (EDAT) pathway. The study also did not explore reasons for not seeking appropriate treatment in case of fever. Further qualitative studies are required to understand the reasons for the same.

Conclusion

To conclude, although there is fair knowledge on transmission and prevention of malaria, there are some misconceptions about the transmission of malaria. Those having poor knowledge about malaria seemed to have poor treatment-seeking behaviour. A considerable number of respondents seek care from informal care providers and seek appropriate care late. There is a need to focus on specific targeted groups, promote awareness on the role of early diagnosis and treatment and address misconceptions about transmission of malaria.

Abbreviations

ACT: Artemisinin based combination therapy; DMR: Department of Medical Research; DMS: Department of Medical Services; DOPH: Department of Public Health; EDAT: Early diagnosis and appropriate treatment; EDTM: Early Diagnosis and Treatment of Malaria; MOHS: Ministry of Health and Sports; NMCP: National Malaria Control Program; PPS: The probability proportionate to size; RAI: Regional Artemisinin Resistance Initiative; STROBE: The Strengthening the Reporting of Observational Studies in Epidemiology; VHV: Village health volunteer; VMW: Voluntary malaria worker; WHO: World Health Organization

Acknowledgements

This research was conducted through the Structured Operational Research and Training Initiative (SORT IT), a global partnership led by the Special Programme for Research and Training in Tropical Diseases at the World Health Organization (WHO/TDR). The model is based on a course developed jointly by the International Union Against Tuberculosis and Lung Disease (The Union) and Medécins sans Frontières (MSF/Doctors Without Borders). The specific SORT IT programme which resulted in this publication was jointly organised and implemented by the following: The Centre for Operational Research, The Union, Paris, France; The Department of Medical Research, Ministry of Health and Sports, Myanmar; The Department of Public Health, Ministry of Health and Sports, Myanmar; The Union Country Office, Mandalay, Myanmar; The Union South-East Asia Office, New Delhi, India; the Operational Research Unit (LUXOR), MSF Brussels Operational Center, Luxembourg; and Burnet Institute, Australia.

Funding

The training programme in which this paper was developed was funded by the Department for International Development (DFID), UK. The funders had no role in study design, data collection and analysis, decision to publish or preparation of the manuscript. The data collection for this survey was funded by Global Fund.

Authors' contributions

The work was conceived and designed by PAN, TMM, JPT, KTW and TO. The field study and data entry was performed by PAN, TMM and AT, and data analysis was done by PAN, TMM and JPT. PAN, TMM, JPT and KTW contributed to writing the paper. All authors read and approved the final manuscript.

Competing interests

The authors declare that they have no competing interests.

Author details

[1]Department of Medical Research, Ministry of Health and Sports, No. 5, Ziwaka Road Dagon Township, Yangon 11191, Myanmar. [2]International Union Against Tuberculosis and Lung Disease, The Union South-East Asia Regional Office, New Delhi, India. [3]National Malaria Control Program, Ministry of Health and Sports, Naypyitaw, Myanmar.

References

1. World Malaria Report 2015. Geneva: World Health Organization; 2015. http://www.who.int/malaria/publications/world-malaria-report-2015/report/en/.
2. Mu TT, Sein AA, Kyi TT, Min M, Aung NM, Anstey NM, Kyaw MP, Soe C, Kyi MM, Hanson J. Malaria incidence in Myanmar 2005–2014: steady but fragile progress towards elimination. Malar J. 2016;15:503.
3. World Health Organization. Malaria Country Profile. 2015.
4. Health in Myanmar 2014 [Internet]. Ministry of Health and Sports, Myanmar; 2014. Available from: www.moh.gov.mm. Accessed 11 Oct 2017.
5. World Health Organization. Guidelines for the treatment of malaria 3rd edition. Geneva: World Health Organization; 2015. http://apps.who.int/iris/bitstream/10665/162441/1/9789241549127_eng.pdf.
6. Ahmed S, Haque R, Haque U, Hossain A, Greenwood BM, Bojang K, Whitty CJM, Targett GA, Marchant T, et al. Knowledge on the transmission, prevention and treatment of malaria among two endemic populations of Bangladesh and their health-seeking behaviour. Malar J. 2009;8:173.
7. Joshi AB, Banjara MR. Malaria related knowledge, practices and behaviour of people in Nepal. J Vector Borne Dis. 2008;45:44–50.
8. Das A, Ravindran TKS, Jena RK, Choudhury RL, Panigrahi BB, Sharma SK, Chattopadhyay R, Chakrabarti K, Ibrahim AM, et al. Factors affecting treatment-seeking for febrile illness in a malaria endemic block in Boudh district, Orissa, India: policy implications for malaria control. Malar J. 2010;9:377.
9. Tobgay T, Pem D, Dophu U, Dumre SP, Na-Bangchang K, Torres CE. Community-directed educational intervention for malaria elimination in Bhutan: quasi-experimental study in malaria endemic areas of Sarpang district. Malar J. 2013;12:132.
10. Najnin N, Bennett CM, Luby SP. Inequalities in care-seeking for febrile illness of under-five children in urban Dhaka, Bangladesh. J Health Popul Nutr. 2011;29:523–31.
11. Aung T, Lwin MM, Sudhinaraset M, Wei C. Rural and urban disparities in health-seeking for fever in Myanmar: findings from a probability-based household survey. Malar J. 2016;15:386.

12. Xu J-W, Xu Q-Z, Liu H, Zeng Y-R. Malaria treatment-seeking behaviour and related factors of Wa ethnic minority in Myanmar: a cross-sectional study. Malar J. 2012;11:417.

13. Mazumdar S. Prevalence, risk factors and treatment-seeking behaviour for malaria: the results of a case study from the Terai region of West Bengal, India. Ann Trop Med Parasitol. 2011;105:197–208.

14. Thandar MM, Kyaw MP, Jimba M, Yasuoka J. Caregivers' treatment-seeking behaviour for children under age five in malaria-endemic areas of rural Myanmar: a cross-sectional study. Malar J. 2015;14:1.

15. Lwin MM, Sudhinaraset M, San AK, Aung T, Snow R, Guerra C, Noor A, Myint H, Mutabingwa T, et al. Improving malaria knowledge and practices in rural Myanmar through a village health worker intervention: a cross-sectional study. Malar J BioMed Central. 2014;13:5.

16. Wikipedia contributors. Myanmar [Internet]. Wikipedia, The Free Encyclopedia. [cited 2016 Aug 26] [Internet]. 2016. Available from: https://en.wikipedia.org/w/index.php?title=Myanmar&oldid=736043272. Accessed 11 Oct 2017.

17. Myanmar Information Management Unit. The 2014 Myanmar Population and Housing Census. [cited 2017 Oct 11] [Internet]. Available at: http://themimu.info/census-data.

18. Annual report 2012. Vector borne disease control programme. Yangon: Ministry of Health and Sports.

19. National Malaria Control Programme. Standard operating procedure for malaria interventions in elimination setting. 2017.

20. Hla-Shein, Than-Tun-Sein, Soe-Soe, Tin-Aung, Ne-Win, Khin-Saw-Aye. The level of knowledge, attitude and practice in relation to malaria in Oo-do village, Myanmar. Southeast Asian J Trop Med Public Health. 1998;29(3):546–9.

21. Kyawt-Kyawt S, Pearson A. Knowledge, attitudes and practices with regard to malaria control in an endemic rural area of Myanmar. Southeast Asian J Trop Med Public Health. 2004;35:53–62.

22. Boland PB. Drug resistance in malaria. World Health Organization Department of Communicable Disease Surveillance and Response [Internet]. 2001 [cited 2017 Sep 20]. Available from: http://www.who.int/csr/resources/publications/drugresist/malaria.pdf. Accessed 11 Oct 2017.

23. McNulty CAM, Boyle P, Nichols T, Clappison P, Davey P. The public's attitudes to and compliance with antibiotics. J Antimicrob Chemother. 2007;60:i63–8.

24. WHO: Scaling up home-based management of malaria. 2004, Geneva: Roll Back Malaria Department/UNICEF/UNDP/World Bank/TDR WHO/HTM/MAL/2004.1096. http://www.who.int/tdr/publications/documents/scaling-malaria.pdf. Accessed 11 Oct 2017.

25. WHO. RBM global strategic plan: roll back malaria 2005–2015. Geneva: Roll Back Malaria Partnership, World Health Organization; 2005.

26. Mitiku I, Assefa A. Caregivers' perception of malaria and treatment-seeking behaviour for under five children in Mandura District, West Ethiopia: a cross-sectional study. Malar J. 2017;16:144.

27. Landier J, Parker DM, Thu AM, Carrara VI, Lwin KM, Bonnington CA, Pukrittayakamee S, Delmas G, Nosten FH. The role of early detection and treatment in malaria elimination. Malar J. 2016;15:363.

28. Nyunt MH, Aye KM, Kyaw MP, Wai KT, Oo T, Than A, Oo HW, Phway HP, Han SS, Htun T, San KK. Evaluation of the behaviour change communication and community mobilization activities in Myanmar artemisinin resistance containment zones. Malar J. 2015;14:522.

29. von Elm E, Altman DG, Egger M, Pocock SJ, Gøtzsche PC, Vandenbroucke JP, Initiative S. The Strengthening the Reporting of Observational Studies in Epidemiology (STROBE) statement: guidelines for reporting observational studies. J Clin Epidemiol. 2008;61:344–9.

14

Evaluations of training programs to improve human resource capacity for HIV, malaria, and TB control: a systematic scoping review of methods applied and outcomes assessed

Shishi Wu[1], Imara Roychowdhury[1] and Mishal Khan[1,2*]

Abstract

Background: Owing to the global health workforce crisis, more funding has been invested in strengthening human resources for health, particularly for HIV, tuberculosis, and malaria control; however, little is known about how these investments in training are evaluated. This paper examines how frequently HIV, malaria, and TB healthcare provider training programs have been scientifically evaluated, synthesizes information on the methods and outcome indicators used, and identifies evidence gaps for future evaluations to address.

Methods: We conducted a systematic scoping review of publications evaluating postgraduate training programs, including in-service training programs, for HIV, tuberculosis, and malaria healthcare providers between 2000 and 2016. Using broad inclusion criteria, we searched three electronic databases and additional gray literature sources. After independent screening by two authors, data about the year, location, methodology, and outcomes assessed was extracted from eligible training program evaluation studies. Training outcomes evaluated were categorized into four levels (reaction, learning, behavior, and results) based on the Kirkpatrick model.

Findings: Of 1473 unique publications identified, 87 were eligible for inclusion in the analysis. The number of published articles increased after 2006, with most (n = 57, 66%) conducted in African countries. The majority of training evaluations (n = 44, 51%) were based on HIV with fewer studies focused on malaria (n = 28, 32%) and TB (n = 23, 26%) related training. We found that quantitative survey of trainees was the most commonly used evaluation method (n = 29, 33%) and the most commonly assessed outcomes were knowledge acquisition (learning) of trainees (n = 44, 51%) and organizational impacts of the training programs (38, 44%). Behavior change and trainees' reaction to the training were evaluated less frequently and using less robust methods; costs of training were also rarely assessed.

(Continued on next page)

* Correspondence: mishal.khan@lshtm.ac.uk
[1]Saw Swee Hock School of Public Health, National University of Singapore, 12 Science Drive 2 #10-01, Singapore, 117549, Singapore
[2]Communicable Diseases Policy Research Group, London School of Hygiene and Tropical Medicine, Keppel St, London WC1E 7HT, United Kingdom

(Continued from previous page)

Conclusions: Our study found that a limited number of robust evaluations had been conducted since 2000, even though the number of training programs has increased over this period to address the human resource shortage for HIV, malaria, and TB control. Specifically, we identified a lack evaluation studies on TB- and malaria-related healthcare provider training and very few studies assessing behavior change of trainees or costs of training. Developing frameworks and standardized evaluation methods may facilitate strengthening of the evidence base to inform policies on and investments in training programs.

Keywords: Scoping review, Training evaluation, Evaluation methods, Tuberculosis, HIV, Malaria

Background

It is becoming increasingly evident that strong human resources for health (HRH) are essential to improve global health, with recent studies showing that health outcomes are strongly correlated with the quality and density of healthcare providers (HCPs) [1, 2]. Despite remarkable increases in financial support to disease-specific prevention and control programs [3, 4], inadequate HRH is still a major impediment in low- and middle-income countries (LMICs), where diseases such as HIV, malaria, and tuberculosis (TB) cause substantial mortality, morbidity, and negative economic impact [1, 5, 6]. In addition to a shortage in the number of HCPs in LMICs [7], lack of training to improve capacity of staff at different service levels, inadequate geographical distribution within countries, dissatisfaction with remuneration, and low motivation along with poor staff retention contribute to the inconsistent and inadequate quality of services provided by HCPs [8]. As a result of the global health workforce crisis, more funding has been invested in strengthening HRH since 2000. Within HIV, malaria, and TB control programs, training of HCPs has been an area of focus [9]. Between 2002 and 2010, the Global Fund to Fight AIDS, TB and Malaria (the Global Fund)—the largest non-governmental funder of human resources—invested US$1.3 billion for human resource development activities, and it is estimated that more than half of this budget was invested in disease-focused training activities [9]. As a result of increasing attention and investment in strengthening HRH in HIV, malaria and TB control programs, in 2014, the Global Fund provided 16 million person-episodes of training for HCPs, which was a tenfold increase compared to the number trained in 2005 [10].

Along with this investment comes a need for evaluations to provide information for international funders and national program managers to determine if a program should continue, improve, end, or scale up, in order to ensure that resources are allocated effectively and efficiently [11]. However, we found no studies that systematically reviewed existing literature on evaluations of HCP training programs. Furthermore, there is no consensus on best practice in terms of evaluation methods applied and outcome indicators assessed; therefore,

summarizing existing literature on evaluations of HCP training is essential.

Among all the frameworks or conceptual models developed to guide conduct of training evaluations, the first and most commonly referenced framework to date is the Kirkpatrick model [12–15]. The Kirkpatrick model has been used in the design of training evaluations in business and industry in the 1960s. It forms the basis of various theories in training evaluation and has had a profound impact on other evaluation models developed subsequently [13, 16–18]. The Kirkpatrick model identifies four levels of training outcomes that can be evaluated: reaction, learning, behavior, and results [19]. The reaction level assesses how well trainees appreciated a particular training program. In practice, evaluators measure trainees' affective response to the quality and the relevance of the training program when assessing reaction [12]. The learning level assesses how well trainees have acquired intended knowledge, skills, or attitudes based on participation in the learning event. It is usually measured in the form of tests [13]. The behavior level addresses the extent to which knowledge and skills gained in training are applied on the job. Lastly, for the results level, evaluators try to capture the impact that training has had at an organizational level; this includes changes in health outcomes [12].

In light of the growing focus on and investment in improving human resource capacity for HIV, malaria, and TB control and the need for evaluations of these investments, we conducted a systematic review to investigate how frequently HIV, malaria, and TB HCP training programs have been scientifically evaluated, synthesize information on the methods and outcome indicators used, and identify areas for improvement in current training evaluation approaches.

Methods

This review was based on the systematic scoping review methodological framework designed by Arksey and O'Malley [20]. The following key steps were included when we conducted the review: (1) identifying the research question, (2) identifying relevant studies, (3) study selection, (4) charting the data, and (5) collating, summarizing, and reporting the results.

Stage 1: identifying research question

The population for this review was HCPs delivering health services related to HIV, TB, or malaria. We included doctors, nurses, healthcare workers, lay health workers, traditional health practitioners, and laboratory technicians in our definition of HCPs. Teachers and other professionals delivering health services outside their routine work were not considered HCPs. The intervention of interest was any training or capacity building activity related to health service delivery. As the purpose of this study is to identify the methods and outcomes used for training evaluations, the study design and outcomes of the included studies were left intentionally broad, and a meta-analysis was not appropriate at this stage.

Stage 2: identifying relevant studies

We conducted a search on articles published after January 1, 2000, in three electronic databases on April 28, 2016: PubMed, Embase, and Cochrane Library. In addition, we searched for relevant gray literature in Google Scholar (first 100 citations) and on six major non-government organizations' (NGOs) websites on July 18, 2016: WHO, Oxfam International, Save the Children, Community Health Workers Central (CHW Central), UNAIDS, and Target TB, UK. The search terms used are summarized in Table 1.

Stage 3: study selection

All citations were imported into EndNote X7 and duplicate citations were removed manually. A two-stage screening process for eligibility was conducted. Articles were eligible for inclusion if the studies met the inclusion and exclusion criteria (Table 2). In the first stage of screening, two researchers independently reviewed titles and abstract of the citations. Results from both researchers were compared, and titles for which an abstract was not available or for which either of the reviewers' suggested inclusion were put forward for subsequent full-text review as part of the second stage of eligibility screening. If the studies did not meet the eligibility criteria, they were excluded at this stage. Articles that could not be obtained through online databases and library searches at the National University of Singapore and London School of Hygiene and Tropical Medicine were also excluded from final analysis.

Stage 4: extracting and analyzing the data

We extracted relevant information from articles included in the final analysis using a pre-designed standardized excel sheet. Table 3 summarizes data extracted and definitions used for categorizing data. For each study, we categorized the training outcomes evaluated into four levels (reaction, learning, behavior, and results) based on the Kirkpatrick model.

Table 1 Search strategy

Database	Search terms in title or abstract	No. of papers retrieved
PubMed	(healthcare workers OR healthcare providers OR healthcare professionals OR healthcare staff OR healthcare practitioners OR health workers OR health providers OR health professionals OR health staff OR health practitioners OR health-care workers OR health-care providers OR health-care professionals OR health-care staff OR health-care practitioners)	131,755
	AND (training OR continuing professional development OR continuing medical education)	16,588
	AND (evaluat* OR assess*)	7518
	AND (tuberculosis OR TB OR HIV OR malaria OR AIDS)	707
	Limit to articles published from January 1, 2000, to April 28, 2016	525
EMBASE	(healthcare workers OR healthcare providers OR healthcare professionals OR healthcare staff OR healthcare practitioners OR health workers OR health providers OR health professionals OR health staff or health practitioners OR health-care workers OR health-care professionals OR health-care providers OR health-care practitioners OR health-care staff)	166,542
	AND (training OR continuing professional development OR continuing medical education)	21,847
	AND (evaluat* OR assess*)	10,544
	AND (malaria OR AIDS OR HIV OR tuberculosis OR TB)	927
	Limit to publication year from 2000 to 2016	806
Cochrane Library	(healthcare workers OR healthcare providers OR healthcare professionals OR healthcare staff OR healthcare practitioners OR health workers OR health providers OR health professionals OR health staff or health practitioners OR health-care workers OR health-care professionals OR health-care providers OR health-care practitioners OR health-care staff)	21,999
	AND (training OR continuing professional development OR continuing medical education)	4984
	AND (evaluat* OR asses*)	3837
	AND (malaria OR AIDS OR HIV OR tuberculosis OR TB)	314
	Limit to publication year from 2000 to 2016	249

Table 2 Inclusion and exclusion criteria

Inclusion criteria	• Study describes evaluations of HIV, malaria, or TB HCP post-graduate training programs • Study contains descriptions of the training program, methods used to evaluate the program and outcomes assessed in the evaluation. • Study was published after January 1, 2000. • Geographic areas of studies are not restricted. • Only published articles will be included.
Exclusion criteria	• Literature reviews with no primary data collection • Study describes framework or methodology proposed for training evaluation without primary data collection and analysis.

Stage 5: collating, summarizing, and reporting the results
Guided by the research question, we summarized the results on characteristics of the included studies using descriptive statistics.

Results

Summary of included studies
We retrieved a total of 1612 citations from the three databases and 400 from the gray literature search. After removing duplicates, we screened titles and abstracts of 1473 unique publications, of which 199 went through to the full-text assessment and 87 met our inclusion criteria for inclusion in the analysis (Fig. 1).

We found that the number of published articles on HCP training evaluation has increased, particularly after 2006 (Table 4). In terms of geographic distribution of studies, most ($n = 57$, 66%) took place in African countries. Compared to the number of studies in Africa, only 16 (18%) evaluation studies took place in Asian countries, and even fewer were conducted in North America ($n = 10$, 11%), Europe ($n = 2$, 2%), and South America ($n = 2$, 2%). The majority of training evaluations—44 studies (51%)—were based on HCPs providing HIV-related health services. Fewer studies were focused on HCPs providing malaria ($n = 28$, 32%) and TB ($n = 23$, 26%) related health services.

Evaluation methods used in the studies
A wide range of training evaluation methods was used. As shown in Fig. 2, the most common method was a

Table 3 Definitions of extracted data

Data extracted	Definition
Year of publication	Year in which the study was published
Study location	Country in which the study took place
Disease area	The disease area that the training program aimed to target (HIV, malaria, or tuberculosis).
Evaluation methods	
Pre- and post-training tests	Trainees were given tests on their knowledge acquisition before and after training sessions. Scores of both tests were compared.
Quantitative survey of trainees	Trainees' feedback, demographic information, or other key information used for evaluation were collected using questionnaires filled out by either trainees or evaluators via one-to-one interviews. Data was analyzed using quantitative methods.
Qualitative interviews	Trainees were interviewed one-to-one by evaluators after training. Information was collected through in-depth or semi-structured interviews. Data was analyzed using qualitative methods.
Review patient records	Patient records were extracted and patient level outcomes were compared before and after the training program or between intervention and control groups. Data sources included medical records at health facilities, patient cards, or local surveillance data.
Patient exit survey	After training programs, patients were surveyed by evaluators after consultations with trainees. A standardized questionnaire was used to record the services received by patients, drugs prescribed, or whether they were satisfied with the consultations.
Observation	Trainees' on-the-job performance was directly observed at their work place and assessed by evaluators or their supervisors.
Standardized patient	Standardized patients refer to people trained to accurately portray a specific medical condition. In this method, trainees' performance was evaluated during clinical encounters without the presence of evaluators.
Focus group discussion	Trainees were gathered in groups after training programs to discuss their experiences, feedback, and reflections on the training programs. The discussion was usually guided by a facilitator.
Cost-effective analysis	The cost of the training program was calculated and compared with the outcomes of the program.
Outcomes evaluated	
Reaction	How trainees react to the training and their perceived value of the training
Learning	To what degree trainees acquire intended knowledge, skills, and attitudes based on participation in the learning event
Behavior	To what degree trainees apply what they learned during training sessions on their job
Results	The downstream organizational outcomes/impacts that occur as a result of the training

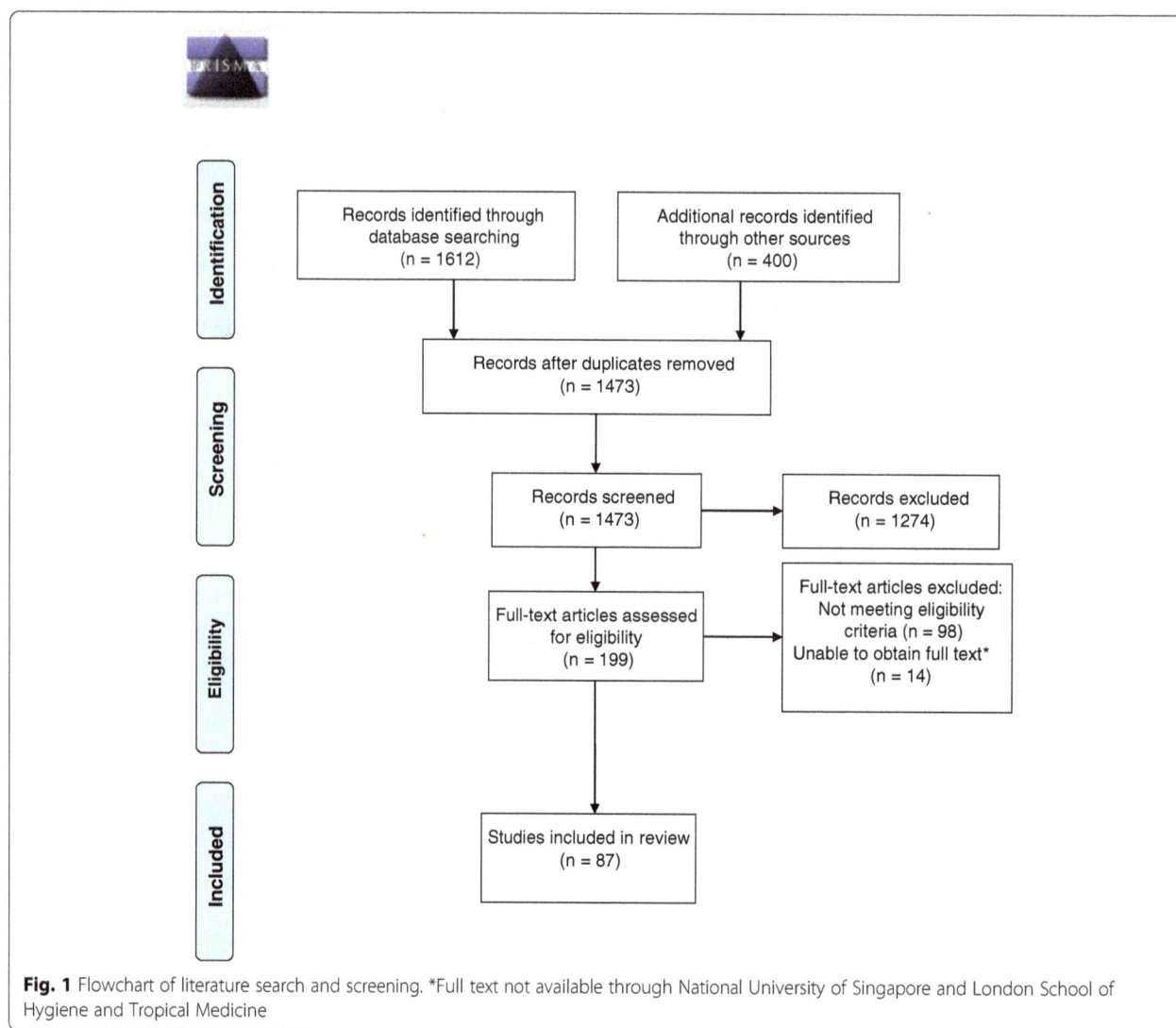

Fig. 1 Flowchart of literature search and screening. *Full text not available through National University of Singapore and London School of Hygiene and Tropical Medicine

quantitative survey of trainees ($n = 29$, 33%). Methods such as reviewing patient records ($n = 27$, 31%) to assess diagnostic and treatment outcomes after HCPs attended training session and pre- and post-training tests ($n = 24$, 28%) were also applied frequently. In contrast, only three studies (3%) evaluated on-the-job behavior change of trainees using standardized patients.

Outcomes assessed in the included studies

In terms of the outcomes evaluated among the included studies, more than half of the included studies ($n = 44$, 51%) evaluated knowledge acquisition (learning) of trainees after training sessions and 38 (44%) studies evaluated downstream results of the training programs. Fewer studies ($n = 16$, 18%) assessed whether trainees liked the program or whether the program was considered useful for trainees (reaction), and 30 (34%) measured the behavior change of trainees after they finished the training and returned to their jobs.

As summarized in Table 5, among the 16 studies evaluating trainees' reaction, more than half ($n = 9$, 56%) conducted a quantitative survey with trainees after training and only two (13%) used pre- and post-training tests to investigate whether trainees liked the training programs or felt the programs were useful to them. In terms of the learning level, the most commonly used method was pre- and post-training tests ($n = 23$, 52%). Qualitative methods such as interviews ($n = 4$, 9%) or focus group discussion ($n = 4$, 9%) were also used, albeit less frequently, when assessing knowledge gain of trainees. Observation was used commonly when assessing behavior change of trainees (11, 37%). Quantitative survey with trainees ($n = 9$, 30%) and qualitative interviews ($n = 7$, 23%) were also used to record self-reported behavior change of trainees after training programs. Additionally, three studies (10%) used standardized patients when evaluating on-the-job performance of trainees after training sessions. Finally, in terms of results on an

Table 4 Summary of included studies

Characteristic	Number of studies (n = 87)	Percentage (%)
Publication year		
2000–2002	2	2
2003–2005	4	5
2006–2008	12	14
2009–2011	25	29
2012–2014	31	36
2015–2016	13	15
Study location		
Africa	57	66
Asia	16	18
Europe	2	2
North America	10	11
South America	2	2
Disease area		
HIV	44	51
TB	23	26
Malaria	28	32

organizational level, review of patient records (n = 26, 68%) was the most commonly used method. Patient exit survey (n = 8, 21%) was also used to assess patients' experiences and satisfaction with the services provided by trainees. Even though cost of the training programs was an important indicator for program managers and policy makers, only eight studies (21%) conducted evaluations on the cost of the programs.

Discussion

Our paper provides the first synthesis of methods applied and outcomes assessed in studies evaluating HCP training for HIV, malaria, and TB service delivery. Overall, we found a fairly limited number of published evaluation studies of HCP training programs, especially in light of the number of training programs implemented

since 2000. Among the 87 training evaluation studies identified, the most commonly applied assessment methods were quantitative surveys and reviews of patient records and the most commonly assessed outcomes were learning and downstream results. Specific gaps in the literature identified were evaluations of TB- and malaria-related HCP training, evaluations conducted in Asian countries with high disease burden, and studies providing objective information on behavior change of trainees or costs of training.

While a substantial proportion (51%) of studies assessed "learning" of trainees, we found that most used pre- and post-training tests. This is likely because tests can be conducted fairly easily after training sessions without further follow-up. However, knowledge assessments using pre- and post-training tests have limitations with many experts in psychology and education stressing that knowledge acquisition is a dynamic process that may not be captured through a simple paper-based assessment [17]. Tests at the end of the training sessions are best suited for testing retention of factual knowledge [21], but for most HCP training programs, improvements in service quality are as important as retained knowledge. Therefore, assessment of behavior change of HCPs after attending training programs is critical in determining whether the objectives of the training interventions have been achieved; our findings revealed that only 30 studies across all three diseases assessed behavior change. Furthermore, behavior change was most commonly assessed through direct observation of trainees' on-the-job performance by evaluators, a method which would result in a high risk of bias because trainees' behavior would likely be altered when evaluators observed their performance during consultations [22]. Surveys and qualitative interviews asking participants if they have applied newly acquired skills were other methods, also subject to bias, commonly used in assessing behavior change of trainees [23]. While self-reporting behavior may vary by cultural context, there is a risk that trainees may not be willing to reveal that

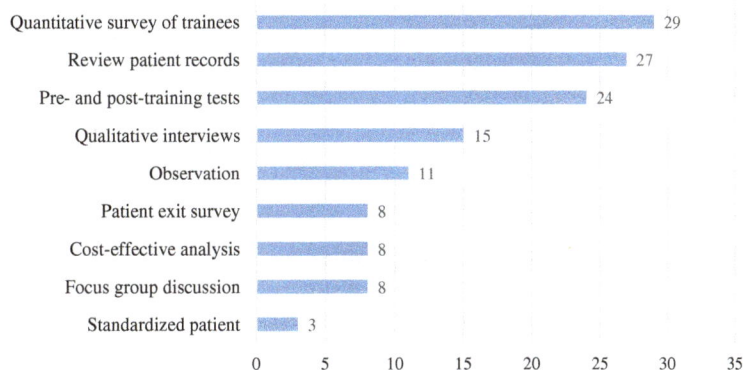
Fig. 2 Number of studies that apply each method

Table 5 Common evaluation methods for each level of the Kirkpatrick model

Level of evaluation	Common methods used	Number of studies[a]	Percentage (%)	References[a]
Reaction (n = 16)	Quantitative survey of trainees	9	56	[23, 32–39]
	Qualitative interview	5	31	[40–44]
	Focus group discussion	4	25	[36, 38, 42, 45]
	Pre- and post-training tests	2	13	[46, 47]
Learning (n = 44)	Pre- and post-training tests	23	52	[27, 33–35, 37, 43, 46–62]
	Quantitative survey	16	36	[23, 45, 63–76]
	Qualitative interview	4	9	[44, 69, 77, 78]
	Focus group discussion	4	9	[51, 56, 78, 79]
Behavior (n = 30)	Observation	11	37	[32, 33, 39, 42, 57, 63, 80–84]
	Quantitative survey of trainees	9	30	[23, 45, 62, 64, 67, 70, 72, 77, 85]
	Qualitative interview	7	23	[44, 69, 77, 78, 86–88]
	Standardized patient	3	10	[56, 89, 90]
	Review patient records	1	3	[85]
	Pre- and post-training tests	1	3	[61]
Results (n = 38)	Review patient records	26	68	[27, 28, 42, 57, 58, 66, 78, 80, 87, 91–107]
	Patient exit survey	8	21	[35, 63, 67, 108–112]
	Cost-effective analysis	8	21	[33, 35, 42, 57, 92, 97, 108, 109]
	Quantitative survey of trainees	2	5	[113, 114]
	Qualitative interview	1	3	[78]

[a]Articles may be double entered in this column

they are not using the skills learned at the training sessions to evaluators, who are often involved in conducting the original training.

An alternative method for assessing the behavior of HCP is through the use of standardized patients, which refers to people trained to accurately portray a specific medical condition [24]. This method—used in some medical schools for evaluating clinical performance—provides a structured way for evaluators to capture trainees' clinical competence and communication skills. Compared to direct observation, it minimizes bias because trainees do not know when a clinical encounter with standardized patients will occur [24, 25]. We found that this assessment method is rarely used in the evaluation of HCP training programs, possibly because it is resource and time consuming to find and train standardized patients.

In addition to assessing learning or knowledge gain, downstream results were also widely evaluated in HCP training programs. As part of these evaluations, researchers typically compared patient-level outcomes before and after training programs or between intervention and control groups by reviewing clinical records of patients who were treated by trainees participated in the training programs. For example, in TB control programs, indicators from standard guidelines, such as treatment success rate and case detection, were used as outcome indicators in evaluation of TB HCP training programs [26]. Likewise, in HIV-related training programs, indicators

such as HIV testing rate and proportion of patients with undetectable viral loads were used as outcome indicators in the training evaluation [27, 28]. However, changes in downstream organizational results, such as improved case detection or treatment success rate used in TB training programs and proportion with undetectable viral loads in HIV training programs, cannot be simply attributed to HCP training programs using, for example, a before-after evaluation approach, because training programs are often embedded within a broader national control strategy with other prevention and control activities ongoing in parallel. Downstream health outcomes are challenging to assess as they are multifactorial and complex. Other factors, such as improved supply of medical equipment or enhanced healthcare infrastructure, may also contribute to better patient outcomes. These evaluations also tend to rely on routine patient records which may vary in accuracy and completeness.

When considering impact on the wider organization or disease control program, costs of training were not widely assessed. Only eight studies assessed the cost of the training programs, even though cost is an important indicator to policymakers in making decisions on resource allocation [29].

In this scoping review, the goal-based Kirkpatrick model was used in categorizing evaluation outcomes of included studies. Even though developed in the 1960s, the Kirkpatrick model is still the most commonly used evaluation framework and formed the foundation for other goal-based evaluation frameworks developed subsequently [12–18]. For example, in the Phillips model, a fifth level, return on investment (ROI), was added to the classic four-level Kirkpatrick model to assess the cost-benefit of the training [16]. Another example is the Hamblin's five-level model, in which the result level in the Kirkpatrick model was split into two: organization and ultimate value [30]. The organization level assesses the impact on organization from the behavior changes of trainees, and the ultimate value measures the financial effects of the training program on the organization and the economy [30]. Apart from the goal-based models for training evaluation, which intend to determine whether the goals set before the start of the training were achieved, system-based models that focus on the assessment of the context and the process of the training program were also developed to guide the evaluation [31]. However, compared to goal-based models, very few system-based models provide detailed description of process involved and outcomes needed to be assessed in each step of the evaluation, which makes them less popular among evaluators [31].

In order to conduct a broad search of gray and published literature, we included three electronic databases, Google scholar, and six NGO websites and did not set language limits to exclude studies published in languages other than English. However, we recognize that we may have missed some HCP training evaluations if the studies were not published or accessible online. Additionally, since we intended to include published peer-reviewed evaluation studies, we did not analyze studies published as conference abstracts or presented as posters at conference in this review. As recognized in other scoping reviews as well, the quality of the included studies was not assessed, because the primary aim was to summarize the range of existing literature in terms of their volume, nature, and characteristics [21]. The lack of rigorous HCP training evaluation studies in current literature may reflect the limited knowledge, experience, and budget available to program managers or researchers in LMICs to conduct training evaluations. A limitation of our study is that we did not analyze qualitative information about challenges with conducting training evaluations mentioned in the studies identified; a further systematic review and analysis of the limitations mentioned in existing training evaluation studies or in interviews with program managers could be conducted in future to investigate barriers and difficulties encountered by evaluators when conducting training evaluations, particularly in LMICs. Such studies would be useful to identify strategies to increase the evidence base in this area. In addition, future studies on development of standardized training evaluation frameworks or methods would also be helpful to minimize biases in

assessment, improve accountability of evaluation results, and make HCP training evaluation more relevant to policymakers.

Conclusions

Evaluations are critical to determine the effectiveness of HCP training in order to inform decisions on future investments. However, our study found limited evidence from robust evaluations conducted since 2000, even though the number of training interventions has increased over this period to address the shortage of HRH for HIV, malaria, and TB control globally. Specifically, we found a limited number of evaluation studies on TB- and malaria-related HCP training and very few studies assessing behavior change of trainees or costs of training. More evidence from well-designed HCP training evaluations is needed, and this may be facilitated by developments in frameworks and standardized methods to assess impacts of training.

Abbreviations
HCP: Healthcare provider; HRH: Human resources for health; LMICs: Low- and middle-income countries; TB: Tuberculosis; The Global Fund: The Global Fund to Fight AIDS, TB and Malaria

Acknowledgements
Not applicable.

Funding
The systematic review was supported by the National University of Singapore.

Authors' contributions
SW designed the search strategy and conducted the literature search. SW and IR screened the titles and abstracts. SW conducted the analysis and drafted the article. MK provided advice at all stages. All authors read and approved the final manuscript.

Competing interests
The authors declare that they have no competing interests.

References
1. Dräger S, Gedik G, Dal Poz M. Health workforce issues and the Global Fund to fight AIDS, tuberculosis and malaria: an analytical review. Hum Resour Health. 2006;4:23.
2. Chen L, Evans T, Anand S, Boufford J, Brown H, Chowdhury M, Cueto M. Human resources for health: overcoming the crisis. Lancet. 2004;364:1984–90.
3. Yu D, Souteyrand Y, Banda MA, Kaufman J, Perriens JH. Investment in HIV/AIDS programs: does it help strengthen health systems in developing countries? Glob Health. 2008;4:8.

4. Ruxin J, Paluzzi J, Wilson P, Tozan Y, Kruk M, Teklehaimanot A. Emerging consensus in HIV/AIDS, malaria, tuberculosis, and access to essential medicines. Lancet. 2005;365:618–21.

5. Victoria M, Granich R, Gilks C, Gunneberg C, Hosseini M, Were W, Raviglione M, Cock K. The global fight against HIV/AIDS, tuberculosis, and malaria. Am J Clin Pathol. 2009;131:844–8.

6. Crisp N, Gawanas B, Sharp I. Training the health workforce: scaling up, saving lives. Lancet. 2008;371:689–91.

7. WHO. The World Health Report 2006: working together for health. Geneva: World Health Organization; 2006. http://www.who.int/whr/2006/whr06_en.pdf?ua=. Accessed 11 Oct 2016.

8. Figueroa-Munoz J, Palmer K, Dal Poz M, Blanc L, Bergström K, Raviglione M. The health workforce crisis in TB control: a report from high-burden countries. Hum Resour Health. 2005;3:2.

9. Bowser D, Sparkes S, Mitchell A, Bossert T, Bärnighausen T, Gedik G, Atun R. Global Fund investments in human resources for health: innovation and missed opportunities for health systems strengthening. Health Policy Plan. 2014;29:986–97.

10. The Global Fund. Results Report 2015. Geneva: The global fund to fight AIDS, tuberculosis and malaria; 2015. https://www.theglobalfund.org/media/2546/results_2015resultsreport_report_en.pdf. Accessed 11 Oct 2016.

11. Habicht J, Victora C, Vaughan J. Evaluation design for adequacy, plausibility and probability of public health programme performance and impact. Int J Epidemiol. 1999;28:10–8.

12. Bates R. A critical analysis of evaluation practice: the Kirkpatrick model and the principle of beneficence. Eval Program Plann. 2004;27:341–7.

13. Alliger G, Tannenbaum S, Bennett W, Traver H, Shotland A. A meta-analysis of the relations among training criteria. Pers Psychol. 1997;50:341–58.

14. Omar M, Gerein N, Tarin E, Butcher C, Pearson S, Heidari G. Training evaluation: a case study of training Iranian health managers. Hum Resour Health. 2009;7:20.

15. Morgan R, Casper W. Examining the factor structure of participant reactions to training: a multidimensional approach. Hum Resour Dev Q. 2000;11:301–17.

16. Phillips P, Phillips J. Symposium on the evaluation of training. Int J Train Dev. 2001;5:240–247.

17. Kraiger K, Ford J, Salas E. Application of cognitive, skill-based, and affective theories of learning outcomes to new methods of training evaluation. J Appl Psychol. 1993;78:311–28.

18. Arthur W, Bennett W, Edens P, Bell S. Effectiveness of training in organizations: a meta-analysis of design and evaluation features. J Appl Psychol. 2003;88:234–45.

19. Kirkpatrick D, Kirkpatrick J. Evaluating training programs: the four levels (3rd Edition). California: Berrett-Koehler Publishers; 2006.

20. Arksey H, O'Malley L. Scoping studies: towards a methodological framework. Int J Soc Res Methodol. 2005;8:19–32.

21. Gagne R. The conditions of learning. New York: Holt, Rine-hart &Winston; 1977.

22. Adair J. The Hawthorne effect: a reconsideration of the methodological artifact. J Appl Psychol. 1984;69:334–45.

23. Cicciò L, Makumbi M, Sera D. An evaluation study on the relevance and effectiveness of training activities in Northern Uganda. Rural Remote Health. 2010;10:1250.

24. Ebbert D, Connors H. Standardized patient experiences: evaluation of clinical performance and nurse practitioner student satisfaction. Nurs Educ Perspect. 2004;25:12–5.

25. Siminoff LA, Rogers HL, Waller AC, Harris-Haywood S, Esptein RM, Carrio FB, Gliva-McConvey G, Longo DR. The advantages and challenges of unannounced standardized patient methodology to assess healthcare communication. Patient Educ Couns. 2011;82:318–24.

26. WHO. Compendium of indicators for monitoring and evaluating national tuberculosis programs. Geneva: World Health Organization; 2004. http://apps.who.int/iris/bitstream/10665/68768/1/WHO_HTM_TB_2004.344.pdf. Accessed 11 Oct 2016.

27. Koyio LN, Sanden WJ, Dimba E, Mulder J, Creugers NH, Merkx MA, van der Ven A, Frencken JE. Oral health training programs for community and professional health care workers in Nairobi East District increases identification of HIV-infected patients. PLoS One. 2014;9:e90927.

28. Fairall L, Bachmann MO, Lombard C, Timmerman V, Uebel K, Zwarenstein M, Boulle A, Georgeu D, Colvin CJ, Lewin S, et al. Task shifting of antiretroviral treatment from doctors to primary-care nurses in South Africa (STRETCH): a pragmatic, parallel, cluster-randomised trial. Lancet. 2012;380:889–98.

29. Johns B, Baltussen R, Hutubessy R. Programme costs in the economic evaluation of health interventions. Cost Eff Resour Alloc. 2003;1:1.

30. Hamblin AC. Evaluation and control of training. New York: McGraw-Hill; 1974.

31. Zinovieff MA, Rotem A. Review and analysis of training impact evaluation methods, and proposed measures to support a United Nations system fellowships evaluation framework prepared. Geneva: WHO's Department of Human Resources for Health; 2008.

32. Bofill L, Weiss SM, Lucas M, Bordato A, Dorigo A, Fernandez-Cabanillas G, Aristegui I, Lopez M, Waldrop-Valverde D, Jones D. Motivational interviewing among HIV health care providers: challenges and opportunities to enhance engagement and retention in care in Buenos Aires, Argentina. J Int Assoc Provid AIDS Care. 2015;14:491–6.

33. Hawkes M, Katsuva JP, Masumbuko CK. Use and limitations of malaria rapid diagnostic testing by community health workers in war-torn Democratic Republic of Congo. Malar J. 2009;8:308.

34. Flys T, Gonzalez R, Sued O, Suarez Conejero J, Kestler E, Sosa N, McKenzie-White J, Monzon II, Torres CR, Page K. A novel educational strategy targeting health care workers in underserved communities in Central America to integrate HIV into primary medical care. PLoS One. 2012;7:e46426.

35. Onwujekwe O, Mangham-Jefferies L, Cundill B, Alexander N, Langham J, Ibe O, Uzochukwu B, Wiseman V. Effectiveness of provider and community interventions to improve treatment of uncomplicated malaria in Nigeria: a cluster randomized controlled trial. PLoS One. 2015;10:e0133832.

36. Sodhi S, Banda H, Kathyola D, Burciul B, Thompson S, Joshua M, Bateman E, Fairall L, Martiniuk A, Cornick R, et al. Evaluating a streamlined clinical tool and educational outreach intervention for health care workers in Malawi: the PALM PLUS case study. BMC Int Health Hum Rights. 2011;11 Suppl 2:S11.

37. Cettomai D, Kwasa J, Birbeck GL, Price RW, Bukusi EA, Meyer AC. Training needs and evaluation of a neuro-HIV training module for non-physician healthcare workers in western Kenya. J Neurol Sci. 2011;307:92–6.

38. Zolfo M, Iglesias D, Kiyan C, Echevarria J, Fucay L, Llacsahuanga E, de Waard I, Suarez V, Llaque WC, Lynen L. Mobile learning for HIV/AIDS healthcare worker training in resource-limited settings. AIDS Res Ther. 2010;7:35.

39. Beach M, Roter D, Saha S, Korthuis P, Eggly S, Cohn J, Sharp V, Moore R, Wilson I. Impact of a brief patient and provider intervention to improve the quality of communication about medication adherence among HIV patients. Patient Educ Couns. 2015;98:1078–83.

40. Gutin SA, Cummings B, Jaiantilal P, Johnson K, Mbofana F, Dawson Rose C. Qualitative evaluation of a Positive Prevention training for health care providers in Mozambique. Eval Program Plann. 2014;43:38–47.

41. Puchalski Ritchie L, Lettow M, Barnsley J, Chan A, Schull M, Martiniuk A, Makwakwa A, Zwarenstein M. Lay health workers experience of a tailored knowledge translation intervention to improve job skills and knowledge: a qualitative study in Zomba district Malawi. BMC Med Educ. 2016;16:54.

42. Dick J, Clarke M, van Zyl H, Daniels K. Primary health care nurses implement and evaluate a community outreach approach to health care in the South African agricultural sector. Int Nurs Rev. 2007;54:383–90.

43. Kamiru HN, Ross MW, Bartholomew LK, McCurdy SA, Kline MW. Effectiveness of a training program to increase the capacity of health care providers to provide HIV/AIDS care and treatment in Swaziland. AIDS Care. 2009;21:1463–70.

44. Felderman-Taylor J, Valverde M. A structured interview approach to evaluate HIV training for medical care providers. J Assoc Nurses AIDS Care. 2007;18:12–21.

45. Blanas DA, Ndiaye Y, Nichols K, Jensen A, Siddiqui A, Hennig N. Barriers to community case management of malaria in Saraya, Senegal: training, and supply-chains. Malar J. 2013;12:95.

46. Magee E, Tryon C, Forbes A, Heath B, Manangan L. The National Tuberculosis Surveillance System training program to ensure accuracy of tuberculosis data. J Public Health Manag Pract. 2011;17:427–30.

47. Collins P, Mestry K, Wainberg M, Nzama T, Lindegger G. Training South African mental health care providers to talk about sex in the era of AIDS. Psychiatr Serv. 2006;57:1644–7.

48. Li L, Wu Z, Liang LJ, Lin C, Guan J, Jia M, Rou K, Yan Z. Reducing HIV-related stigma in health care settings: a randomized controlled trial in China. Am J Public Health. 2013;103:286–92.

49. Vanden Driessche K, Sabue M, Dufour W, Behets F, Van Rie A. Training health care workers to promote HIV services for patients with tuberculosis in the Democratic Republic of Congo. Hum Resour Health. 2009;7:23.

50. Chang LW, Kadam DB, Sangle S, Narayanan S, Borse RT, McKenzie-White J, Bowen CW, Sisson SD, Bollinger RC. Evaluation of a multimodal, distance

learning HIV management course for clinical care providers in India. J Int Assoc Physicians AIDS Care (Chic). 2012;11:277–82.

51. Vaz M, Page J, Rajaraman D, Rashmi D, Silver S. Enhancing the education and understanding of research in community health workers in an intervention field site in South India. Indian J Public Health Res Dev. 2014;5:178–82.

52. Rakhshani F, Mohammadi M. Improving community health workers' knowledge and behaviour about proper content in malaria education. J Pak Med Assoc. 2009;59:3995–8.

53. van der Elst E, Smith A, Gichuru E, Wahome E, Musyoki H, Muraguri N, Fegan G, Duby Z, Bekker L, Bender B, et al. Men who have sex with men sensitivity training reduces homoprejudice and increases knowledge among Kenyan healthcare providers in coastal Kenya. J Int AIDS Soc. 2013;16(Suppl 3):18748.

54. Awaisu A, Mohamed M, Noordin N, Abd. Aziz N, Sulaiman S, Muttalif A, Mahayiddin A. Potential impact of a pilot training program on smoking cessation intervention for tuberculosis DOTS providers in Malaysia. J Public Health. 2010;18:279–288.

55. Wu PS, Chou P, Chang NT, Sun WJ, Kuo HS. Assessment of changes in knowledge and stigmatization following tuberculosis training workshops in Taiwan. J Formos Med Assoc. 2009;108:377–85.

56. Renju J, Andrew B, Nyalali K, Kishamawe C, Kato C, Changalucha J, Obasi A. A process evaluation of the scale up of a youth-friendly health services initiative in northern Tanzania. J Int AIDS Soc. 2010;13:32.

57. Kyabayinze DJ, Asiimwe C, Nakanjako D, Nabakooza J, Bajabaite M, Strachan C, Tibenderana JK, Van Geertruyden JP. Programme level implementation of malaria rapid diagnostic tests (RDTs) use: outcomes and cost of training health workers at lower level health care facilities in Uganda. BMC Public Health. 2012;12:291.

58. Ssekabira U, Bukirwa H, Hopkins H, Namagembe A, Weaver MR, Sebuyira LM, Quick L, Staedke S, Yeka A, Kiggundu M, et al. Improved malaria case management after integrated team-based training of health care workers in Uganda. Am J Trop Med Hyg. 2008;79:826–33.

59. Weaver MR, Crozier I, Eleku S, Makanga G, Mpanga Sebuyira L, Nyakake J, Thompson M, Willis K. Capacity-building and clinical competence in infectious disease in Uganda: a mixed-design study with pre/post and cluster-randomized trial components. PLoS One. 2012;7:e51319.

60. Capital Ka Cyrilliciriazova TK, Neduzhko OO, Kang Dufour M, Culyba RJ, Myers JJ. Evaluation of the effectiveness of HIV voluntary counseling and testing trainings for clinicians in the Odessa region of Ukraine. AIDS Behav. 2014;18 Suppl 1:S89–95.

61. Mulligan R, Seirawan H, Galligan J, Lemme S. The effect of an HIV/AIDS educational program on the knowledge, attitudes, and behaviors of dental professionals. J Dent Educ. 2006;70:857–68.

62. Kabra SK, Mukherjee A, Vani SA, Sinha S, Sharma SK, Mitsuyasu R, Fahey JL. Continuing medical education on antiretroviral therapy in HIV/AIDS in India: needs assessment and impact on clinicians and allied health personnel. Natl Med J India. 2009;22:257–60.

63. Rowe AK, de Leon GF, Mihigo J, Santelli AC, Miller NP, Van-Dunem P. Quality of malaria case management at outpatient health facilities in Angola. Malar J. 2009;8:275.

64. Alam N, Mridha MK, Kristensen S, Vermund SH. Knowledge and skills for management of sexually transmitted infections among rural medical practitioners in Bangladesh. Open J Prev Med. 2015;5:151–8.

65. Wu Z, Detels R, Ji G, Xu C, Rou K, Ding H, Li V. Diffusion of HIV/AIDS knowledge, positive attitudes, and behaviors through training of health professionals in China. AIDS Educ Prev. 2002;14:379–90.

66. Operario D, Wang D, Zaller ND, Yang MF, Blaney K, Cheng J, Hong Q, Zhang H, Chai J, Szekeres G, et al. Effect of a knowledge-based and skills-based programme for physicians on risk of sexually transmitted reinfections among high-risk patients in China: a cluster randomised trial. Lancet Glob Health. 2016;4:e29–36.

67. Ouma PO, Van Eijk AM, Hamel MJ, Sikuku E, Odhiambo F, Munguti K, Ayisi JG, Kager PA, Slutsker L. The effect of health care worker training on the use of intermittent preventive treatment for malaria in pregnancy in rural western Kenya. Trop Med Int Health. 2007;12:953–61.

68. Domarle O, Randrianarivelojosia M, Duchemin JB, Robert V, Ariey F. Atelier paludisme: an international malaria training course held in Madagascar. Malar J. 2008;7:80.

69. O'Malley G, Beima-Sofie K, Feris L, Shepard-Perry M, Hamunime N, John-Stewart G, Kaindjee-Tjituka F, Brandt L, group Ms. "If I take my medicine, I will be strong": evaluation of a pediatric HIV disclosure intervention in Namibia. J Acquir Immune Defic Syndr. 2015;68:e1–7.

70. Poudyal A, Jimba M, Murakami I, Silwal R, Wakai S, Kuratsuji T. A traditional healers' training model in rural Nepal: strengthening their roles in community health. Trop Med Int Health. 2003;8:956–60.

71. Heunis C, Wouters E, Kigozi G, van Rensburg-Bonthuyzen Janse E, Jacobs N. TB/HIV-related training, knowledge and attitudes of community health workers in the Free State province, South Africa. Afr J AIDS Res. 2013;12:113–9.

72. Peltzer K, Mngqundaniso N, Petros G. A controlled study of an HIV/AIDS/STI/TB intervention with traditional healers in KwaZulu-Natal, South Africa. AIDS Behav. 2006;10:683–90.

73. Peltzer K, Nqeketo A, Petros G, Kanta X. Evaluation of a safer male circumcision training programme for traditional surgeons and nurses in the Eastern Cape, South Africa. Afr J Tradit Complement Altern Med. 2008;5:346–54.

74. Matsabisa M, Spotose T, Hoho D, Javu M. Traditional health practitioners' awareness training programme on TB, HIV and AIDS: a pilot project for the Khayelitsha area in Cape Town, South Africa. J Med Plant Res. 2009;3:142–7.

75. Adams LV, Olotu R, Talbot EA, Cronin BJ, Christopher R, Mkomwa Z. Ending neglect: providing effective childhood tuberculosis training for health care workers in Tanzania. Public Health Action. 2014;4:233–7.

76. Köse S, Mandiracioglu A, Kaptan F, Gülsen M. Improving knowledge and attitudes of health care providers following training on HIV/AIDS related issues: a study in an urban Turkish area. J Med Sci. 2012;32:94–103.

77. Hanass-Hancock J, Alli F. Closing the gap: training for healthcare workers and people with disabilities on the interrelationship of HIV and disability. Disabil Rehabil. 2015;37:2012–21.

78. Downing J, Kawuma E. The impact of a modular HIV/AIDS palliative care education programme in rural Uganda. Int J Palliat Nurs. 2008;14:560–8.

79. van der Elst EM, Gichuru E, Omar A, Kanungi J, Duby Z, Midoun M, Shangani S, Graham SM, Smith AD, Sanders EJ, Operario D. Experiences of Kenyan healthcare workers providing services to men who have sex with men: qualitative findings from a sensitivity training programme. J Int AIDS Soc. 2013;16 Suppl 3:18741.

80. Skarbinski J, Ouma PO, Causer LM, Kariuki SK, Barnwell JW, Alaii JA, de Oliveira AM, Zurovac D, Larson BA, Snow RW, et al. Effect of malaria rapid diagnostic tests on the management of uncomplicated malaria with artemether-lumefantrine in Kenya: a cluster randomized trial. Am J Trop Med Hyg. 2009;80:919–26.

81. Brentlinger PE, Assan A, Mudender F, Ghee AE, Vallejo Torres J, Martinez Martinez P, Bacon O, Bastos R, Manuel R, Ramirez Li L, et al. Task shifting in Mozambique: cross-sectional evaluation of non-physician clinicians' performance in HIV/AIDS care. Hum Resour Health. 2010;8:23.

82. Mukanga D, Babirye R, Peterson S, Pariyo GW, Ojiambo G, Tibenderana JK, Nsubuga P, Kallander K. Can lay community health workers be trained to use diagnostics to distinguish and treat malaria and pneumonia in children? Lessons from rural Uganda. Trop Med Int Health. 2011;16:1234–42.

83. Namagembe A, Ssekabira U, Weaver MR, Blum N, Burnett S, Dorsey G, Sebuyira LM, Ojaku A, Schneider G, Willis K, Yeka A. Improved clinical and laboratory skills after team-based, malaria case management training of health care professionals in Uganda. Malar J. 2012;11:44.

84. Counihan H, Harvey SA, Sekeseke-Chinyama M, Hamainza B, Banda R, Malambo T, Masaninga F, Bell D. Community health workers use malaria rapid diagnostic tests (RDTs) safely and accurately: results of a longitudinal study in Zambia. Am J Trop Med Hyg. 2012;87:57–63.

85. Bruno TO, Hicks CB, Naggie S, Wohl DA, Albrecht H, Thielman NM, Rabin DU, Layton S, Subramaniam C, Grichnik KP, et al. VISION: a regional performance improvement initiative for HIV health care providers. J Contin Educ Health Prof. 2014;34:171–8.

86. Atchessi N, Ridde V, Haddad S. Combining user fees exemption with training and supervision helps to maintain the quality of drug prescriptions in Burkina Faso. Health Policy Plan. 2013;28:606–15.

87. Tadesse Y, Yesuf M, Williams V. Evaluating the output of transformational patient-centred nurse training in Ethiopia. Int J Tuberc Lung Dis. 2013;17:9–14.

88. Lalonde B, Uldall KK, Huba GJ, Panter AT, Zalumas J, Wolfe LR, Rohweder C, Colgrove J, Henderson H, German VF, et al. Impact of HIV/AIDS education on health care provider practice: results from nine grantees of the Special Projects of National Significance Program. Eval Health Prof. 2002;25:302–20.

89. Li L, Lin C, Guan J. Using standardized patients to evaluate hospital-based intervention outcomes. Int J Epidemiol. 2014;43:897–903.

90. Aung T, Longfield K, Aye NM, San AK, Sutton TS, Montagu D, Group PHUGH. Improving the quality of paediatric malaria diagnosis and treatment by rural providers in Myanmar: an evaluation of a training and support intervention. Malar J. 2015;14:397.

91. Talukder K, Salim MA, Jerin I, Sharmin F, Talukder MQ, Marais BJ, Nandi P, Cooreman E, Rahman MA. Intervention to increase detection of childhood tuberculosis in Bangladesh. Int J Tuberc Lung Dis. 2012;16:70–5.

92. Vaca J, Peralta H, Gresely L, Cordova R, Kuffo D, Romero E, Tannenbaum TN, Houston S, Graham B, Hernandez L, Menzies D. DOTS implementation in a middle-income country: development and evaluation of a novel approach. Int J Tuberc Lung Dis. 2005;9:521–7.

93. Christie CD, Steel-Duncan J, Palmer P, Pierre R, Harvey K, Johnson N, Samuels LA, Dunkley-Thompson J, Singh-Minott I, Anderson M, et al. Paediatric and perinatal HIV/AIDS in Jamaica an international leadership initiative, 2002–2007. West Indian Med J. 2008;57:204–15.

94. Park PH, Magut C, Gardner A, O'Yiengo DO, Kamle L, Langat BK, Buziba NG, Carter EJ. Increasing access to the MDR-TB surveillance programme through a collaborative model in western Kenya. Trop Med Int Health. 2012;17:374–9.

95. Zurovac D, Githinji S, Memusi D, Kigen S, Machini B, Muturi A, Otieno G, Snow RW, Nyandigisi A. Major improvements in the quality of malaria case-management under the "test and treat" policy in Kenya. PLoS One. 2014;9:e92782.

96. Puchalski Ritchie LM, Schull MJ, Martiniuk AL, Barnsley J, Arenovich T, van Lettow M, Chan AK, Mills EJ, Makwakwa A, Zwarenstein M. A knowledge translation intervention to improve tuberculosis care and outcomes in Malawi: a pragmatic cluster randomized controlled trial. Implement Sci. 2015;10:38.

97. Fairall L, Bachmann MO, Zwarenstein M, Bateman ED, Niessen LW, Lombard C, Majara B, English R, Bheekie A, van Rensburg D, et al. Cost-effectiveness of educational outreach to primary care nurses to increase tuberculosis case detection and improve respiratory care: economic evaluation alongside a randomised trial. Trop Med Int Health. 2010;15:277–86.

98. Clarke M, Dick J, Zwarenstein M, Lombard CJ, Diwan VK. Lay health worker intervention with choice of DOT superior to standard TB care for farm dwellers in South Africa: a cluster randomised control trial. Int J Tuberc Lung Dis. 2005;9:673–9.

99. Lewin S, Dick J, Zwarenstein M, Lombard CJ. Staff training and ambulatory tuberculosis treatment outcomes: a cluster randomized controlled trial in South Africa. Bull World Health Organ. 2005;83:250–9.

100. Manabe YC, Zawedde-Muyanja S, Burnett SM, Mugabe F, Naikoba S, Coutinho A. Rapid improvement in passive tuberculosis case detection and tuberculosis treatment outcomes after implementation of a bundled laboratory diagnostic and on-site training intervention targeting mid-level providers. Open Forum Infect Dis. 2015;2:ofv030.

101. Ngasala B, Mubi M, Warsame M, Petzold MG, Massele AY, Gustafsson LL, Tomson G, Premji Z, Bjorkman A. Impact of training in clinical and microscopy diagnosis of childhood malaria on antimalarial drug prescription and health outcome at primary health care level in Tanzania: a randomized controlled trial. Malar J. 2008;7:199.

102. Eriksen J, Mujinja P, Warsame M, Nsimba S, Kouyate B, Gustafsson LL, Jahn A, Muller O, Sauerborn R, Tomson G. Effectiveness of a community intervention on malaria in rural Tanzania—a randomised controlled trial. Afr Health Sci. 2010;10:332–40.

103. Mubi M, Janson A, Warsame M, Martensson A, Kallander K, Petzold MG, Ngasala B, Maganga G, Gustafsson LL, Massele A, et al. Malaria rapid testing by community health workers is effective and safe for targeting malaria treatment: randomised cross-over trial in Tanzania. PLoS One. 2011;6:e19753.

104. Mbonye MK, Burnett SM, Burua A, Colebunders R, Crozier I, Kinoti SN, Ronald A, Naikoba S, Rubashembusya T, Van Geertruyden JP, et al. Effect of integrated capacity-building interventions on malaria case management by health professionals in Uganda: a mixed design study with pre/post and cluster randomized trial components. PLoS One. 2014;9:e84945.

105. Weaver MR, Burnett SM, Crozier I, Kinoti SN, Kirunda I, Mbonye MK, Naikoba S, Ronald A, Rubashembusya T, Zawedde S, Willis KS. Improving facility performance in infectious disease care in Uganda: a mixed design study with pre/post and cluster randomized trial components. PLoS One. 2014;9:e103017.

106. Morris MB, Chapula BT, Chi BH, Mwango A, Chi HF, Mwanza J, Manda H, Bolton C, Pankratz DS, Stringer JS, Reid SE. Use of task-shifting to rapidly scale-up HIV treatment services: experiences from Lusaka, Zambia. BMC Health Serv Res. 2009;9:5.

107. Audet CM, Gutin SA, Blevins M, Chiau E, Alvim F, Jose E, Vaz LM, Shepherd BE, Dawson Rose C. The impact of visual aids and enhanced training on the delivery of positive health, dignity, and prevention messages to adult patients living with HIV in rural north central Mozambique. PLoS One. 2015; 10:e0130676.

108. Mangham-Jefferies L, Wiseman V, Achonduh OA, Drake TL, Cundill B, Onwujekwe O, Mbacham W. Economic evaluation of a cluster randomized trial of interventions to improve health workers' practice in diagnosing and treating uncomplicated malaria in Cameroon. Value Health. 2014;17:783–91.

109. Wiseman V, Mangham-Jefferies L, Achonduh O, Drake T, Cundill B, Onwujekwe O, Mbacham W. Economic evaluation of interventions to improve health workers' practice in diagnosing and treating uncomplicated malaria in Cameroon. Am J Trop Med Hyg. 2014;91(5 Suppl. 1):268.

110. Mbacham WF, Mangham-Jefferies L, Cundill B, Achonduh OA, Chandler CI, Ambebila JN, Nkwescheu A, Forsah-Achu D, Ndiforchu V, Tchekountouo O, et al. Basic or enhanced clinician training to improve adherence to malaria treatment guidelines: a cluster-randomised trial in two areas of Cameroon. Lancet Glob Health. 2014;2:e346–58.

111. Nyandigisi A, Memusi D, Mbithi A, Ang'wa N, Shieshia M, Muturi A, Sudoi R, Githinji S, Juma E, Zurovac D. Malaria case-management following change of policy to universal parasitological diagnosis and targeted artemisinin-based combination therapy in Kenya. PLoS One. 2011;6:e24781.

112. Rose CD, Courtenay-Quirk C, Knight K, Shade SB, Vittinghoff E, Gomez C, Lum PJ, Bacon O, Colfax G. HIV intervention for providers study: a randomized controlled trial of a clinician-delivered HIV risk-reduction intervention for HIV-positive people. J Acquir Immune Defic Syndr. 2010;55:572–81.

113. Bin Ghouth AS. Availability and prescription practice of anti-malaria drugs in the private health sector in Yemen. J Infect Dev Ctries. 2013;7:404–12.

114. Ohkado A, Pevzner E, Sugiyama T, Murakami K, Yamada N, Cavanaugh S, Ishikawa N, Harries AD. Evaluation of an international training course to build programmatic capacity for tuberculosis control. Int J Tuberc Lung Dis. 2010;14:371–3.

15

Real-time observation of pathophysiological processes during murine experimental *Schistosoma japonicum* infection using high-resolution ultrasound imaging

Katsumi Maezawa[1][*] , Rieko Furushima-Shimogawara[1], Akio Yasukawa[2], Nobuo Ohta[1,3] and Shiro Iwanaga[1]

Abstract

Background: Hepatosplenic lesion formation is one of the typical clinical symptoms of schistosomiasis japonica. Although it is established that circum-oval granuloma formation mediated by T lymphocytes is the key event triggering the formation of hepatic lesions, the time-course kinetics of disease progression remains to be fully elucidated.

Methods: The real-time process of the pathophysiology of schistosomiasis japonica from the early to late clinical phase was non-invasively observed in a murine experimental infection model using high-resolution ultrasonography. Together with clinical parameters, including body weight and the levels of serum markers of hepatic damage or fibrosis, ultrasonography was used to assess changes in the liver parenchyma and diameter of the portal vein and portal blood flow velocity. In parallel, parasitological parameters were observed, including egg number in the feces and maturation of parasites.

Results: Abnormal high-echo spot patterns in the liver parenchyma, reflecting hepatic fibrosis in ultrasonography, appeared in the liver at 4 weeks post-infection and the pattern became more enlarged and severe over time. This finding was concordant with parasite maturation and initial egg excretion. The serum M2BPGi level markedly increased from 8 weeks post-infection, suggesting sharp deterioration of hepatic fibrosis. At the same time, the diameter of the portal vein, reflecting portal hypertension, became enlarged and reached the peak level at 8 weeks post-infection. Ascites were apparent around the spleen at 9 weeks post-infection, and dilatation of the splenic vein was noted at 10 weeks post-infection. Live adult worms seemed to be detected in the portal vein at 4 weeks post-infection by ultrasonography.

Conclusions: We obtained real-time imaging of the development of hepatosplenic lesions of schistosomiasis japonica in mice. The time-course kinetics of the onset, development, and modulation of each symptom was uncovered. These results are expected to provide new clues for understanding the pathophysiology of human schistosomiasis japonica.

Keywords: *Schistosoma japonicum*, Schistosomiasis, Ultrasonography, Non-invasive observation, Liver fibrosis, Portal hypertension, Real-time imaging

* Correspondence: yrl00232katsumi@gmail.com
[1]Department of Environmental Parasitology, Tokyo Medical and Dental University Graduate School of Medical and Dental Sciences, 1-5-45 Yushima, Bunkyo-ku, Tokyo 113–8519, Japan
Full list of author information is available at the end of the article

Background

Schistosomiasis is caused by the intravenous trematode *Schistosoma* sp., and is endemic to more than 70 countries, putting 218 million people at risk of infection. *Schistosoma japonicum* infection is endemic in Asian countries, including China, the Philippines, and Indonesia; as a zoonotic pathogen, control of *S. japonicum* infection is more complicated and difficult compared with that of other schistosome species [1, 2]. Schistosomiasis is divided into two clinical types, intestinal and urinary, and *S. japonicum* causes the former type. Schistosomiasis japonica is characterized by severe hepatosplenic lesions with circum-oval granuloma formation, hepatic fibrosis, portal hypertension, and so forth [3–5].

The immunopathology of schistosomiasis has been well characterized; several studies have shown that the T cell response to egg antigens triggers the symptoms. Parasite eggs discharged inside blood vessels are trapped in the capillary vessels, which induces granuloma formation around the vessels under the control of egg antigen-specific T cell responses [6–8]. Cercariae, the infective larvae of schistosome parasites, penetrate the host skin and mature in the mesenteric/portal vein. In a murine experimental infection model, adult *S. japonicum* start egg production around 4 weeks post-infection (PI), and thus, the hepatosplenic lesion develops as of 4 weeks PI [9]. The peak response is observed around 8 weeks PI, and then, the granulomatous response is subsequently downregulated due to initiation of an immunomodulation mechanism [10]. Discussion on the time-course development of pathology has mainly been based on cross-sectional observations because the samples were obtained from sacrificed animals at the time of observation. However, continuous changes during the infection process have not yet been studied because of the lack of available non-invasive equipment for small experimental animals. High-resolution ultrasonography is a recently available technology, which has now become applicable for studies with mice [11, 12]. As a non-invasive approach, it is possible to conduct continuous observations of disease progress in the same mouse using high-resolution ultrasonography [13, 14]. There is no direct evidence that the clinicopathological changes observed in a mouse model are comparable to those in human infection; however, the pathophysiology of schistosomiasis in humans seems to be similar to findings in the murine model. Thus, research on the pathophysiology of human schistosomiasis would be greatly promoted with the possibility to conduct longitudinal, but not cross-sectional, observations in mice.

Accordingly, the aim of the present study was to conduct real-time observations of the progress of schistosomiasis japonica using high-resolution ultrasonography in a murine model of infection. The main goal of our study was to continuously observe the time-course development of hepatosplenic lesions in a non-invasive manner in the same group of mice to obtain more detailed and dynamic information on the pathophysiology of schistosomiasis japonica. The results were compared with information obtained by conventional parasitological and/or pathological tools. Based on this new source of information, we discuss the process of disease development and modulation and the future applicability of this approach.

Methods

Animals

Female BALB/c mice (5 weeks old) were used in this study (Crea Japan, Tokyo). The mice were maintained at 23 °C with a 12-h light/12-h dark cycle with free access to food and water.

Parasite infection

For short to mid-term observations up to 13 weeks PI (group 1, $n = 12$), 5-week-old mice (body weight 18–21 g) were infected with 25 cercariae of the Yamanashi strain of *S. japonicum* under intraperitoneal anesthesia with 50 mg/kg of pentobarbital as described elsewhere [15]. In parallel, another group of mice (group 2, $n = 10$) was infected with 10 cercariae for longer term observation for up to 1 year. Mice that were not infected were used as negative controls.

Body weight and egg number per gram (EPG) counts

Body weight of the infected mice of group 1 was measured up to 13 weeks PI except for 3 weeks PI and 6 weeks PI. Worm eggs were gathered from the mice feces of each week in order, fixed the eggs with formalin, melted the residue with ethyl acetate, and then collected by MDL modification method in which the eggs were precipitated by centrifugation. Thereafter, the number of the eggs per 1 g in feces was calculated by microscopic examination (EPG). EPG was determined at 7, 8, 9, and 11 weeks PI.

Ultrasonographic observation

Ultrasonic examination was continuously performed weekly for weeks from 3 to 13 weeks, randomly selected from group 1. For the mice randomly selected, the same individuals were used until the end of the experiment to see changes in intraperitoneal cavity and EPG over time. The mice were fixed on a platform after being anesthetized with Somnopentyl® or Isoflurane®, and ultrasonographic observation was performed while keeping the mouse in a fixed position with a conditioned temperature and stable circulation. The echo jelly warmed with hot water was applied to the same site, and the optimal position for intraperitoneal retrieval was used. For the mice in group 2, the observation was performed at 1 year PI.

We used an ALOKA Noblus (linear probe for humans, 18–4 MHz; Hitachi Corporation, Tokyo, Japan) or Prospect 3.0 ultrasound imaging apparatus for small animals (50 MHz, resolution 30 µm; Nepagene, Chiba). The ALOKA machine was used for observations over a wide range of tissues, including the liver, spleen, portal vein, intestine, and ascites. The spleen depth was measured in the middle portion of the organ. The diameter of the portal vein trunk was measured at the porta hepatis, and the diameter of the splenic vein was measured near the branch from the portal vein. The Prospect 3.0 machine was used for measuring the angle of the liver edge and portal blood flow.

Blood markers of liver function and fibrosis

A mouse different from the mouse used in the ultrasonic examination was sacrificed by injection of a lethal dose of pentobarbital. Blood samples were obtained at 0, 6, 7, 8, 10, 13, and 23 weeks PI.

After macroscopic aspects of the livers and other abdominal organs were recorded, blood was collected from the posterior vena cava and the alanine amino transferase (ALT), albumin/globulin ratio (A/G), and Mac-2 binding protein glycosylation isomer (M2BPGi) [16–18] values were measured as indicators of liver function and hepatic fibrosis. ALT and A/G were inspected by Oriental Yeast Co., Tokyo and M2BPGi was inspected with Possible Co., Gifu.

Statistical analysis

Statistical analysis was performed with Student's t test. P values < 0.05 were regarded as statistically significant.

Results

Body weight and EPG

There was no difference in body weight up to 6 weeks PI, but differences in body weight became apparent between infected mice and control mice as of 7 weeks PI (Fig. 1). Although the difference was only statistically marginal, this trend suggests the progression of general symptoms as of 6 weeks PI. An increase of EPG was also observed on the infected mice at 7 weeks PI, and EPG continuously increased over time (Fig. 1).

Blood parameters

The ALT values increased as of 6 weeks PI, and the maximum values were noted around 7 weeks PI. The M2BPGi level, as a marker of hepatic fibrosis, was increased from 8 weeks PI. After that, it decreased markedly at 13 weeks, again high at 23 weeks. The A/G ratio decreased gradually up to 6 weeks PI and was stable thereafter. Together, these results suggested that failure of liver function was most apparent around 6–8 weeks PI (Fig. 2).

Ultrasonography

Liver

In the control mice, there was no particular signal in the liver, and the strength of the signal was almost at the same level between the liver and kidney through the study period. In group 1 mice, no particular change was detected before 3 weeks PI, but diffuse spots of a high-echo signal were detected at 4 weeks PI and after. These spots then increased in number, a thin linear shadow appeared at 8 weeks PI, and the spots were fused to each other and expanded in size at 10 weeks PI. These linear high-echo signal areas became more intensified and spread over the whole liver. A similar tendency was

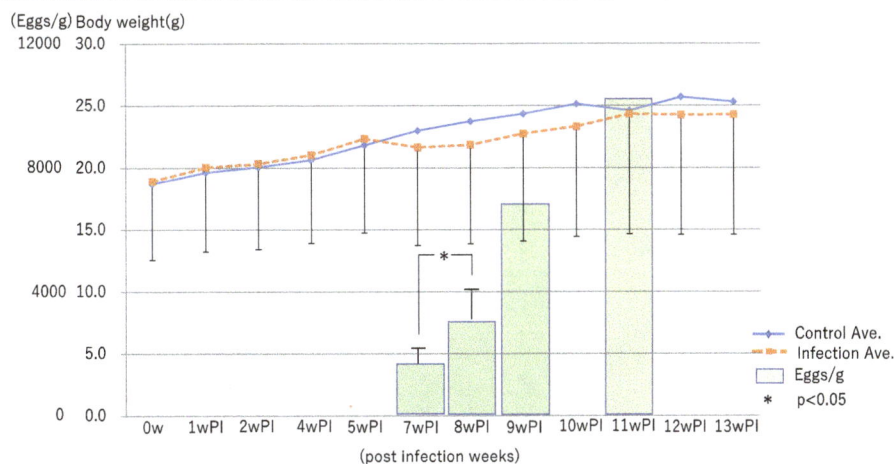

Fig. 1 Observation of body weight and EPG. Dotted line lines indicate changes in body weight of infected mice and solid line lines indicate control mice. The bars showed EPG. Differences in body weight seemed to be apparent between infected mice and control mice after 7 weeks PI. However, there was no significant difference between control and infected mice

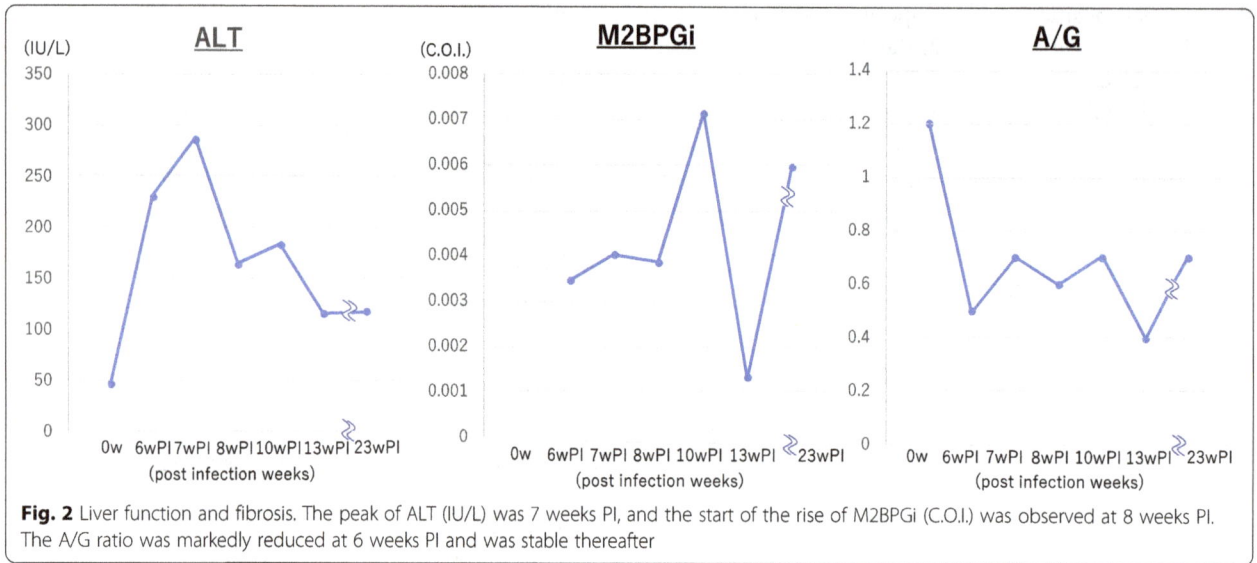

Fig. 2 Liver function and fibrosis. The peak of ALT (IU/L) was 7 weeks PI, and the start of the rise of M2BPGi (C.O.I.) was observed at 8 weeks PI. The A/G ratio was markedly reduced at 6 weeks PI and was stable thereafter

detected in the livers of group 2 mice, and the linear high-echo spots were even further intensified (Fig. 3).

Along with the progression of infection, the angle of the periphery of the liver became gradually obtuse, indicating the appearance of hepatic hypertrophy and/or atrophy (Fig. 4).

Portal vein and splenic vein

The diameter of the portal vein of the control mice was 0.7–0.8 mm, which was enlarged in group 1 mice. Such enlargement continued until 8 weeks PI, but then gradually recovered to the normal range. The mice in group 2 (at 1 year PI) showed a portal vein diameter that was similar to that of the control mice. The blood flow of the portal vein temporally slowed down at 6 weeks PI,

but returned back to the control level thereafter (Fig. 5). Of note, an unidentified image was observed inside the portal vein at 4 weeks PI and thereafter. The image was independent of the heart beat and moved slowly, suggesting that it was a live worm body.

The diameter of the splenic vein was approximately 0.3 mm in control mice at the site of divergence from the portal vein and then doubled by 10 weeks PI (Fig. 6). A similar degree of dilatation was observed at 12 weeks PI, but it was difficult to clearly detect in the mice at 1 year PI due to the influence of intestinal flatulence.

Other findings of the peritoneal cavity

The depth of the spleen became gradually enlarged from 4 weeks PI (Fig. 7). A low level of ascites was noted at

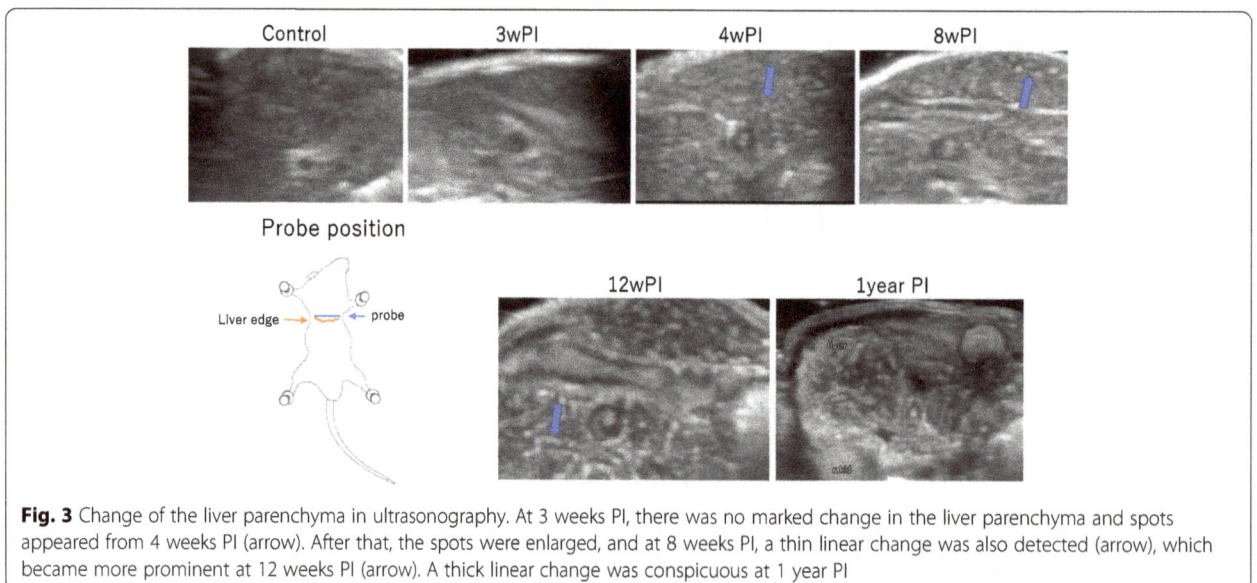

Fig. 3 Change of the liver parenchyma in ultrasonography. At 3 weeks PI, there was no marked change in the liver parenchyma and spots appeared from 4 weeks PI (arrow). After that, the spots were enlarged, and at 8 weeks PI, a thin linear change was also detected (arrow), which became more prominent at 12 weeks PI (arrow). A thick linear change was conspicuous at 1 year PI

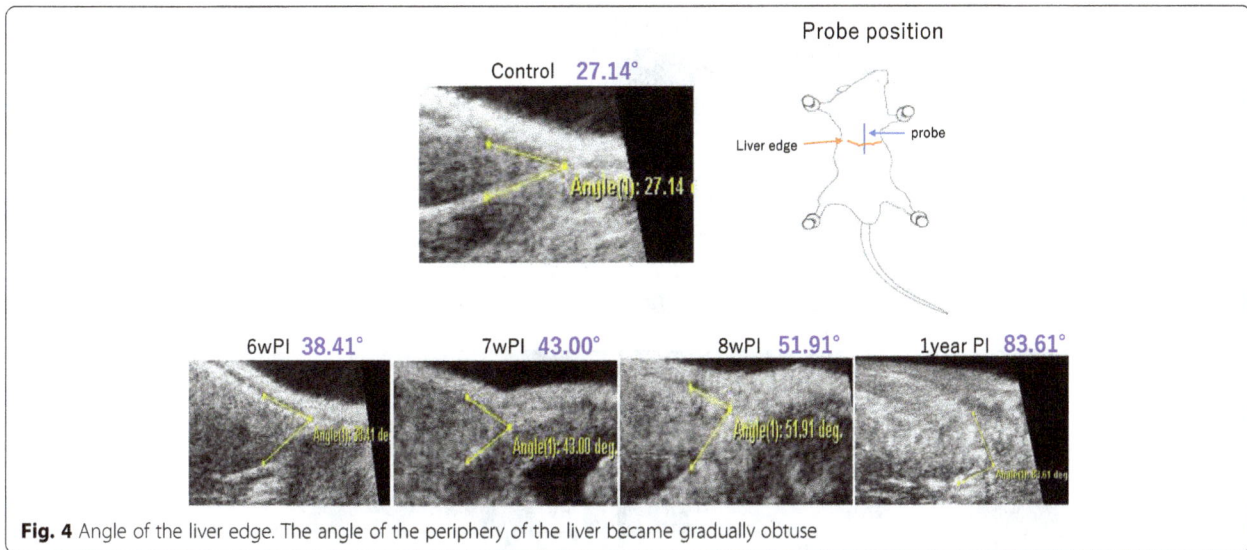

Fig. 4 Angle of the liver edge. The angle of the periphery of the liver became gradually obtuse

9 weeks PI, which increased gradually at 10 weeks PI and thereafter. The mice at 1 year PI showed more intense ascites (Fig. 8). Observation of the intestinal wall suggested loss of flexibility as of 6 weeks PI because a high-echo signal was noted in the intestinal wall thickening, which increased in intensity over time (Fig. 9).

Discussion

Recent developments of tools for bioimaging have provided the opportunity to conduct real-time observations of various biological phenomena and track the responses occurring inside living bodies [19, 20]. High-resolution ultrasonography is one such tool for real-time bioimaging and has been applied in various fields of clinical medicine for diagnosis and/or clinical evaluation. High-resolution ultrasonography is already widely applied in

the field of veterinary medicine, and improvement of the tools has facilitated their application in experimental mice for research.

The profiles of parasitic diseases are outcomes of complicated host–parasite interactions and require continuous/longitudinal observation rather than conventional cross-sectional observations, to provide information for gaining a more profound understanding of the pathophysiology. Although it has been elucidated that hepatic fibrosis, portal hypertension, splenomegaly, ascites, and other characteristics are typical findings of schistosomiasis japonica [21–23], the underlying pathophysiology remains somewhat of a jigsaw puzzle because each piece appears to be somewhat independent and this information has been obtained using different sample sources and approaches.

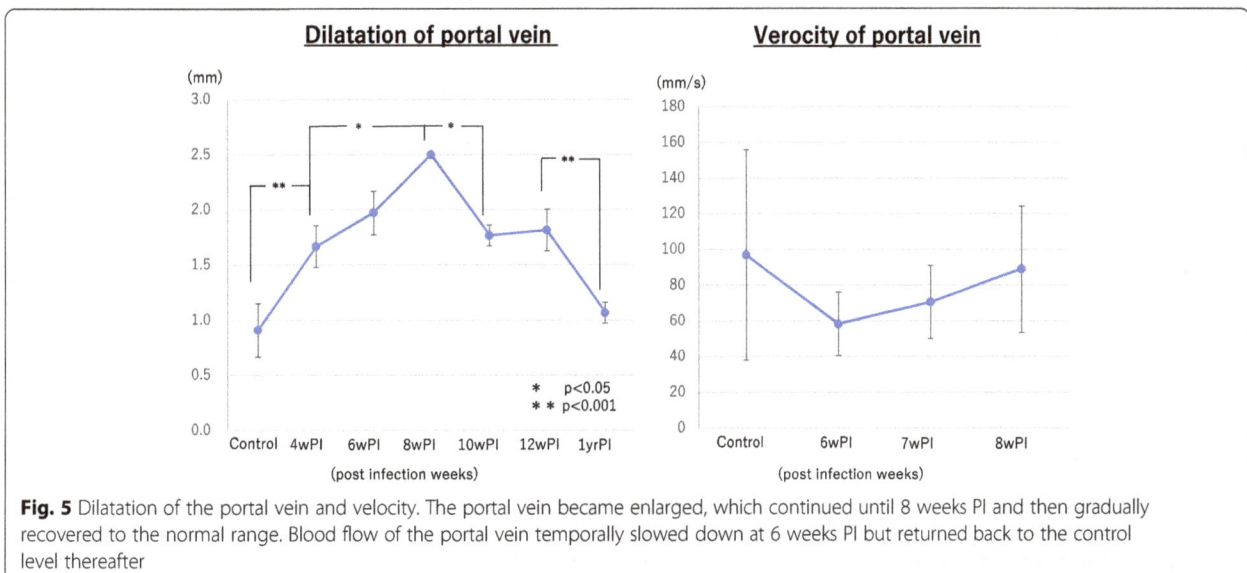

Fig. 5 Dilatation of the portal vein and velocity. The portal vein became enlarged, which continued until 8 weeks PI and then gradually recovered to the normal range. Blood flow of the portal vein temporally slowed down at 6 weeks PI but returned back to the control level thereafter

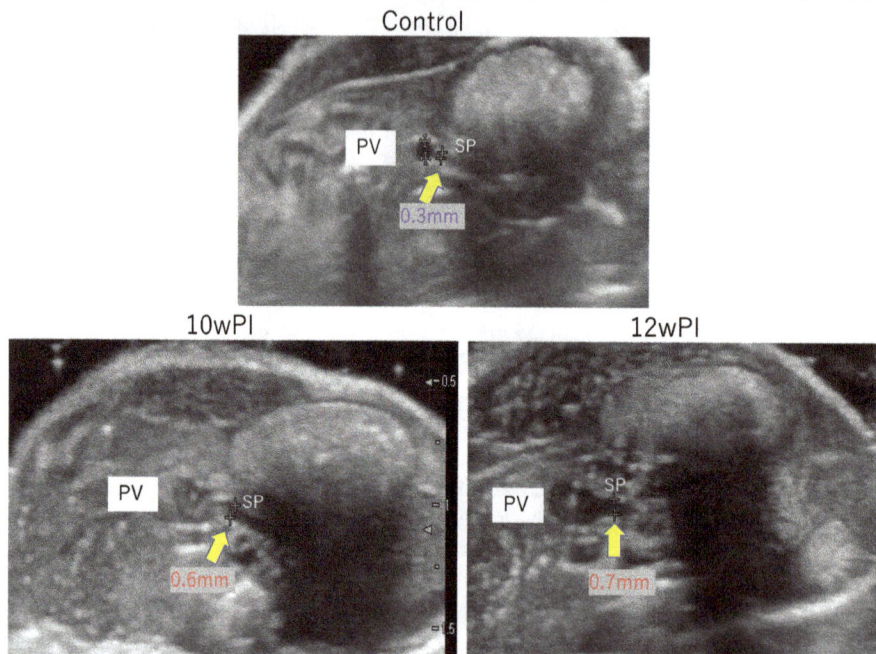

Fig. 6 Dilatation of the splenic vein. The diameter of the splenic vein (SP) was around 0.3 mm in control mice at the site of divergence from the portal vein (PV) but doubled in size at 10 and 12 weeks PI

In the present study, we adopted high-resolution ultrasonography to determine the time-course changes of hepatosplenic lesions formed during *S. japonicum* infection in mice, and the findings and their detailed order of each clinical sign are summarized in Fig. 10. In brief, liver dysfunction due to embolized eggs was the first response, followed by hepatic fibrosis. Hepatic fibrosis was enhanced without modulation, and thickening of the intestinal wall appeared at around the same time or slightly earlier. The thickening of the intestinal wall is more likely to be due to embolism by worm eggs [24, 25]. Portal hypertension was observed later, and the peak level was detected at around 8 weeks PI. Ascites and dilatation of the splenic vein were the final events detected; after that time point, the portal hypertension and liver function impairment returned to the control levels.

Hepatic fibrosis is one of the typical symptoms of schistosomiasis japonica. Spotty echo was detected in the liver parenchyma of infected mice at 4 weeks PI and after, which was similar to the "starry-sky"-like pattern of changes in the human liver described by the World Health Organization (WHO) [26–28]. In the WHO guidelines, the extent of liver parenchyma in

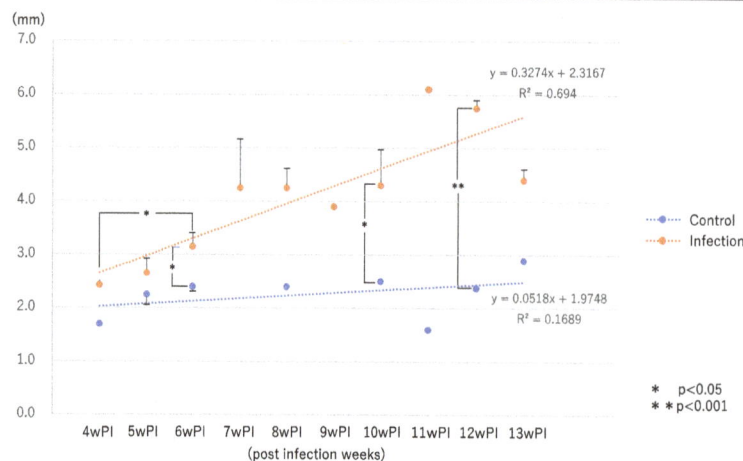

Fig. 7 Depth of the spleen. The depth of the spleen was gradually enlarged from 4 weeks PI and then continued to increase

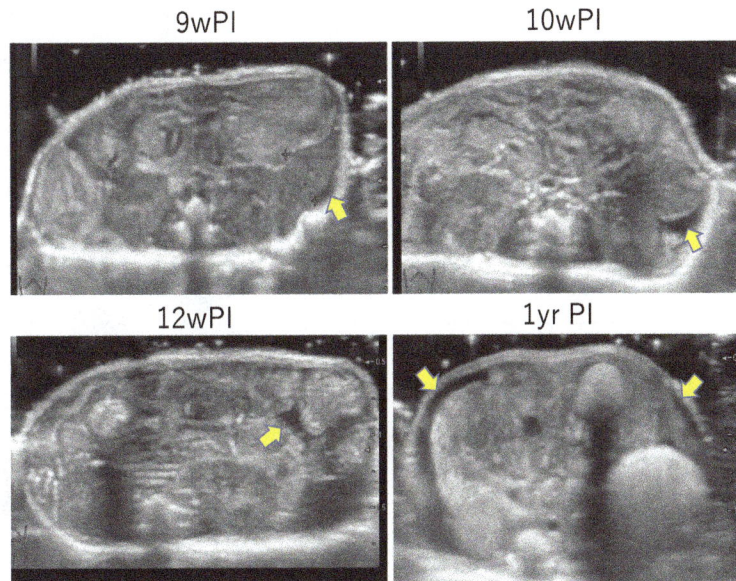

Fig. 8 Ascites. Low-level ascites were noted at 9 weeks PI and increased gradually at 10 weeks PI and thereafter. Mice at 1 year PI showed more intense ascites. (arrow; ascites)

ultrasonography is scored and used for evaluating the severity of schistosomiasis japonica, in the order of a "starry-sky," "rings and pipe-stems," "ruff" around portal bifurcation, "patches," and "bird's claw" pattern. In the present study, starry-sky-like lesions were observed as of 4 weeks PI, which might indicate egg granuloma formation and fibrosis of Glisson's sheath [9]. This finding was concordant with the timing of oviproduction and egg embolism in the microcapillary vessels in Glisson's sheath. The fibrotic pattern observed in the late phase in mice seemed to be equivalent to the "network pattern" of fibrosis observed in cases of human schistosomiasis [29–31]. Our observation of mice at 1 year PI revealed more severe fibrotic patterns, although the other parameters returned to almost normal levels.

Along with hepatic fibrosis, hypertrophy or atrophy of the liver was promoted, suggesting that the liver damage had already been promoted in the earlier phase of infection. The liver dysfunction was caused by microembolism of the eggs, resulting in a circulatory disturbance, and hepatic function was impaired from the beginning of infection. Although liver function was impaired during the phase of hepatic fibrosis, it recovered in spite of the continuous progression of hepatic fibrosis. Progress of hepatic fibrosis on ultrasound images was not a parallel trend to the transition of M2BPGi level. M2BPGI level may be similar to markers such as IL-17 and TGF-β [9].

With regard to portal hypertension, the hepatic arterial blood flow rate has been reported to increase to

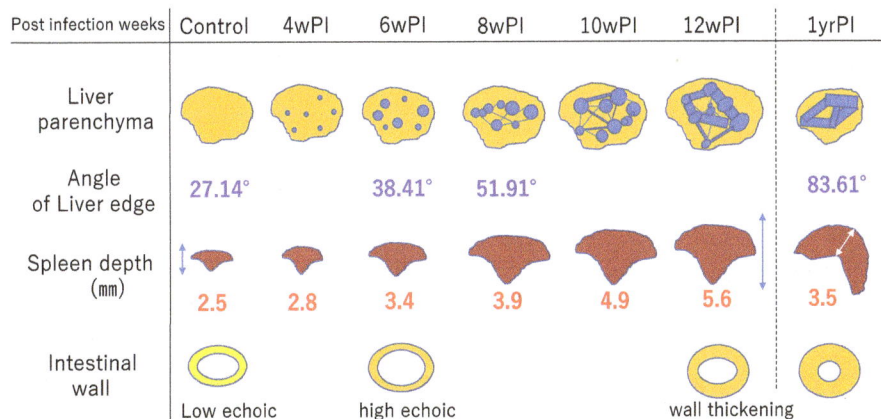

Fig. 9 Schema of hepatosplenomegaly and intestinal lesions. Along with changes in the liver parenchyma and changes in the spleen cross-section, a high-echo signal was noted indicating intestinal wall thickening, which increased in intensity over time

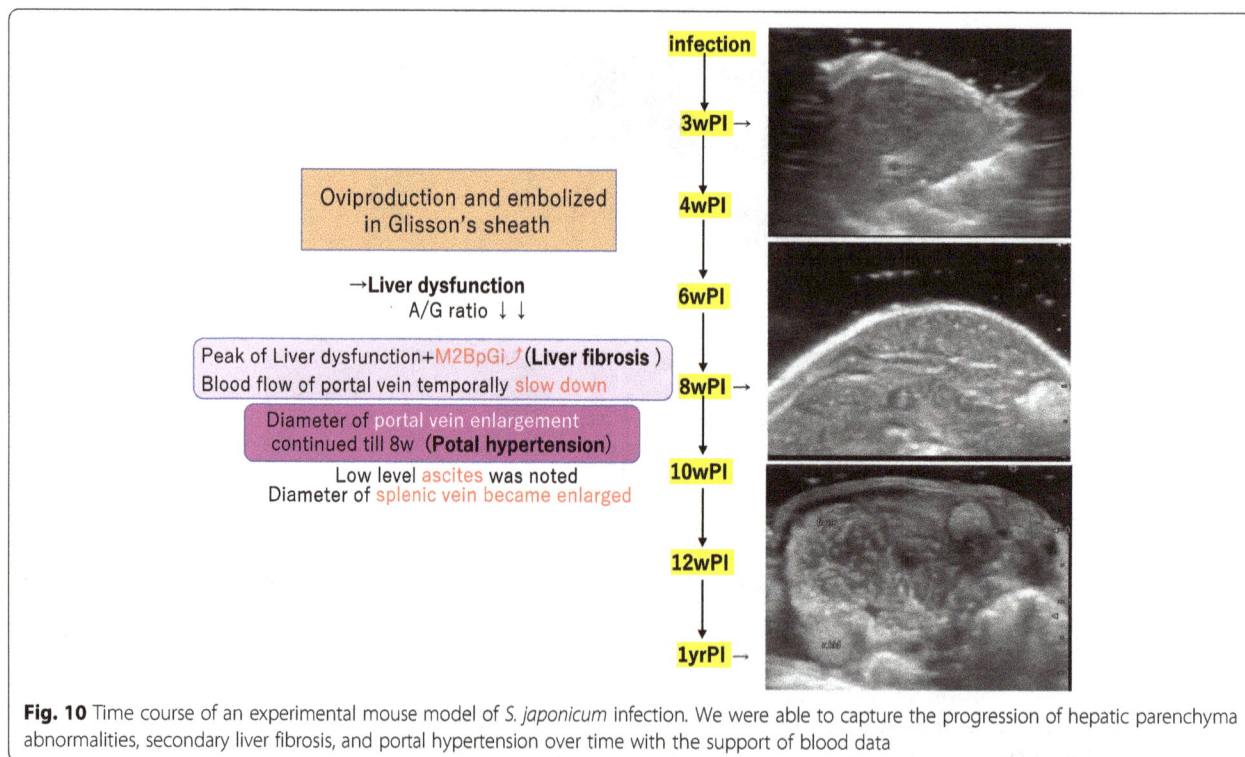

Fig. 10 Time course of an experimental mouse model of *S. japonicum* infection. We were able to capture the progression of hepatic parenchyma abnormalities, secondary liver fibrosis, and portal hypertension over time with the support of blood data

compensate for the decreased portal blood flow [32–34]; however, this was not apparent in our present observations. The diameter and blood flow of the portal vein suggested that the diameter and portal pressure were associated in the early phase of infection. However, hepatic fibrosis was at the maximum level around 8 weeks PI and then gradually decreased, reaching almost normal levels (despite the presence of severe hepatic fibrosis) at 1 year PI. There are various explanations for this finding. For example, portal hypertension reached the maximum level at the time point of maximum egg granuloma formation, or blood flow continued through bypass routes to eliminate the portal hypertension. As the dilatation of the splenic vein was clearly detected at 10 weeks PI, a change in hemodynamics similar to that of human portal hypertension could have occurred, which was not captured on the ultrasound during our observations. It is thus possible to speculate that portal hypertension and the degree of hepatic fibrosis are not necessarily parallel responses to infection.

It is interesting to note that our high-resolution ultrasonographic observation seemed to detect the presence of a live parasite in the portal vein. The image moved spontaneously and slowly, and the length was comparable to the size of adult *S. japonicum*. If this image was indeed an adult worm, and if it would be possible to obtain more clear images, high-resolution ultrasonography can emerge as a new diagnostic approach. From the perspective of parasitology, it is still not clear how the schistosomulae move from the host lung to the mesenteric/portal vein. Thus, real-time bioimaging might be a useful tool for resolving this long-standing question.

The real-time bioimaging of the pathophysiology of schistosomiasis japonica can also provide a new tool for research on vaccine/new drug development. Currently, the efficacies of a vaccine and/or new drug with respect to reduction in the worm burden or alleviation of the pathological damage are analyzed with conventional approaches. It is expected that new information would become available by conducting imaging analysis with ultrasonography, especially with respect to how and when the worms are killed or the pathology becomes modified in experimental murine schistosomiasis. This would further help to expand strategies of vaccine/drug development and make such control tools more feasible in the near future [35].

Conclusions

We successfully conducted the real-time imaging of the development of hepatosplenic lesions of schistosomiasis japonica in mice. It is expected that new information will become available using imaging analysis with ultrasonography as to how and when the worms are killed or the pathology is modified in experimental murine schistosomiasis.

Abbreviations
A/G: Albumin/globulin ratio; ALT: Alanine amino transferase; EPG: Egg number per gram of feces; M2BPGi: Mac-2 binding protein glycosylation isomer; PI: Post-infection

Acknowledgements
The authors give thanks to Dr. A. Hino for her suggestions and technical advice. Also, I would like to express my gratitude to Dr. K. Uemura for providing us with equipment.

Funding
Not applicable

Authors' contributions
KM and RFS conceived and designed the study. AY contributed to the ultrasonographic analysis. NO and SI were involved in planning the study and data analysis. All authors read and approved the final manuscript.

Competing interests
The authors declare that they have no competing interests.

Author details
[1]Department of Environmental Parasitology, Tokyo Medical and Dental University Graduate School of Medical and Dental Sciences, 1-5-45 Yushima, Bunkyo-ku, Tokyo 113–8519, Japan. [2]Nishiogi Veterinary Medical Hospital, 4-9-2 Nishiogikita, Suginami-ku, Tokyo 167–0042, Japan. [3]Depertment of Clinical Nutrition, Faculty of Health Science, Suzuka University of Medical Science, 1001-1, Kishioka-cyo, Suzuka-shi, Mie 510-0293, Japan.

References
1. Chitsulo L, Engels D, Montresor A, Savioli L. The global status of schistosomiasis and its control. Acta Trop. 2000;77:41–51.
2. Fernandez TJ Jr, Pettila T, Banez B. An epidemiological study on *Schistosoma japonicum* in domestic animals in Leyte, Philippines. Southeast Asian J Trop Med Public Health. 1982;13:575–9.
3. Barsoum RS, Esmat G, El-Baz T. Human schistosomiasis: clinical perspective: review. J Adv Res. 2013;4:433–44.
4. Weerakoon KGAD, Gobert GN, Cai P, McManus DP. Advances in the diagnosis of human schistosomiasis. Clin Microbiol Rev. 2015;28:939–67.
5. Zhang BB, Cai WM, Tao J, Zheng M, Liu RH. Expression of Smad proteins in the process of liver fibrosis in mice infected with *Schistosoma japonicum*. Chinese J Parasitol Parasit Dis. 2013;31:89–94. [Article in Chinese]
6. Bartley PB, Ramm GA, Jones MK, Ruddell RG, Li Y, McManus DP. A contributory role for activated hepatic stellate cells in the dynamics of *Schistosoma japonicum* egg-induced fibrosis. Int J Parasitol. 2006;36: 993–1001.
7. Wynn TA, Cheever AW. Cytokine regulation of granuloma formation in schistosomiasis. Curr Opin Immunol. 1995;7:505–11.
8. Wilson MS, Mentink-Kane MM, Pesce JT, Ramalingam TR, Thompson R, Wynn TA. Immunopathology of schistosomiasis. Immunol Cell Biol. 2007;85: 148–54.
9. Zhang Y, Chen L, Gao W, Hou X, Gu Y, Huang D, et al. IL-17 neutralization significantly ameliorates hepatic granulomatous inflammation and liver damage in *Schistosoma japonicum* infected mice. Eur J Immunol. 2012;42: 1523–35.
10. Jenkins SJ, Hewitson JP, Jenkins GR, Mountford AP. Modulation of the host's immune response by schistosome larvae. Parasite Immunol. 2005;27:385–93.
11. Foster FS, Zhang MY, Zhou YQ, Liu G, Mehi J, Cherin E, et al. A new ultrasound instrument for in vivo microimaging of mice. Ultrasound Med Biol. 2002;28:1165–72.
12. Han A, Erdman JW, Simpson DG. Early detection of fatty liver disease in mice via quantitative ultrasound. IEEE International Ultrasonics Symposium. 2014, 2014; https://doi.org/10.1109/ULTSYM.2014.0589.
13. Fernández-Domínguez I, Echevarria-Uraga JJ, Gómez N, Luka Z, Wagner C, Lu SC, et al. High-frequency ultrasound imaging for longitudinal evaluation of non-alcoholic fatty liver disease progression in mice. Ultrasound Med Biol. 2011;37:1161–9.
14. Chen W, Chen JY, Tung YT, Chen HL, Kuo CW, Chuang CH, et al. High-frequency ultrasound imaging to evaluate liver fibrosis progression in rats and Yi Guan Jian herbal therapeutic effects. Evid Based Complement Altern Med. 2013;2013:302325.
15. Tucker MS, Karunaratne LB, Lewis FA, Freitas TC, Liang YS. Schistosomiasis, 103. Curr Protoc Immunol, Unitas. 2013;19(1) https://doi.org/10.1002/0471142735.im1901s28.
16. Hisashi N. Development of M2BPGi: a novel fibrosis serum glyco-biomarker for bchronic hepatitis/cirrhosis diagnostics. Expert Rev Proteomics. 2015;12: 683–93.
17. Wei B, Feng S, Chen E, Li D, Wang T, Gou Y, et al. M2BPGi as a potential diagnostic tool of cirrhosis in Chinese patients with hepatitis B virus infection. J Clin Lab Anal. 2017; https://doi.org/10.1002/jcla.22261.
18. Xu H, Kong W, Liu L, Chi X, Wang X, Wu R, et al. Accuracy of M2BPGi, compared with Fibro Scan®, in analysis of liver fibrosis in patients with hepatitis C. BMC Gastroenterol. 2017;17:62.
19. Marcello M, Emilia V, Giuliana S, Adelaide G, Giancarlo T, Andrea A, et al. Morphological ultrasound microimaging of thyroid in living mice. Endocrinology. 2009;150:4810–5.
20. Hartono S, Thng CH, Chuang KH, Hung H, Koh TS. Dynamic contrast-enhanced MRI of mouse liver: a feasibility study using a dual-input two-compartment tracer kinetic model. JBiomedical Science and Engineering. 2015;8:90–7.
21. Gryseels B, Polman K, Clerinx J, Kestens L. Human schistosomiasis. Lancet. 2006;368:1106–18.
22. Dessein A, Arnaud V, He H, Li J, Dessein H, Hou X, et al. Genetic analysis of human predisposition to hepatosplenic disease caused by schistosomes reveals the crucial role of connective tissue growth factor in rapid progression to severe hepatic fibrosis. Pathol Biol. 2013;61:3–10.
23. Dunn MA, Kamel R. Hepatic schistosomiasis. Hepatology. 1981;1:653–61.
24. Aki T. Examination of the findings with intestinal wall thickening in patients of liver cirrhosis on ultrasonography. Japanese J Med Ultrasound Technol. 2014;39:359–66.
25. Strickland GT. Gastrointestinal manifestations of schistosomiasis. Gut. 1994; 35:1334–7.
26. Silva LCS, Andrade LM, Queiroz LC, Voieta I, Azeredo LM, Antunes CM, et al. *Schistosoma mansoni* magnetic resonance analysis of liver fibrosis according to WHO patterns for ultrasound assessment of schistosomiasis-related morbidity. Mem Inst Oswaldo Cruz. 2010;105:467–70.
27. King CH, Magak P, Salam EA, Ouma JH, Kariuki HC, Blanton RE, World Health Organization. Measuring morbidity in schistosomiasis mansoni: relationship between image pattern, portal vein diameter and portal branch thickness in large-scale surveys using new WHO coding guidelines for ultrasound in schistosomiasis. Tropical Med Int Health. 2003;8:109–17.
28. Richter J, Hatz C, Campagne G, Bergquist NR, Jenkins JM. Ultrasound in schistosomiasis: a practical guide to the standardised use of ultrasonography for the assessment of schistosomiasis-related morbidity. World Health Organization 2000. http://www.who.int/iris/handle/10665/66535.
29. Richter J. Evolution of schistosomiasis-induced pathology after therapy and interruption of exposure to schistosomes: a review of ultrasonographic studies. Acta Trop. 2000;77:111–31.
30. Doehring-Schwerdtfeger E, Kardorff R. Ultrasonography in schistosomiasis in Africa. Mem Inst Oswaldo Cruz. 1995;90:141–5.
31. Catalano OA, Sahani DV, Forcione DG, Czermak B, Liu CH, Soricelli A, et al. Biliary infections: spectrum of imaging findings and management. Radiographics. 2009;29:2059–80.
32. Cheever AW, Warren KS. Hepatic blood flow in mice with acute hepato-splenic schistosomiasis mansoni. Trop Med Hyg. 1964;58:406–12.
33. Bosch J, Groszmann RJ, Shah VH. Evolution in the understanding of the pathophysiological basis of portal hypertension: how changes in paradigm are leading to successful new treatments. J Hepatol. 2015;62:S121–30.
34. Bloch EW, Wahab MFA, Warren KS. In vivo microscopic observations of the pathogenesis and pathophysiology of hepatosplenic schistosomiasis in the mouse liver. Am J Trop Med Hyg. 1972;21:546–57.
35. You H, McManus DP. Vaccines and diagnostics for zoonotic schistosomiasis japonica. Parasitology. 2015;142:271–89.

16

Wuchereria bancrofti infection at four primary schools and surrounding communities with no previous blood surveys in northern Uganda: the prevalence after mass drug administrations and a report on suspected non-filarial endemic elephantiasis

Emmanuel Igwaro Odongo-Aginya[1]*, Alex Olia[1], Kilama Justin Luwa[2], Eiji Nagayasu[3], Anna Mary Auma[4], Geoffrey Egitat[4], Gerald Mwesigwa[4], Yoshitaka Ogino[5,6], Eisaku Kimura[7] and Toshihiro Horii[7]

Abstract

Background: A prevalence study of *Wuchereria bancrofti* infection was carried out in 2014 at 4 study sites in northern Uganda using antigen and microfilaria tests. Each study site consists of a primary school and surrounding communities. These sites are inside the filariasis endemic area and have been covered by mass drug administration under the national elimination programme. However, no prevalence study had been conducted there before the present study. Without information on past and present endemicity levels, our study was meant to be an independent third-party investigation to know the latest filariasis situation.

Results: A total of 982 people including 570 schoolchildren (7–19 years) and 412 community people (7–25 years) were examined, all of them for filarial antigen and 695 for microfilariae. The study revealed that all subjects were negative by both methods.

Conclusions: It was considered that annual mass drug administrations together with anti-malarial activities such as indoor residual spraying had contributed to the reduction of the filarial infection. However, based on the past data obtained near our study sites, we cannot exclude the possibility that filarial prevalence rates in our study sites were very low or even zero originally. During the study, we encountered several patients with lower leg edema and pachydermic (elephant skin-like), mossy skin lesion of the foot. Judging from clinical features and bare-footed life-style of people in the area, non-filarial elephantiasis, possibly podoconiosis, was suspected. This elephantiasis has been reported in areas where filariasis is not endemic.

Keywords: *Wuchereria bancrofti*, Prevalence, Mass drug administration, Podoconiosis, Uganda

* Correspondence: eiodongoaginya@gmail.com
[1]Department of Microbiology and Immunology, Faculty of Medicine, Gulu University, P.O. Box 166, Gulu, Uganda
Full list of author information is available at the end of the article

Background

Lymphatic filariasis (LF), which is one of the neglected tropical diseases (NTDs) in the world, is caused by *Wuchereria bancrofti* in Africa and transmitted mostly by *Anopheles* and *Culex* mosquitoes [1]. The adult worms parasitize the human lymphatic system and cause dilation of lymph vessels. The vessel dilation accompanied by inflammation impairs the normal drainage of lymph fluid and leads to the accumulation of the fluid or lymphedema. The edematous skin is liable to bacterial infections which can trigger an acute febrile symptom or fever attack, and repeated attacks will result in thickening of the skin and eventually disfiguring lesions known as elephantiasis [2, 3]. In the scrotum, dead adult worms may block the lymph vessel and cause accumulation of lymph fluid in the tunica vaginalis, a membranous pouch surrounding the testis. This will produce a swelling of the scrotum or hydrocele [4].

Before 2010, it was estimated that 120 million people in 81 countries were infected with LF and 40 million incapacitated or disfigured by lymphedema (including elephantiasis) and/or hydrocele [5], and World Health Organization (WHO) ranked LF as the no. 2 cause of permanent and long-term disability [6]. The Global Programme to Eliminate Lymphatic Filariasis was launched by WHO in 2000 targeting the elimination by 2020. The strategy is to give 4–6 annual mass drug administrations (MDAs) with ivermectin (or diethylcarbamazine) and albendazole covering all eligible people living in endemic areas regardless of filarial infection. An endemic area was defined as having an infection rate of ≥1% using antigen (or microfilaria) test. Approximately 1.34 billion people globally were expected to participate in the annual treatment [5].

Uganda is one of the countries in Africa, south of the Sahara, with extensive elimination activities for LF. The first epidemiological study was conducted in 1998 in Lira, Soroti, and Katakwi districts of northern and eastern Uganda. The antigen and microfilaria (*mf*) prevalence rates for the three districts were reported to be 18.3–30.1% and 9.7–25.5%, respectively. Similarly, the prevalence rates of hydrocele and limb elephantiasis in adults aged ≥20 years were 7.0–28.7% and 3.7–9.7%, respectively [7]. A countrywide distribution of LF in Uganda was subsequently assessed in Oct. 2000–Apr. 2003 with schoolchildren at 76 locations based on antigen assay. The survey showed that *W. bancrofti* infections were concentrated in the north of the Victoria Nile and the Lake Kyoga. Utilizing the same data, the first nation-wide filariasis distribution and prevalence map was prepared for the national elimination program. Further analysis, based on the map and the population (2002) data, estimated that 8.7 million people (35.3% of the national population) live in areas where antigen-positive rate of school-aged children is >1% [8].

In our study sites, which are under the national filariasis elimination program, no filariasis survey had been done before this study. A pre-treatment *mf* survey carried out in 2008 at two sites which are located relatively close to our study sites documents that no positives were found (unpublished report). An attempt to predict the pre-treatment prevalence based on published prevalence maps was not successful because the results varied so much by map. Also, we could not obtain enough information on regular annual MDAs and drug coverage and actual intake at local government offices. Under these circumstances, it was considered important to conduct an independent study, which is separate from the government initiative, to determine recent prevalence and intensity of infection. Another impetus to start this study was unconfirmed information by local medical officers that they see many cases of elephantiasis.

Meanwhile, in a study conducted in Oct./Nov. 1998 in the Mt. Elgon area of Uganda, the presence of non-filarial elephantiasis, most likely podoconiosis, was reported [9]. The disease is found in the high mountain area, where filariasis does not exist. Three cases of podoconiosis were also reported in the south-western highland in Uganda [10]. In the course of the study, we encountered several "unusual" elephantiasis cases among people walking barefoot. The findings are documented in this report.

Methods

Study sites

The study was carried out at four study sites selected one from each of four districts of Oyam, Nwoya, Amuru, and Gulu in northern Uganda (Fig. 1). Each study site consists of a primary school and surrounding village communities. Before the site selection, the information on LF situation and elimination activities was first collected at each District Office with assistance of the District Health Officer (DHO) and District Vector Control Officer (DVCO), and one sub-county, 4–16 of which constitute one district in this study area, was selected. Then, at the sub-county office, 5–7 candidate schools were listed for blood test. All the candidate schools were visited and 4th to 7th grade schoolchildren were questioned as a class and recorded individually for their knowledge of drugs used for MDA, actual intake of the drugs and the number of clinical cases in their villages. Finally, based on summarized answers, one study school with relatively more clinical cases and lower drug intake rate was selected for the antigen and *mf* survey. Several communities surrounding the selected school were also included as part of the study site with advice from village leaders, village health team, and teachers. Hereafter, the study sites are thus designated using the names of

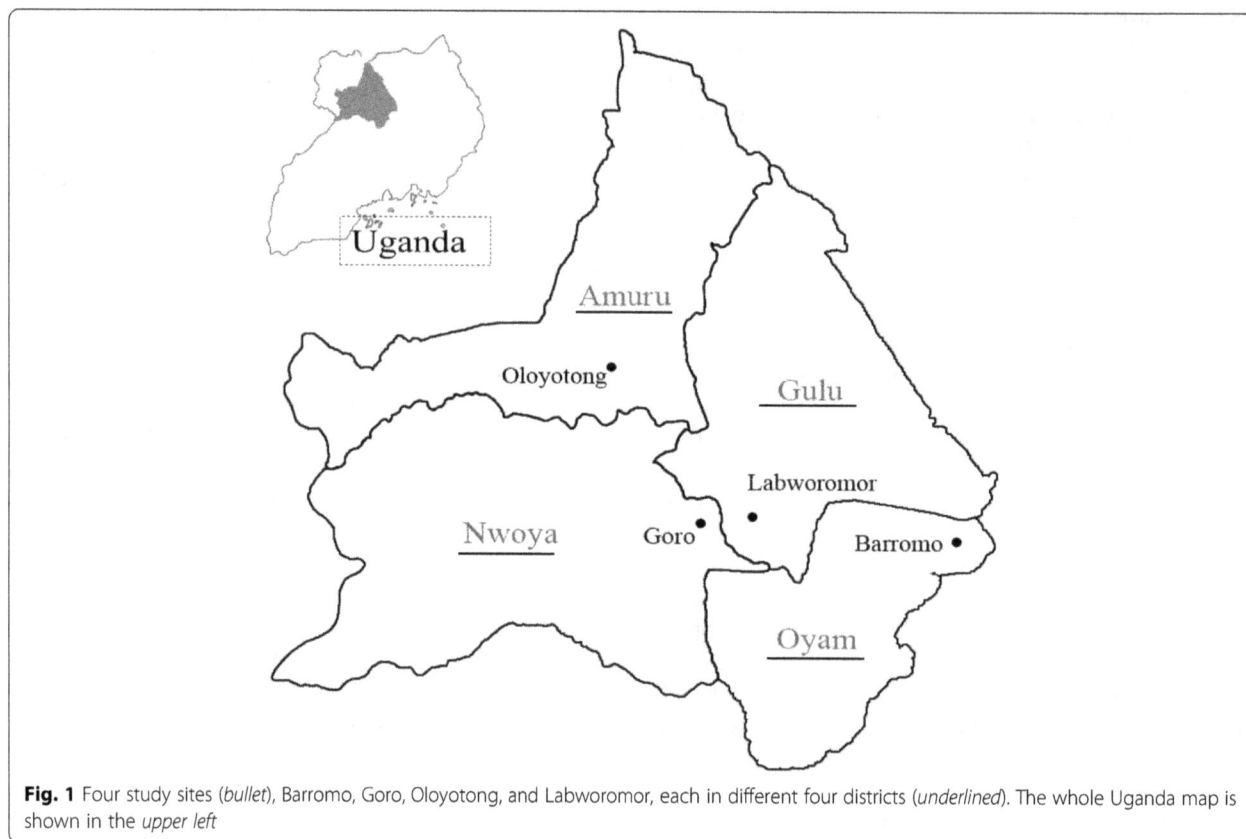

Fig. 1 Four study sites (*bullet*), Barromo, Goro, Oloyotong, and Labworomor, each in different four districts (*underlined*). The whole Uganda map is shown in the *upper left*

the selected schools: Barromo, Goro, Oloyotong, and Labworomor (Fig. 1).

Study subjects

At the selected school, male and female children of grades 1–7 were recruited. A minimum of 20 children per grade were sampled by drawing individually Yes/No lots of folded papers to get a total of >140 subjects/school. The official age to start schooling is at 6 years old, but in reality, the age per grade varies widely. In this study, children's ages ranged from 7 to 19 years. The lowest age of 7 years was fixed by us. In the communities, >50 children aged 7–13 years, who do not go to school, and >60 people aged 14–25 years were targeted. Thus, >250 subjects/study site or >1000 subjects for the whole study were included. The subjects were first examined for antigen and only those checked for antigen were included in the *mf* study.

Diagnostic methods

Blood collections were carried out at each of the selected school for enrolled children and a convenient point for community people. For antigen test, BinaxNow® Filariasis antigen test (AlereScarborough, Inc.) was used in the daytime following manufacturer's instructions: 100 µl of heparinized finger-prick blood was applied to the

sample pad and the result was read after 10 min. For *mf* test, approximately 60 µl of blood was collected after 8:30 pm, smeared on a glass slide which was later stained with 10% Giemsa for 10 min.

Results

The field study was carried out in Oct.–Nov. 2014. This is in the rainy season in northern Uganda, and the work was often interrupted with strong showers. A total of 982 volunteer subjects (570 schoolchildren and 412 community people) were examined for the filarial antigen in the four study sites (Table 1A). Analyzed by age, 94.6% ($n = 539$) of schoolchildren were 7–15 years, and the rest between 16–19 years. Adults aged 20–25 years accounted for 26.5% ($n = 109$) of all community subjects. The results of the antigen test were unexpected: all of the subjects were negative.

For *mf* test, a total of 695 subjects, which is 70.8% of those tested for antigen, were examined at night from 8:30 pm to midnight (Table 1B). Schoolchildren and community children aged 7–13 years participated in the *mf* survey at the rates of 76.3 and 74.4%, respectively, but for community youths and adults (14–25 years), participation was only 55.0% of the total tested for antigen. Only 29 adults (20–25 years) were examined for *mf*. All slides examined were negative for *W. bancrofti mf*, and

Table 1 Results of *W. bancrofti* antigen (A) and microfilaria (B) tests according to study site which includes a primary school and surrounding communities

Study site	Sex	Barromo		Goro		Oloyotong		Labworomor		Total exam.
		No. exam.	No. positive	No. exam.	No. positive	No. exam.	No. positive	No. exam.	No. positive	
A										
Schoolchildren (7–19 years)	M	85	0	77	0	71	0	67	0	300
	F	55	0	64	0	76	0	75	0	270
	Total	140	0	141	0	147	0	142	0	570
Community children (7–13 years)	M	24	0	21	0	22	0	18	0	85
	F	23	0	36	0	15	0	13	0	87
	Total	47	0	57	0	37	0	31	0	172
Community people (14–25 years)	M	28	0	38	0	39	0	33	0	138
	F	25	0	22	0	22	0	33	0	102
	Total	53	0	60	0	61	0	66	0	240
Community total		100	0	117	0	98	0	97	0	412
All subjects		240	0	258	0	245	0	239	0	982
B										
Schoolchildren (7–19 years)	M	72	0	46	0	62	0	48	0	228
	F	39	0	45	0	65	0	58	0	207
	Total	111	0	91	0	127	0	106	0	435
Community children (7–13 years)	M	19	0	12	0	19	0	16	0	66
	F	17	0	23	0	12	0	10	0	62
	Total	36	0	35	0	31	0	26	0	128
Communitypeople (14–25yrs)	M	20	0	29	0	19	0	10	0	78
	F	15	0	13	0	13	0	13	0	54
	Total	35	0	42	0	32	0	23	0	132
Community total		71	0	77	0	63	0	49	0	260
All subjects		182	0	168	0	190	0	155	0	695

In community surveys by the antigen and microfilaria tests, schoolchildren are excluded

no *mf* of another species, *Mansonella perstants*, which is distributed in Uganda [11], were found in any of the blood smears either.

During the blood surveys, about 7–8 male and female adults visited us asking advice for their "filarial" elephantiasis. The lesions were basically similar: lower leg edema, and fine pachydermic (which is like a rough elephant skin) or mossy skin change on the feet. The photographs of three cases (a, b, and c) are shown in Fig. 2. The edema is slight or moderate and confined below the knee (Fig. 2a1–c1). The skin lesion, which is typically bilateral and severer at one side, is most prominent around toes (Fig. 2a2–c2). In case a, some toe nails are unrecognizable (Fig. 2a2, arrows). In case b, a pachydermic lesion is observed along the side of the foot (Fig. 2b). Most people in these areas walk and work barefooted. Based on this life style, clinical picture and negative antigen/*mf* results (with the assumption that our sites are non-endemic originally), we conclude that a possibility of non-filarial endemic elephantiasis, podoconiosis, should be considered.

Discussion

A total of 982 people were examined with the antigen test, and 695 of them (70.8%) were also examined for *mf*, despite the fact that the second blood collection was done at night with unpredictable downpours. The results of the blood tests turned out to be all negative. This can be explained, in general, by the effect of anti-filarial MDAs. They have been implemented in Oyam district since 2005 when the district was a part of Apac district and in the other three districts since 2009. Before our study in 2014, 8, 4, and 3 rounds of annual MDAs were conducted by the national program in Oyam, Amuru and Gulu, and Nwoya districts, respectively. The treatment coverage was satisfactory (>65%) in Oyam, Amuru and Nwoya, but in Gulu three of four rounds resulted in low coverage rates of 34–58%. However, specific rates

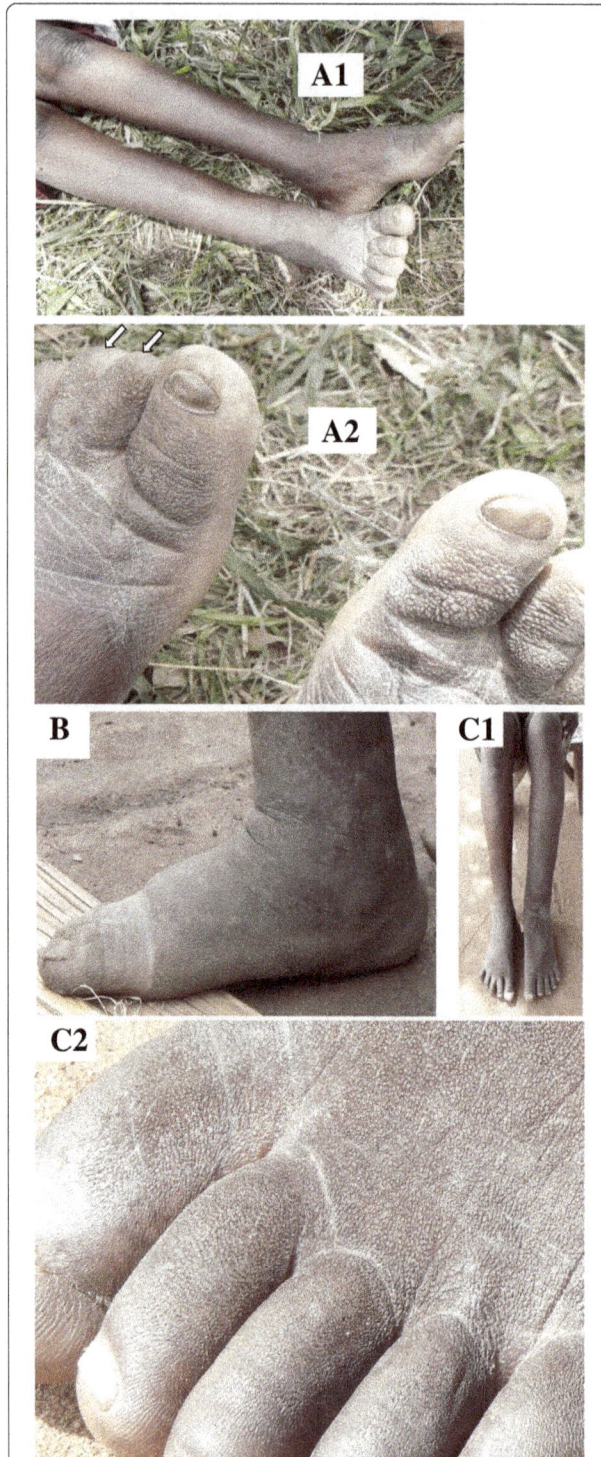

Fig. 2 Three cases (**A**, **B**, and **C**) with leg edema and pachydermic skin changes. In case **A**, the *right lower* leg is slightly edematous and the dorsal skin of the *right* foot is whitish in appearance (**A1**). The skin of the foot is pachydermic and mossy: the skins of the *right* toes are rather spiny, and the nails of the *left* 2nd and 3rd toes are unrecognizable (*arrows*) (**A2**). In case **B**, foot edema and pachydermic skin change along the side of the foot are recognized (**B**). Mild edema is observable in the *left lower* leg of case **C** (**C1**), and the skin around the *left* toes is pachydermic (**C2**)

for our study sites are unknown. Various anti-malarial activities might have also influenced the result, though quantitative effects of these interventions to reduce the prevalence of filarial infection are unknown. Between 2009 and 2014, our four districts were covered by the intensive indoor residual spraying (IRS) program for malaria control [12]. It is reported that five rounds of IRS, especially using bendiocarb, reduced malaria morbidity significantly in Apac district [13], implying that IRS would reduce FL transmission as the two different parasites share the same vector species of *Anopheles*. A mass distribution campaign of long-lasting insecticidal nets (LLINs) initially focused on pregnant women and children under 5 years in 2009–2010 and then expanded in 2013–2014 to nationwide universal distribution of LLINs. In Mid-North region including our study districts, each household was reported to own an average of 2.7 LLINs [12, 14]. The possible supportive effect of LLINs in anti-filarial MDAs is reported [15].

To understand the totally negative results, crucial information is the pre-MDA infection level in our study sites. In order to have rough estimates of the pre-MDA rates, the geographical positioning system (GPS) data of our study sites (recorded at the schools) were first plotted on the antigen prevalence map made by Onapa et al. [8], which gave a rate of >5% at all four sites (Fig. 3a). Since the map by Onapa et al. was created based on a limited number of samples ($n = 76$) scattered across the whole country, the prevalence map could not be accurate for our purpose. However, based on the predicted estimate (>5%), we still anticipated some positives in our study even after treatment. As for the comparability between predicted rates from the map and antigen rates by our study, the average number of subjects examined and the age range in Onapa et al. [8] are 231 persons/school and 5–19 years, and ours are 218 persons/site and 7–19 years excluding adults aged 20–25 years. Interestingly, by the use of a newly published (2015) pre-MDA antigen prevalence map for Uganda [16], we predicted high rates of 21–30% in Barromo and 11–20% in the other three sites (Fig. 3b). Surprisingly, another filariasis distribution map of Uganda published in 2007 for the integrated control of NTDs [17] excludes three of our districts, Nwoya, Amuru, and Gulu from the LF endemic area (Fig. 3c). In fact, in the pre-treatment *mf* survey carried out in July–October 2008 by the national elimination program, no positives were recorded for two sites, Koch Goma in Nwoya district ($n = 442$) and Opit in Gulu district ($n = 354$) [previously mentioned unpublished report]. The former site is located 10 km from our Goro site and the latter 29 km from our Labworomor site. Then it could be inferred, based on the relative proximity, that our two sites had very low infection rates when MDA started or that the sites are non-

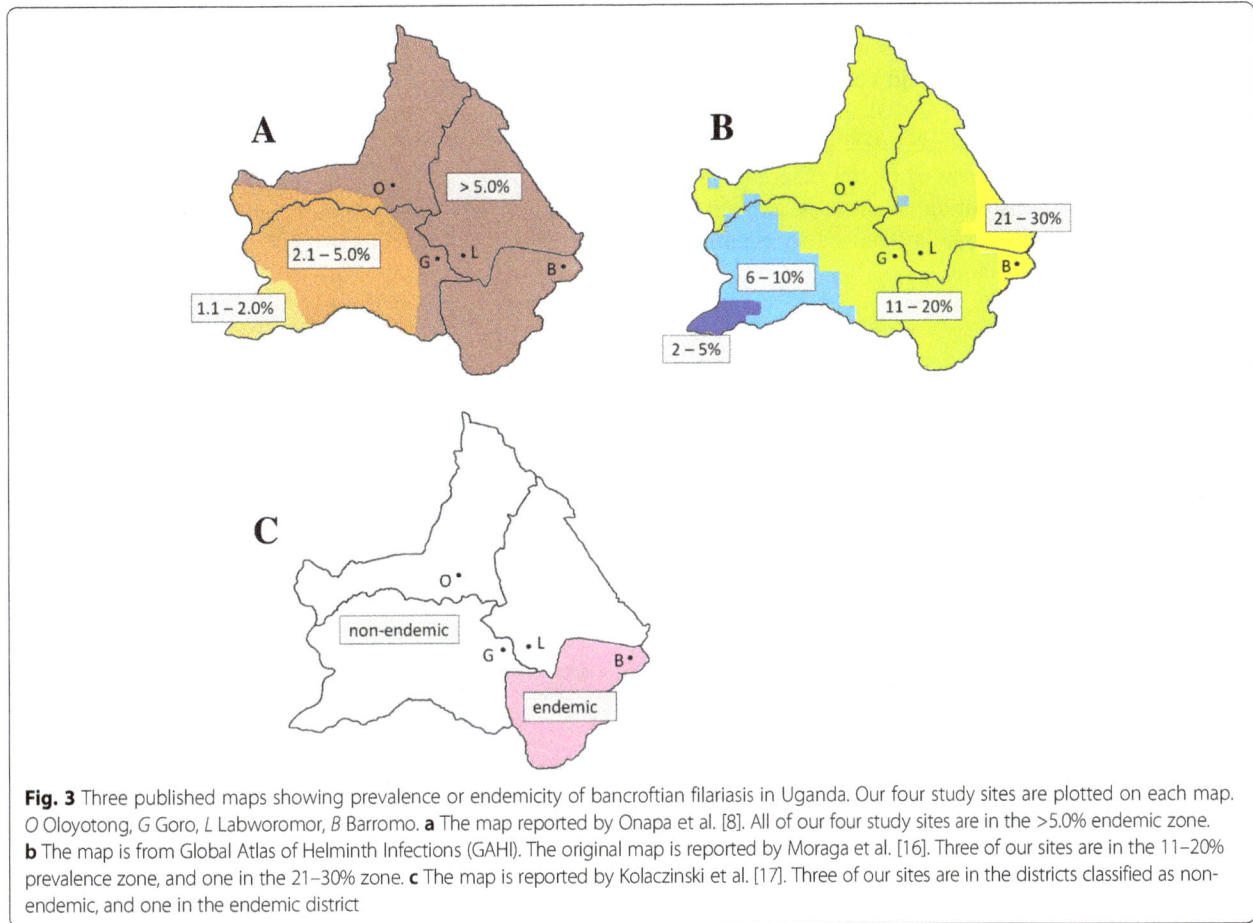

Fig. 3 Three published maps showing prevalence or endemicity of bancroftian filariasis in Uganda. Our four study sites are plotted on each map. *O* Oloyotong, *G* Goro, *L* Labworomor, *B* Barromo. **a** The map reported by Onapa et al. [8]. All of our four study sites are in the >5.0% endemic zone. **b** The map is from Global Atlas of Helminth Infections (GAHI). The original map is reported by Moraga et al. [16]. Three of our sites are in the 11–20% prevalence zone, and one in the 21–30% zone. **c** The map is reported by Kolaczinski et al. [17]. Three of our sites are in the districts classified as non-endemic, and one in the endemic district

endemic from the beginning. This conclusion, if confirmed, will be a challenge to the reliability of computer-based mapping. Barromo site belongs to a more endemic region, and its pre-treatment prevalence might be higher than those of the other three sites. Prolonged and more intensive MDAs could explain the zero prevalence we obtained there.

During this study, we encountered patients with unique elephantiasis: the leg edema is mild and restricted below the knee, but mossy skin change around their toes is obvious. We also noticed that most people walk and work barefooted. Thus, non-filarial elephantiasis such as podoconiosis was suspected. Podoconiosis is a well-known non-filarial endemic elephantiasis found in high mountain areas (1000–2800 m) in Ethiopia, where weathered volcanic ash containing silicon predominates in soil and people live barefoot in a cool and relatively rainy (annual precipitation of >1000 mm) environment [18]. A pathological study revealed amorphous and crystalline silicon compounds in macrophages of femoral lymph nodes [19]. In Uganda, podoconiosis cases were reported from highlands of >1500 m [9, 10], while LF distribution was limited in areas lower than 1300 m [8]. In Ethiopia, however, potential distribution overlap of

these two different types of elephantiasis is reported at an altitude of 1225–1698 m [20], and one report clearly mentions the co-endemicity in western Ethiopia [21]. Our study sites are located at 1086–1119 m, which is lower than the reported endemic range. However, a recent report that quartz, crystallized silicon dioxide, is closely related to the occurrence of podoconiosis [22] may suggest wider distribution of podoconiosis because quartz is ubiquitous in the environment, and its microscopic particles may be absorbed through the foot skin. Another supportive reason to suspect podoconiosis is found in the previously mentioned unpublished report from Koch Goma and Opit of 931 people examined clinically, 13 elephantiasis (1.40%), and 1 hydrocele (0.11%) cases were found ($p < 0.002$). It is quite unusual to have a significantly higher elephantiasis rate than a hydrocele rate in LF endemic areas [23, 24]. In 2011, WHO identified podoconiosis as one of NTDs and its elimination has been considered [25], and it will be important for us to confirm the diagnosis, though the definite diagnosis of podoconiosis is not easy [26]. If we can confirm the absence of LF in the area, it can be a strong supportive evidence for podoconiosis, and for this, *W. bancrofti* antibody test may be valuable.

Although silicon compounds play an essential role, the exact pathogenesis of podoconiosis is yet unknown. The skin lesions we observed are mild compared with those reported in various articles [27–29]. It may be possible that we encountered early stage cases. It is also possible that the skin lesion is influenced by the difference in the concentration and constitution of silicon compounds in soil. The severity may also be influenced by genetic difference between people/population [30].

Conclusions

Two of the computer-based maps predicted relatively high prevalence of LF infections in our study sites, but no antigen/*mf* positives were detected by our study. Also, in another study carried out in nearby areas before MDAs, no *mf* positives were found. Thus, we suspected the possibility that our area was originally non-endemic (or very low endemic). The present study also suggests a possibility that non-filarial elephantiasis or probable podoconiosis could be co-endemic with filarial elephantiasis in Uganda. It is necessary to confirm the diagnosis and investigate the clinical and epidemiological significance of "unusual" elephantiasis in Uganda.

Abbreviations

IRS: Indoor residual spraying; LF: Lymphatic filariasis; LLINs: Long-lasting insecticidal nets; MDAs: Mass drug administrations; *Mf*: Microfilaria; NTDs: Neglected tropical diseases; WHO: World Health Organization

Acknowledgements

We would thank schoolchildren and the communities in our study sites for their cooperation in blood collection, especially late at night. Without hard work by school teachers, village health team members, and community leaders, the study could not have been done. We are grateful for the assistance by the District Health Officers and District Education Officers. District Vector Control Officers worked always with us until late at night.

Funding

This work was supported by funds for Integrated Promotion of Social System Reform and Research and Development (MEXT: Strategic Promotion of International Cooperation to Accelerate Innovation in Africa) (15651988); Grant for Translational Research Network Program (AMED) and Global Health Innovative Technology Fund (G2013-105; G2014-109) to TH.

Authors' contributions

EIOA, EK, planed and designed the study. TH provided the fund for the study. AO, KJL, EIOA, EN, YO, EK, AMA, GE, GM mobilized and recruited the schoolchildren and the community in the study. AMA, GE, GM performed the antigen tests and made smears for microfilaria. AO and EIOA stained and examined the slides. EN and YO checked the records and analyzed the data. EIOA and EK drafted the manuscript, and all the authors read and approved it for submission.

Ethics approval and consent to participate

Ethical approval for the study was obtained from St. Mary's Hospital Lacor Institutional Research and Ethics Committee (LHIREC 011/03/14). Uganda National Council for Science and Technology (UNCST) also approved the study (HS 1629), and the Research Secretariat in the Office of the President wrote an introductory letter (ADM154/212/01) to the Resident District Commissioners (RDCs) in the proposed sites allowing us to carry out the study. The field work was carried out per district with cooperation of the RDC. At each school, the headmaster signed and stamped consent form to allow us to study the pupils in the school. Schoolchildren aged ≥18 years consented to the study, while for those <18 years, their older brothers or sisters in the same school, or their guardians/parents consented to participate in the study in addition to personal assent. In the community, written consent/assent was obtained individually.

Competing interests

The authors declare that they have no competing interests.

Author details

[1]Department of Microbiology and Immunology, Faculty of Medicine, Gulu University, P.O. Box 166, Gulu, Uganda. [2]Department of Biology, Faculty of Science, Gulu University, P.O.Box 166, Gulu, Uganda. [3]Division of Parasitology, Department of Infectious Diseases, Faculty of Medicine, University of Miyazaki, Miyazaki 889-1692, Japan. [4]Vector Control Division, Ministry of Health, P.O.Box 1661, Kampala, Uganda. [5]Department of Parasitology, Kochi Medical School, Kochi University, Nankoku, Kochi 783-8505, Japan. [6]Department of Haematology and Respiratory Medicine, Kochi Medical School, Kochi University, Nankoku, Kochi 783-8505, Japan. [7]Department of Molecular Protozoology, Research Institute for Microbial Diseases, Osaka University, Suita, Osaka 565-0871, Japan.

References

1. WHO (WHO/HTM/NTD/PCT/2013.10). Lymphatic filariasis: a handbook of practical entomology for national lymphatic filariasis elimination programmes; 2013.
2. Dreyer G, Addiss D, Roberts J, Norões J. Progression of lymphatic vessel dilatation in the presence of living adult *Wuchereria bancrofti*. Trans R Soc Trop Med Hyg. 2002;96:157–61.
3. Dreyer G, Medeiros Z, Netto MJ, Leal NC, de Castro LG, Piessens WF. Acute attacks in the extremities of persons living in an area endemic for bancroftian filariasis: differentiation of two syndromes. Trans R Soc Trop Med Hyg. 1999;93:413–7.
4. Norões J, Addiss D, Cedenho A, Figueredo-Silva J, Lima G, Dreyer G. Pathogenesis of filarial hydrocele: risk associated with intrascrotal nodules caused by death of adult *Wuchereria bancrofti*. Trans R Soc Trop Med Hyg. 2003;97:561–6.
5. WHO (WHO/HTM/NTD/PCT/2010.6). Progress report 2000-2009 and strategic plan 2010-2020 of the global programme to eliminate lymphatic filariasis: halfway towards eliminating lymphatic filariasis; 2010.
6. WHO. The World Health Report 1995: The report of The Director General (http://www.who.int/whr/1995/en/). Bridging the gaps. Geneva; 1995
7. Onapa AW, Simonsen PE, Pedersen EM, Okello DO. Lymphatic filariasis in Uganda: baseline investigations in Lira, Soroti and Katakwi Districts. Trans R Soc Trop Med Hyg. 2001;95:161–7.
8. Onapa AW, Simonsen PE, Baehr I, Pedersen EM. Rapid assessment of the geographical distribution of lymphatic filariasis in Uganda, by screening of schoolchildren for circulating filarial antigens. Ann Trop Med Parasitol. 2005;99:141–53.
9. Onapa AW, Simonsen PE, Pedersen EM. Non-filarial elephantiasis in the Mt. Elgon area (Kapchorwa district) of Uganda. Acta Trop. 2001;78:171–6.
10. Dwek P, Kong LY, Wafer M, Cherniak W, Pace R, Malhamé I, et al. Case report and literature review: podoconiosis in southwestern Uganda. Int J Trop Dis Health. 2015;9:1–7.
11. Stensgaard AS, Vounatsou P, Onapa AW, Utzinger J, Pedersen EM, Kristensen TK, et al. Ecological drivers of *Mansonella perstans* infection in Uganda and

patterns of co-endemicity with lymphatic filariasis and malaria. PLoS Negl Trop Dis. 2016;10:e0004319.

12. Yeka A, Gasasira A, MpimbazaA, Nsobya S, Staedke SG et al. Malaria in Uganda: Challenges to control on the long road to elimination;1. Epidemiology and current control effort. Acta Trop. 2012;121(3):184–95.

13. Kigozi R, Baxi SM, Gasasira A, Sserwanga A, Kakeeto S, Nasr S, et al. Indoor residual spraying of insecticide and malaria morbidity in a high transmission intensity area of Uganda. PLoS ONE. 2012;7:e42857.

14. The Republic of Uganda. Universal coverage of LLINs in Uganda—insights into the campaign implementation; 2014.

15. Ashton RA, Kyabayinze DJ, Opio T, Auma A, Edwards T, Matwale G, et al. The impact of mass drug administration and long-lasting insecticidal net distribution on Wuchereria bancrofti infection in humans and mosquitoes: an observational study in northern Uganda. Parasit Vectors. 2011;4:134.

16. Global Atlas of Helminth Infections (GAHI). Predicted antigenaemia prevalence and probability that prevalence is >1% prior to large-scale MDA-based interventions (1990-onwards) Uganda. Based on Moraga P, Cano J, et al. Modelling the distribution and transmission intensity of lymphatic filariasis in sub-Saharan Africa prior to scaling up interventions: integrated use of geostatistical and mathematical modelling. Parasit Vectors. 2015;8:560.

17. Kolaczinski JH, Kabatereine NB, Onapa AW, Ndyomugyenyi R, Kakembo ASL, Brooker S. Neglected tropical diseases in Uganda: the prospect and challenge of integrated control. Trends Parasitol. 2007;23:485–93.

18. Deribe K, Cano J, Newport MJ, Golding N, Pullan R, Sime H, et al. Mapping and modelling the geographical distribution and environmental limits of podoconiosis in Ethiopia. PLoS Negl Trop Dis. 2015;9:e0003946.

19. Price EW, Henderson WJ. Silica and silicates in femoral lymph nodes of barefooted people in Ethiopia with special reference to elephantiasis of the lower legs. Trans R Soc Trop Med Hyg. 1979;73:640–7.

20. Sime H, Deribe K, Assefa A, Newport MJ, Enquselassie F, Gebretsadik A, et al. Integrated mapping of lymphatic filariasis and podoconiosis: lessons learnt from Ethiopia. Parasit Vectors. 2014;7:397.

21. Yimer M, Hailu T, Mulu W, Abera B. Epidemiology of elephantiasis with special emphasis on podoconiosis in Ethiopia: a literature review. J Vector Borne Dis. 2015;52:111–5.

22. Molla YB, Wardrop NA, Le Blond JS, Baxter P, Newport MJ, Atkinson PM, et al. Modelling environmental factors correlated with podoconiosis: a geospatial study of non-filarial elephantiasis. Int J Health Geogr. 2014;13:24.

23. Gyapong JO, Webber RH, Bennett S. The potential role of peripheral health workers and community key informants in the rapid assessment of community burden of disease: the example of lymphatic filariasis. Trop Med Int Health. 1998;3:522–8.

24. Meyrowitsch DM, Simonsen PE, Makunde WH. Bancroftian filariasis: analysis of infection and disease in five endemic communities of north-eastern Tanzania. Ann Trop Med Parasitol. 1995;89:653–63.

25. Deribe K, Wanji S, Shafi O, Tukahebwa EM, Umulisa I, Molyneux DH, et al. The feasibility of eliminating podoconiosis. Bull World Health Organ. 2015;93:712–8.

26. Padovese V, Marrone R, Dassoni F, Vignally P, Barnabas GA, Morrone A. The diagnostic challenge of mapping elephantiasis in the Tigray region of northern Ethiopia. Int J Dermatol. 2016;55:563–70.

27. Wendemagegn E, Tirumalae R, Böer-Auer A. Histopathological and immunohistochemical features of nodular podoconiosis. J Cutan Pathol. 2015;42:173–81.

28. Morrone A, Padovese V, Dassoni F, Pajno MC, Marrone R, Franco G, et al. Podoconiosis: an experience from Tigray, northern Ethiopia. J Am Acad Dermatol. 2011;65:214–5.

29. Visser BJ, Korevaar DA, van der Zee J. Images in Clinical Tropical Medicine: a 24-year-old Ethiopian farmer with burning feet. Am J Trop Med Hyg. 2012;87:583.

30. Ayele FT, Adeyemo A, Finan C, Hailu E, Sinnott P, Burlinson ND, et al. HLA class II locus and susceptibility to podoconiosis. N Engl J Med. 2012;366:1200–8.

17

Mosquito arbovirus survey in selected areas of Kenya: detection of insect-specific virus

Hanako Iwashita[1,2*] (iD), Yukiko Higa[1], Kyoko Futami[1], Peter A. Lutiali[3], Sammy M. Njenga[4], Takeshi Nabeshima[5] and Noboru Minakawa[1]

Abstract

Background: Many arboviral outbreaks have occurred in various locations in Kenya. Entomological surveys are suitable methods for revealing information about circulating arboviruses before human outbreaks are recognized. Therefore, mosquitoes were collected in Kenya to determine the distribution of arboviruses.

Methods: Various species of mosquitoes were sampled from January to July 2012 using several collection methods. Mosquito homogenates were directly tested by reverse transcription-polymerase chain reaction (RT-PCR) using various arbovirus-targeted primer pairs.

Results: We collected 12,569 mosquitoes. Although no human-related arboviruses were detected, Culex flavivirus (CxFV), an insect-specific arbovirus, was detected in 54 pools of 324 *Culex quinquefasciatus* individuals collected during the rainy season. Of these 54 positive pools, 96.3% (52/54) of the mosquitoes were collected in Busia, on the border of western Kenya and Uganda. The remaining two CxFV-positive pools were collected in Mombasa and Kakamega, far from Busia. Phylogenetic analysis revealed minimal genetic diversity among the CxFVs collected in Mombasa, Kakamega, and Busia, even though these cities are in geographically different regions. Additionally, CxFV was detected in one mosquito pool collected in Mombasa during the dry season. In addition to *Culex* mosquitoes, *Aedes* (*Stegomyia*) and *Anopheles* mosquitoes were also positive for the *Flavivirus* genus. Cell fusing agent virus was detected in one pool of *Aedes aegypti*. Mosquito flavivirus was detected in three pools of *Anopheles gambiae* s.l. collected in the dry and rainy seasons.

Conclusions: Although no mosquitoes were positive for human-related arbovirus, insect-specific viruses were detected in various species of mosquitoes. The heterogeneity observed in the number of CxFVs in *Culex* mosquitoes in different locations in Kenya suggests that the abundance of human-related viruses might differ depending on the abundance of insect-specific viruses. We may have underestimated the circulation of any human-related arbovirus in Kenya, and the collection of larger samples may allow for determination of the presence of human-related arboviruses.

Keywords: Arbovirus, Insect-specific virus, Culex flavivirus, *Aedes* mosquito, *Culex* mosquito, *Anopheles* mosquito, Busia, Kakamega, Mombasa, Kenya

* Correspondence: hanako@med.u-ryukyu.ac.jp
[1]Department of Vector Ecology and Environment, Institute of Tropical Medicine, Nagasaki University, 1-12-4 Sakamoto, Nagasaki 852-8523, Japan
[2]Department of Bacteriology, Graduate School of Medicine, University of the Ryukyus, 207 Uehara, Nishiharacho, Okinawa 903-0125, Japan
Full list of author information is available at the end of the article

Background

Emergence and re-emergence of vector-borne diseases are crucial public health problems worldwide [1, 2]. In Kenya, many sporadic outbreaks have been reported in geographically different areas [3]. For example, an outbreak of dengue (DEN) fever occurred in the coastal towns of Malindi and Kilifi in 1982 [4], and in 1992–1993, an outbreak of yellow fever (YF) occurred in Rift Valley Province [5]. There were outbreaks of Rift Valley fever (RVF) in 1997 and 2006 [6–8], and an outbreak of chikungunya (CHIK) fever occurred in 2004 in the coastal area of Kenya [9, 10]. In Uganda, an epidemic of o'nyong'nyong (ONN) started in early 1959 and spread to Kenya [11, 12].

In general, febrile diseases caused by viruses are still confused with non-viral diseases, such as malaria [2]. Moreover, cases can remain unnoticed because some arboviral infections are mild and self-limiting during the early stage. Therefore, the number of human arboviral cases might be much higher than has been reported. Even in the absence of clinical outbreaks, historic serosurveys in Kenya can provide important clues about circulating arboviruses in various environments [13]. For instance, Mease et al. in [14] assessed the prevalence of IgG against yellow fever virus (YFV), West Nile virus (WNV), dengue virus (DENV), and chikungunya virus (CHIKV) using serum samples from healthy Kenyans. According to their data, 46.6% of the people in all study areas had antibodies against at least one of these arboviruses [14]. As historic serosurveys in Kenya have documented several arboviruses in geographically different areas [15], a large epidemic of arbovirus can occur anywhere at any time because, as demonstrated recently, many factors such as demographic, geographic environmental and climate change factors can complicate and worsen the situation [16]. Many studies have revealed that a threat of arboviral transmission is present throughout Kenya, regardless of the officially announced reports of outbreaks [17, 18].

Controlling arboviral diseases is difficult because of the complex environment and ecology, including relationships among viruses, vectors, and humans [2, 16, 19]. Multiple vector species are often involved in an arboviral disease, and a single vector can also transmit several diseases. Moreover, primary vectors vary among geographical areas, and the level of vector competence may also vary among species depending on each area [20]. Mosquitoes are known to carry not only human-related viruses but also insect-specific viruses, such as Culex flavivirus and Aedes flavivirus [21]. In addition, interactions between many types of viruses and many other organisms may affect vector competence inside the mosquito [22]. For example, the presence of co-infection with insect-specific virus and WNV has been reported [23]. In this case, co-infection

might be considered a factor for the emergence of arbovirus, though the function of insect-specific viruses remains unclear. Assessing the potential for arbovirus outbreaks at the local level can be facilitated by identifying all patterns of relationships, including triangular relationships (human-vector-arbovirus environment), in each area [24]. Moreover, entomological baseline data may contribute to estimations of disease risk and allow precautionary measures to be taken against virus activity. In this study, we mainly selected collection sites where other researchers had previously found or suspected arbovirus activity. For example, border areas are suspected to be areas of potential arbovirus infection because busy transportation hubs may provide many opportunities for human-vector contact [25]. Although the presence of arboviruses has not yet been reported in some indigenous forests in Kenya, many species of mosquitoes can serve as bridge vectors of arboviruses, easily spreading sylvatic arboviruses such as sylvatic YF and sylvatic DENV from forests to human environments in these areas in Kenya [26]. We suspected that arboviruses were silently circulating, without outbreak detection. Therefore, an active survey was undertaken in border areas, including coastal boundaries and indigenous forests. The aim of this study was to obtain data regarding the presence of arboviruses in mosquitoes in selected areas of Kenya. Our additional goal was to recognize the main vector species of arboviruses.

Methods
Study areas
Mosquito sampling was performed in eastern (Mombasa and Kwale) and western (Kakamega and Busia) Kenya, which included a variety of areas, such as urban coastal border, land border, and rural areas next to a forest where there is suspected arbovirus activity (Fig. 1). The sampling was conducted in two different seasons: the rainy season and a season other than the rainy season; March to June in Kenya generally constitutes the rainy season. We initiated this study in January 2012, before the rainy season, which we conventionally termed the dry season. Between January 18 and 26, 2012 (representing dry-season sampling), we conducted a preliminary survey only in eastern Kenya. Between May 9 and June 8, 2012 (representing rainy-season sampling), we conducted the same survey in both eastern and western Kenya.

Eastern Kenya: Mombasa (the center: 4°3.509'S; 39°40.363'E)
This busy port town includes the urban coastal border with high levels of human activity. Dengue cases have been reported here for approximately the last 30 years [4]. We suspected that due to human activity, arboviral mosquitoes can be easily transported outside this area. Mosquitoes were collected in resident areas in the 2012

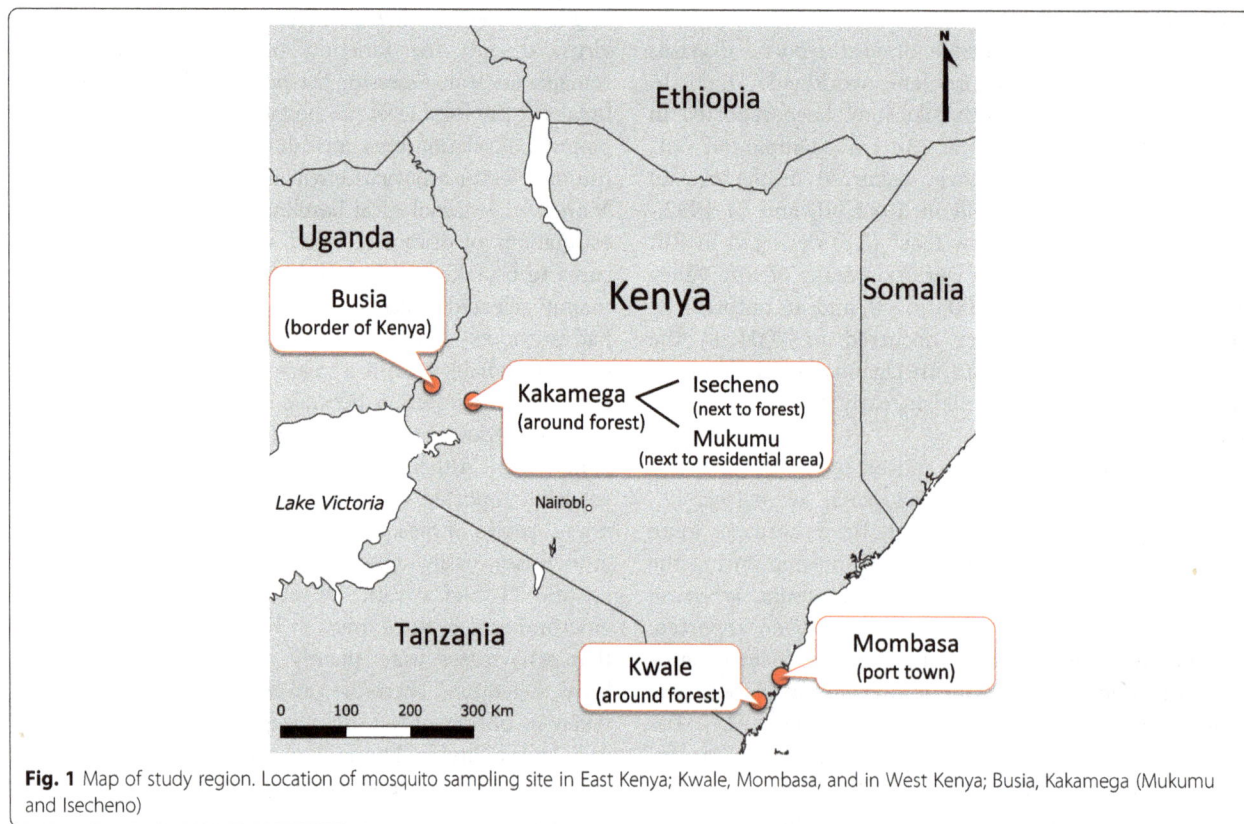

Fig. 1 Map of study region. Location of mosquito sampling site in East Kenya; Kwale, Mombasa, and in West Kenya; Busia, Kakamega (Mukumu and Isecheno)

dry season (from January 24 to January 26) and in the 2012 rainy season (from May 15 to May 17).

Eastern Kenya: Kwale (the center: 4°10.525'S; 39°27.087'E)

In this rural area, patches of indigenous forests (Shimba Hills National Reserve) exist next to the residential area. The edge of the indigenous forest can act as a border cross which arboviral mosquitoes can be transported from the forest to the residential area. Mosquitoes were sampled from houses in the 2012 dry season (from January 18 to January 20) and in the 2012 rainy season (from May 9 to May 12).

Western Kenya: Kakamega (the center: 0°16.923'N; 34°45.234'E)

Kakamega forest has a remarkable diversity of insects, birds and animals, which can serve as reservoir hosts of arboviruses [27]. We selected two areas: one exactly next to the indigenous forest (Isecheno), and another, a residential area (Mukumu) along the main road in this region. The edge of the indigenous forest is considered to be a dangerous border of arboviral activity, similar to Kwale. We suspect that the area is easily penetrable by arboviral mosquitoes from forests to residential areas and vice versa. The main road is also regarded as a border, which may encourage transmission of arboviruses. Mosquitoes were collected in Mukumu from June 2 to June 4 and in Isecheno from June 6 to June 8.

Western Kenya: Busia (the center: 0°27.914'N; 34°5.979')

Busia is in the western land border (Kenya and Uganda) area, including a busy town with high human activity. Serological surveys were conducted and revealed a high positive rate of antibodies against arboviruses in healthy residents [14]. In this area, many residents may have already suffered from arboviral diseases, with or without symptoms. Transmission between humans and mosquitoes may have been underestimated due to the complicated human activity. Mosquito surveillance can provide other information to show the actual circulation of arboviruses. Mosquitoes were collected from May 25 to May 27.

Mosquito sampling

In each area, mosquitoes were collected for 3 consecutive days from 13 selected houses within approximately 0.5 km² in each targeted area, except one area (for 4 consecutive days in Kwale in the rainy season). A systematic sampling method was applied for selecting study houses in each targeted area [28]. For example, in Kakamega, the main intersection (0°16.923'N; 34°45.234'E) on Kisumu-Kakamega Road was used as the starting point for the systematic sampling of houses. From this point, we established 13 sampling points at 250-m intervals. The nearest house from each point was then selected. The house belongs to a large family (> 5 people), and it was suggested because our study targets human-related arboviruses. Another house was selected if the household head or guardian was not willing to participate in the study. The same method was performed in other areas. Collection methods used the following traps: (i) CDC light traps, (ii) CDC gravid traps, and (iii) BG sentinel traps. Additionally, indoor resting mosquito collection with hand aspirators was performed in all houses. To use 20 traps effectively, we placed 2 types of traps randomly within each of the 13 study houses. We intended to collect as many mosquitoes as possible because arbovirus transmission is usually maintained at a low level in a mosquito population [29]. When the number of mosquitoes collected was insufficient, the position of the traps or type of traps was randomly changed. We used the most effective collection combination with positioning and type of traps at each study site.

In our study, the position of the traps depended on the structure of the house. CDC light traps were suspended > 1.5 m above the ground inside and outside of the houses but not near any other sources of artificial light. CDC gravid traps were placed in a stable area somewhere inside or outside the house where nothing could upset the medium in the pan, for example, under eaves. BG sentinel traps were placed in the house with enough space or outside of the house. CDC light traps were operated from dusk to dawn, whereas other traps were operated for 3–4 days continuously. Resting mosquito collection was performed using oral aspirators by three persons in all rooms of the selected houses in the early morning for 15 min each day; this occurred during all collection periods when the house was visited to remove the mosquito-sampling bags from the traps. To prevent RNA degradation, the captured mosquitoes were kept alive during transfer to the laboratory.

Mosquito identification

At the laboratory, the collected mosquitoes were killed at – 20 °C and placed on white filter paper in a Petri dish placed on a chill table and identified morphologically to the species level under a stereoscopic microscope using published keys [30–33]. For accurate identification, *Aedes aegypti*, *Culex quinquefasciatus*, *Anopheles funestus*, and *An. rivulorum* were confirmed by polymerase chain reaction (PCR) using specific primers (Table 1).

Mosquito processing

A maximum of 30 individuals were pooled according to species, sex, physiological status, (i.e., unfed, blood fed, or gravid), and collection site and then were frozen in liquid nitrogen. For virus detection, we used all pools collected during the dry season, with each category (male, unfed, fed and gravid) examined separately. In contrast, for the pools collected during the rainy season, only unfed and gravid mosquito pools of *Ae. aegypti*, *An.*

funestus, *An. gambiae s.l.*, and *Cx. quinquefasciatus* were used. Moreover, both unfed and gravid mosquitoes were combined for some pools of each species. Blood-fed mosquitoes were excluded to prevent contamination of the virus contained in a blood meal, though we did utilize blood-fed mosquitoes collected during the dry season because of the small sample size. For the samples collected during the rainy season, we concentrated on detecting viruses in only female pools, excluding those that were blood-fed.

Pooled specimens were placed in a 1.5-ml microcentrifuge tube with 300 µl of minimal essential medium (MEM) (minimum essential medium containing 10% foetal bovine serum, L-glutamine, penicillin, streptomycin, and amphotericin B). The mosquitoes were ground in MEM, and the homogenate was centrifuged; 200 µl of the supernatant was collected and kept at – 80 °C for future use (for cell culture). To maintain approximately 100 µl of the suspension, 75 µl of lysis buffer was added. The homogenates were prepared using sterile, RNase-free utensils.

Total RNA extraction and virus identification by reverse transcription-PCR

Total RNA was extracted from each pool of mosquitoes using an extraction kit (SV Total RNA Isolation System, Promega, Tokyo, Japan) according to the manufacturer's instructions. RNA was eluted in 50 µl of sterile distilled water. Reverse transcription reactions were performed to synthesize first-strand cDNA using RNA to cDNA EcoDry Premix (Random Hexamers) (Clontech Laboratories, Inc., Mountain View, CA, USA). The cDNA was amplified by PCR using an AccuPower™ PCR Premix Kit (Bioneer Co., Daejon, Korea) with virus-specific primers (Table 1), and the products were evaluated by 1.5% agarose gel electrophoresis. For all positive samples, products of the expected size were extracted from the gel and were purified using a MonoFas DNA Purification Kit (GL Sciences, Tokyo, Japan). Purified amplicons were bidirectionally sequenced using a BigDye Terminator version 3.1 Cycle Sequencing Kit (Applied Biosystems, Foster City, CA, USA) and analyzed with an ABI3130 Genetic Analyzer (Applied Biosystems). Nucleic acid sequences were compared with those in the GenBank database using the BLAST program.

The process was repeated for three universal primers for flavivirus (the main targets are DENV, YFV, and WNV), two universal primers for alpha viruses (the main targets are ONN virus and CHIKV) and single primer sets for RVFV (phlebovirus) (Table 1). For flaviviruses and alpha viruses, we prepared multiple primer sets to detect not only a well-known virus but also novel viruses. In the case of flavivirus detection, all pools were initially screened for flavivirus RNA by using universal flavivirus primer sets cFD2 and MAMD, which target the non-structural protein 5 (NS5) gene. To identify

Table 1 Primers used to detect and to sequence arbovirus from mosquito pools in Kenya

Target	Primer name	Nucleotide sequence (5′ to 3′)	Polarity	Product (bp)	Cycle condition	Reference
Universal primers for flavivirus	MAMD	AACATGATGGGRAARAGRGARAA	Forward	252	94°C, 2 min, 1 cycle; 94°C, 1 min, 53°C, 1 min, 72°C, 1 min, 35 cycles; 72°C, 5 min, 1 cycle	Scaramozzino et al. (2001) [48]
	cFD2	GTGTCCCAGCCGGCGGTGTCATCAGC	Reverse			
Universal primers for flavivirus	FLAVI-1	AATGTACGCTGATGACACAGCTGGCT GGGACAC	Forward	854–863	94°C, 5 min, 1 cycle; 94°C, 1 min, 58°C, 1 min, 72°C, 90 s, 45 cycles; 72°C, 10 min, 1 cycle	Ayers et al.(2006) [49]
	FLAVI-2	TCCAGACCTTCAGCATGTCTTCTGTTGT CATCCA	Reverse			
Universal primers for flavivirus (mainly YF)	YF-1	GGTCTCCTCTAACCTCTAG	Forward	675	94°C, 2 min, 1 cycle; 94°C, 30 s, 53°C, 30 s, 72°C, 1 min, 35 cycles; 72°C, 5 min, 1 cycle	Tanaka et al. (1993) [50]
	YF-3	GAGTGGATGACCACGGAAGACATGC	Reverse			
Universal primers for alpha viruses (mainly chikungunya and o'nyong'nyong viruses)	nsP1-S	TAGAGCAGGAAATTGATCC	Forward	354	94°C, 2 min, 1 cycle; 94°C, 30 s, 53°C, 30 s, 72°C, 45 s, 35 cycles; 72°C, 5 min, 1 cycle	Hasebe et al. (2002) [51]
	nsP1-C	CTTTAATCGCCTGGTGGTA	Reverse			
Universal primers for alpha viruses (mainly chikungunya and o'nyong'nyong viruses)	E1-S	TACCCATTCATGTGGGG	Forward	294	94°C, 2 min, 1 cycle; 94°C, 30 s, 53°C, 30 s, 72°C, 45 s, 35 cycles; 72°C, 5 min, 1 cycle	Hasebe et al. (2002) [51]
	E1-C	GCCTTTGTACACCACGAT	Reverse			
Rift Valley virus	RVF009	CCAAATGACTACCAGTCAGC	Forward	400–500	94°C, 2 min, 1 cycle; 94°C, 30 s, 50°C, 30 s, 72°C, 1 min, 35 cycles; 72°C, 5 min, 1 cycle	Jupp et al. (2000) [52] (modified)
	RVF007	GACAAATGAGTCTGGTAGCA	Reverse			
Mosquito RNA marker	Act-2F	ATGGTCGGYATGGGNCAGAAGGACTC	Forward	683	94°C, 2 min, 1 cycle; 94°C, 30 s, 54°C, 30 s, 72°C, 45 s, 35 cycles; 72°C, 5 min, 1 cycle	Staley et al. (2010) [53]
	Act-8R	GATTCCATACCCAGGAAGGADGG	Reverse			
Culex quinquefaciatus	ACEpip	GGAAACAACGACGTATGTACT	Forward	610	94°C, 5 min, 1 cycle; 94°C, 30 s, 54°C, 30 s, 72°C, 1 min, 35 cycles; 72°C, 5 min, 1 cycle	Kasai et al. (2008) [39]
	ACEquin	CCTTCTTGAATGGCTGTGGCA	Forward	274		
	B1246s	TGGAGCCTCCTCTTCACGG	Reverse			
Aedes aegypti	18SFHIN	GTAAGCTTCCTTTGTACACACCGCCCGT	Forward	550	97°C, 4 min, 1 cycle; 96°C, 30 s, 48°C, 30 s, 72°C, 2 min, 30 cycles; 72°C, 4 min, 1 cycle	Higa et al. (2010) [54]
	aeg.r1	TAACGGACACCGTTCTAGGCCCT	Reverse			
Anopheles funestus, Anopheles rivulorum	UV	TGTGAACTGCAGGACACAT	Forward		94°C, 2 min, 1 cycle; 94°C, 30 s, 45°C, 30 s, 72°C, 40 s, 30 cycles; 72°C, 5 min, 1 cycle	Koekemoer et al. (2002) [55]
	FUN	GCATCGATGGGTTAATCATG	Reverse	505		
	RIV	CAAGCCGTTCGACCCTGATT	Reverse	411		

Note: Each 25 μl reaction mixture contained. (Accupower TM PCR PreMix kit with 2 μl template, 15.2 μl sterile water, and 1.4 μl of 100 pmol/μl each of primers)

human-related flaviviruses, such as DENV, YFV, and WNV, all pools were screened with primer sets YF-1 and YF-3. To generate a larger NS5 cDNA segment for sequencing, putative positive samples detected using previous primer sets (cFD2 and MAMD) were again screened for flavivirus RNA using another universal flavivirus primer set (FLAVI1 and FLAVI2) targeting the NS5 gene. Confirmed bands of approximately 860 bp were sequenced as described above. In the case of alpha virus detection, primer sets (nsP1-S and nsP1-C; E1-S and E1-C) designed based on the genes non-structural protein 1 (nsP1) and glycoprotein E1 (E1) were used for amplification.

The following inactivated viruses available in the laboratory were used as positive controls: DEN-1 (Hawaii strain), YFV (17D strain, attenuated live vaccine strain), WNV (NY99 strain), CHIKV (S27 strain, African prototype), RVFV (Smithburn strain, attenuated live vaccine strain) (All positive controls were kindly provided by Dr. S Inoue). As a quality control for the detection step, each cDNA was checked by PCR using the mosquito β-actin primer.

Calculation of infection rates

We calculated the minimum infection rate (MIR) of arboviruses in each mosquito species at each site using the Poolscreen2 program [34]. MIR is expressed as the number of pools infected per 1000 mosquitoes tested, and it assumes that only one mosquito is positive in a pool. To determine the number of flavivirus-positive samples, the results using primer sets cFD2 and MAMD were employed. MIR was calculated when at least 100 mosquitoes were tested per species per site.

Phylogenetic analysis

For virus species identification, the collected sequences were confirmed by an alignment search in gene databases using MEGA6 with the ClustalW method [35]. Phylogenetic and molecular evolutionary analyses were conducted by using the p-distance option with the neighbor-joining (NJ) method. Bootstrap analyses were performed with 1000 replicates. Representative flavivirus sequences were used in the phylogenetic analysis as outgroup sequences.

Results

Mosquito collection

During the dry season in eastern Kenya (Table 2)

In Kwale (January 18–20, 2012), we employed a cumulative number of 39 trap sessions (per day per house) in 13 houses for 3 days (total numbers of each trap session

Table 2 Summary of mosquitoes collected in the dry season in East Kenya

Study site		Kwale			Mombasa		
Collection methods employed (number of trap sessions)[#]		As; 39, BG; 12, CDC; 15, GT; 12			As; 39, BG; 12, CDC; 15, GT; 12		
Methods collected mosquitoes (number of trap sessions)[#]		As; 7, BG; 3, CDC; 10, GT; 6			As; 33, BG; 7, CDC; 14, GT; 12		
Collection period		January 18–20, 2012 (3 days)			January 24–26, 2012 (3 days)		
Number of houses		13 houses			13 houses		
Species	Physiological status	No. collected	Pools	Positive pool	No. collected	Pools	Positive pool
Ae. aegypti	Fed				2	1	0
	Unfed	3	3	0	16	2	0
An. coustani	Fed	1	1	0			
An. funestus	Fed	1	1	0			
An. gambiae s.l.	Fed	3	1	0			
	Unfed	8	1	1	2	1	1
An. longipulpis	Fed	1	1	0			
An. rivulorum	Fed	4	1	0			
Anopheles sp.	Male	1	1	0			
Cx. cinereus	Gravid	1	1	0			
Cx. decens	Unfed	2	1	0			
	Gravid	4	1	0			
Cx. quinquefasciatus	Male	15	1	0	235	10	1
	Fed	30	2	0	105	6	0
	Unfed	19	1	0	375	13	0
	Gravid	64	4	0	129	7	0
Cx. laticinctus	Gravid	5	1	0			
Cx. simpsoni	Male	1	1	0			
	Unfed				2	1	0
Cx. univiittetus	Unfed				2	1	0
Culex sp.	Male				1	1	0
	Unfed	1	1	0	3	1	0
Mansonia sp.	Fed	2	1	0			
	Unfed	8	1	0			
Others	Male	2					
	Unfed	3					
Total		179	26	1	872	44	2

[#]Abbreviations of collection methods are *As* aspirator, *BG*: BG sentinel trap, *CDC*:CDC light trap, *GT* CDC gravid trap per day per house were 12 BG sentinel, 15 CDC light, and 12 CDC gravid trap sessions) and a cumulative number of 39 aspirator catch sessions (per day per house) in 13 houses for 3 days using a 3-person aspirator catch team in each house. We collected 179 mosquitoes in the following subset of attempts: 3 BG sentinel trap sessions, 10 CDC light trap sessions, 6 CDC gravid trap sessions, and 7 aspirator catches. In Mombasa (January 24–26, 2012), we collected 872 mosquitoes by the same cumulative number of trap sessions as in Kwale. The collection methods entailed 7 BG sentinel trap sessions, 14 CDC light trap sessions, 12 CDC gravid trap sessions, and 33 aspirator catches. The total number of mosquitoes collected in Kwale and Mombasa was 1051. Of these mosquitoes, 796 (75.7%) were identified as females. For these samples collected during the dry season, all species were tested, including males of each species (70 pools) (Table 2). Only five mosquitoes were not identified and were excluded.

During the rainy season in eastern and western Kenya (Table 3)

In Kwale (May 9–12, 2012), we employed a cumulative number of 57 trap sessions (per day per house) in 13 houses for 4 days (total numbers of each trap session per day per house were 30 BG sentinel, 16 CDC light, and 22 CDC gravid trap sessions) and a cumulative number of 48 aspirator catches (per day per house) in 13 houses for 4 days using a 3-person aspirator catch team in each house. We collected 2592 mosquitoes in the following subset of attempts: 25 BG sentinel trap sessions, 11 CDC light trap sessions, 22 CDC gravid trap sessions, and 42 aspirator catches. In Mombasa (May 15–17, 2012), we employed a cumulative number of 42 trap sessions (per day per house) in 13 houses for 3 days (total numbers of trap sessions were 13 BG sentinel traps, 12 CDC light traps, and 17 CDC gravid traps) and a cumulative number of 30 aspirator catch sessions (per day per house) in 13 houses for 3 days using a 3-person aspirator catch team in each house. We collected 1974 mosquitoes in the following subset of attempts: 12 BG sentinel trap sessions, 11 CDC light trap sessions, 17 CDC gravid trap sessions, and 28 aspirator catches. In Busia (May 25–27, 2012), we employed a cumulative number of 45 trap sessions (per day per house) in 13 houses for 3 days (total numbers of trap sessions were 18 BG sentinel, 12 CDC light, and 15 CDC gravid trap sessions) and a cumulative number of 36 aspirator catch sessions (per day per house) in 13 houses for 3 days using 3-person aspirator catch team in each house. We collected 4598 mosquitoes in the following subset of attempts: 17 BG sentinel trap sessions, 12 CDC light trap sessions, 15 CDC gravid trap sessions, and 36 aspirator catches. In Kakamega (Mukumu) (June 2–4, 2012), we

employed a cumulative number of 51 trap sessions (per day per house) in 13 houses for 3 days (total numbers of each trap sessions per day per house were 15 BG sentinel, 18 CDC light, and 18 CDC gravid trap sessions) and a cumulative number of 39 aspirator catches (per day per house) in 13 houses for 3 days using 3-person aspirator catch team in each house. We collected 2087 mosquitoes in the following subset of attempts: 13 BG sentinel trap sessions, 16 CDC light trap sessions, 15 CDC gravid trap sessions, and 34 aspirator catches. In Kakamega (Isecheno) (June 6–8, 2012), we employed a cumulative number of 57 trap sessions (per day per house) in 13 houses for 3 days (total numbers of trap sessions per day per house were 15 BG sentinel, 21 CDC light, and 21 CDC gravid trap sessions) and a cumulative number of 39 aspirator catch sessions (per day per house) in 13 houses for 3 days using a 3-person aspirator catch team in each house. We collected 267 mosquitoes in the following subset of attempts: 8 BG sentinel trap sessions, 11 CDC light trap sessions, 17 CDC gravid trap sessions, and 20 aspirator catches.

In total, we collected 11,518 mosquitoes at all sampling sites. Of these mosquitoes collected during the rainy season, 8663 (75.2%) were identified as female. Only unfed and gravid female mosquitoes (414 pools) were used for virus detection in samples collected during the rainy season (Table 4). The number of mosquitoes collected in Kakamega (Isecheno) was one order of magnitude lower than that collected at the other study sites.

Arbovirus detection

Overall, 484 pools consisting of 7788 mosquitoes were tested. The selected species collected in both seasons for the detection of arbovirus were *Ae. aegypti* (41 pools), *An. funestus* (8 pools), *An. gambiae* s.l. (47 pools), *An. rivulorum* (5 pools), and *Cx. quinquefasciatus* (368 pools). The following species of mosquitoes collected during only the dry season from East Kenya were also used for detection: *An. coustani* (1 pool), *An. longipalpis* (1 pool), *Cx. cinereus* (1 pool), *Cx. decens* (2 pools), *Cx. laticinctus* (1 pool), *Cx. simpsoni* (2 pool), *Cx. univittatus* (1 pool), *Anopheles* sp. (1 pool), *Culex* sp. (3 pools) and *Mansonia* sp. (2 pools). Although we collected 2 individuals of *Cx. decens* (1 male and 1 female from Isecheno), *Cx. simpsoni* (1 female from Busia), and *Cx. univittatus* (1 female from Busia) during the rainy season, we did not use these specimens for detection because of their small sample numbers compared to all other pools during the rainy season.

Human-related arboviruses from all mosquitoes

All pools were negative for human-related arboviruses, such as DENV, YFV, WNV, ONN, and CHINV.

Table 3 Summary of mosquitoes collected in the rainy season in East and West Kenya

Study area		East Kenya			East Kenya			West Kenya			West Kenya			West Kenya		
Study site		Kwale			Mombasa			Busia			Kakamega (Mukumu)			Kakamega (Isecheno)		
Collection methods employed (number of trap sessions)#		As; 48, BG; 30, CDC; 16, GT; 22			As; 30, BG; 13, CDC; 12, GT; 17			As; 36, BG; 18, CDC; 12, GT; 15			As; 39, BG; 15, CDC; 18, GT; 18			As; 39, BG; 15, CDC; 21, GT; 21		
Methods collected mosquitoes (number of trap sessions)#		As; 42, BG; 25, CDC; 11, GT; 22			As; 28, BG; 12, CDC; 11, GT; 17			As; 36, BG; 17, CDC; 12, GT; 15			As; 34, BG; 13, CDC; 16, GT; 15			As; 20, BG; 8, CDC; 11, GT; 17		
Collection period (days)		May 9–12, 2012 (4 days)			May 15–17, 2012 (3 days)			May 25–27, 2012 (3 days)			June 2–4, 2012 (3 days)			June 6–8, 2012 (3 days)		
Number of houses		13 houses			13 houses			13 houses			13 houses			13 houses		
Species	Physiological status	No. collected	Pool	Positive pool	No. collected	Pool	Positive pool	No. collected	Pool	Positive pool	No. collected	Pool	Positive pool	No. collected	Pool	Positive pool
Aedes sp.	Male				2											
	Unfed	3			2									1		
Ae. aegypti	Male				2											
	Unfed	11	8	0	49	14	1*	4	8	0	3	3	0	2	2	0
	Gravid	2			7			6			1			1		
An. brumripes	Unfed	1												2		
An. funestus	Male							3								
	Fed							5								
	Unfed							59	7	0						
	Gravid							2								
An. gambiae s.l.	Male							22						3		
	Fed	2						37						3	3	0
	Unfed	18	3	0				402	34	1	3	4	0	3		
	Gravid							9			1					
An. garnhami	Fed										1					
	Unfed	6														
An. parensis	Unfed	1														
An. rivulorum	Unfed							4	3	0	1	1	0			
	Gravid										1					
Anopheles sp.	Male	1														
	Fed	2														
	Unfed	6						2			1					
	Gravid													1		
Cx. decens	Male													1		
	Gravid													1		

Table 3 Summary of mosquitoes collected in the rainy season in East and West Kenya (Continued)

Study area		East Kenya			East Kenya			West Kenya			West Kenya			West Kenya		
Cx. quinquefasciatus	Male	355			540			1554			332			38		
	Fed	202			351			331			840			79		
	Unfed	106	106	0	443	52	1*	1243	113	52***	472	46	1**	53	7	0
	Gravid	1867			554			906			431			79		
Cx. simpsoni	Unfed							1								
Cx. univittetus	Unfed							1								
Culex sp.	Male	3			3											
	Fed	1			1											
	Unfed	4			2						1			0		
	Gravid	1			1									3		
Lutzia	Gravid				2						2					
Others	Male	2														
	Unfed	1			15			3								
	Gravid							1								
Total		2592	117	0	1974	66	2	4598	165	53	2087	54	1	267	12	0

Note: We used only unfed and gravid mosquitoes for the pools to detect arboviruses. Unfed and gravid mosquitoes were separated into each category, but some of them were combined into one pool.
*The pool comprised only gravid mosquitoes
**The pool comprised only unfed mosquitoes
***Pools consisted of unfed and gravid mosquitoes
#Abbreviations of "collection methods" are As aspirator, BG BG sentinel trap, CDC CDC light trap, GT CDC gravid trap

Table 4. Information of positive samples for insect specific arbovirus

Places	Season	Species of mosquito	No. of mosquitoes	Physiological status of used pools	No. pools	No. positive pools	MIR*	MIR Lower-upper limits	Physiological status of positive pool
Ae. aegypti mosquito pools									
Kwale	Dry	*Ae. aegypti*	3	Unfed	3	0	NA	NA	
Kwale	Rain	*Ae. aegypti*	13	Unfed, gravid	8	0	NA	NA	
Mombasa	Dry	*Ae. aegypti*	18	Fed, unfed	3	0	NA	NA	
Mombasa	Rain	*Ae. aegypti*	56	Unfed, gravid (♂; excluded)	14	1	NA	NA	Female, gravid
Busia	Rain	*Ae. aegypti*	10	Unfed, gravid	8	0	NA	NA	
Kakamega (Mukumu)	Rain	*Ae. aegypti*	4	Unfed, gravid	3	0	NA	NA	
Kakamega (Isecheno)	Rain	*Ae. aegypti*	3	Unfed, gravid	2	0	NA	NA	
Cx. quinquefasciatus mosquito pools									
Kwale	Dry	*Cx. quinquefasciatus*	128	♂, fed, unfed, gravid	8	0	NA	NA	
Kwale	Rain	*Cx. quinquefasciatus*	1973	Unfed, gravid (♂, fed; excluded)	106	0	NA	NA	
Mombasa	Dry	*Cx. quinquefasciatus*	844	♂, fed, unfed, gravid	36	1	1.18	0.07–5.75	♂
Mombasa	Rain	*Cx. quinquefasciatus*	997	Unfed, gravid (♂, fed; excluded)	52	1	1.01	0.06–4.89	Female, gravid
Busia	Rain	*Cx. quinquefasciatus*	2149	Unfed, gravid (♂, fed; excluded)	113	52	32.26	24.42–42.12	Female, unfed + gravid
Kakamega (Mukumu)	Rain	*Cx. quinquefasciatus*	903	Unfed, gravid (♂, fed; excluded)	46	1	1.11	0.06–5.37	Female, unfed
Kakamega (Isecheno)	Rain	*Cx. quinquefasciatus*	132	Unfed, gravid (♂, fed; excluded)	7	0	NA	NA	
An. gambiae mosquito pools									
Kwale	Dry	*An. gambiae*	11	Fed, unfed	2	1	NA	NA	Female, unfed
Kwale	Rain	*An. gambiae*	18	Unfed, (fed; excluded)	3	0	NA	NA	
Mombasa	Dry	*An. gambiae*	2	Unfed	1	1	NA	NA	Female, unfed
Mombasa	Rain	*An. gambiae*	0		0	0	NA	NA	
Busia	Rain	*An. gambiae*	411	Unfed, gravid (♂, fed; excluded)	34	1	2.44	0.14–11.87	Female, unfed
Kakamega (Mukumu)	Rain	*An. gambiae*	4	Unfed, gravid	4	0	NA	NA	
Kakamega (Isecheno)	Rain	*An. gambiae*	3	Unfed (fed; excluded)	3	0	NA	NA	

*Minimum infection rate

Mosquito-related arboviruses from *Culex quinquefasciatus*

Using the primer sets cFD2 and MAMD, PCR bands were observed for 54 female *Cx. quinquefasciatus* pools during the rainy season and 1 male *Cx. quinquefasciatus* pool during the dry season in Mombasa (Tables 2 and 3). The nucleotide sequences for positive PCR reactions amplified using the primer sets cFD2 and MAMD from all these pools were compared with the GenBank database (BLAST), and sequencing results of all samples were 99% identical to the homologous region of Culex flavivirus (CxFV) strain Uganda08 (GQ165808.1). When we limited our analysis to female mosquitoes only, Busia yielded the most positive pools (52 pools) followed by Bamburi (1 pool) and Mukumu (1 pool).

To generate a larger NS5 cDNA segment for sequencing to be used in phylogenetic analyses, only pools that were positive for flavivirus using the primer sets cFD2 and MAMD were amplified with the primer sets FLAVI1 and FLAVI2. Bands of approximately 860 nt (597 nt was used) were observed, and nucleotide sequencing was successful for 22 pools of *Cx. quinquefasciatus* (21 female pools and 1 male pool) among 55 pools (54 female pools and 1 male pool). The genomic sequences obtained using both primer sets (FLAVI1 and FLAVI2) share similar nucleotide sequence identity (99%) with CxFV from Uganda (GenBank: GQ165808.1). This result was the same as that using the primer sets cFD2 and MAMD. A phylogenetic tree was constructed with the NJ method using NS5 gene sequences of 22 CxFV strains by adding CxFV NS5 gene sequences from Uganda (GenBank: GQ165808.1) and Guatemala (GenBank: EU805806) obtained from BLAST. Additionally, NS5 gene sequences of human-related flaviviruses, such as WNV (GenBank: DQ118127.1, GenBank: AF202541), DNV (GenBank: AY099336.1, GenBank: AF326825.1, GenBank: U87411.1), and Japanese encephalitis virus (GenBank: M18370.1), were included as outgroup sequences. The NS5 gene sequences of our samples from Kenya clustered with CxFV NS5 gene sequences from Uganda and Guatemala. Although Busia, Kakamega, and Mombasa are in completely different regions of Kenya, the phylogenetic tree shows sequence similarity (Fig. 2).

Mosquito-related arboviruses from *Ae. aegypti* and *An. gambiae*

The PCR products using the primer sets FLAVI1 and FLAVI2 for one pool of *Ae. aegypti* were shown to correspond to cell-fusing agent virus (CFAV) (NC_001564.1, 96% BLAST identity). In terms of *An. gambiae* s.l. pools, PCR products using the same primer sets as above were observed for three female pools, consisting of one pool from Kwale and one pool from Mombasa (both collected during the dry season) and one pool from Busia (collected during the rainy season). The nucleotide sequencing results of the two samples collected in Kwale and Mombasa were similar to mosquito flavivirus sequences (KM088036.1 and KM088037.1, 99% BLAST identity) reported from Kenya. The sequence of the sample collected from one pool from Busia was moderately divergent from the other two, being most similar a sequence of Anopheles flavivirus (KX148546.1, 85% BLAST identity) reported from Liberia. According to Kuno et al., a viral species is defined as the same group of viruses with > 84% nucleotide sequence identity among them [36]. Our sequence analysis demonstrated slightly higher nucleotide sequence identity than this cut-off. Therefore, the viruses from *An. gambiae* s.l. collected in Busia represent a variant of the closely related Anopheles flavivirus. The phylogenetic analyses including arboviruses from *Cx. quinquefasciatus* are presented in Fig. 2.

Minimum infection rate (MIR)

Although our study sites were geographically limited, MIR for *Cx. quinquefasciatus* showed a heterogeneous distribution for this species among the selected sites. Busia was the region with the highest MIR among all *Cx. quinquefasciatus* pools collected in Kenya (Table 4).

Other *Cx. quinquefasciatus* pools revealed only one positive pool, with an MIR of approximately 1.0 (Table 4). Furthermore, taking into account differences in sampling efficiency among the study sites, seasons and traps, the *Cx. quinquefasciatus* specimens collected in Busia showed a higher MIR (MIR = 32.26; 95% CI = 24.42–42.12) than those collected in Mombasa during the rainy season (MIR = 1.01; 95% CI = 0.06–4.89) and during the dry season (MIR = 1.18; 95% CI = 0.07–5.75), and those collected in Kakamega during the rainy season (MIR = 1.11; 95% CI = 0.06–5.37). CxFV was detected in Mombasa during the dry season in a male pool as well as in female pools; however, there were no positive samples found in female pools during the dry season. No differences in MIR were found between the dry and rainy seasons in Mombasa, even though the pools of male and fed mosquitoes collected in the rainy season were not tested. Because of the limited number of samples, it is uncertain whether heterogeneity exists among *Ae. aegypti* and *An. gambiae* MIRs.

Discussion

In this study in Kenya, we did not detect any human-related arboviruses, and the main vector species of arboviruses were not found. Instead, we did detect mosquito-specific arboviruses from many types of mosquitoes. In particular, high prevalence of CxFV is *Cx. quinquefasciatus* was found in Busia, and this strain of CxFV is similar to one reported in Uganda by Cook et al. [37, 38]. Additionally, a similar CxFV was detected in each female pool from Mombasa and Kakamega. These areas in Kenya are separated by great distances. Additional sampling in the area between Busia and Kakamega in western Kenya and in the area between Kakamega and Mombasa in middle to eastern Kenya will likely increase the precision of the data regarding CxFV prevalence and geographic variation in Kenya. At present, the consequences of this geographic variation in Kenya are not clear. Moreover, we detected CxFV in one male pool collected in Mombasa. This result suggests that vertical maintenance may be common, even though Mombasa is an area with a lower positive rate compared to Busia.

Although many studies have reported mosquito-specific flavivirus detection in *Culex* and *Aedes* [39], there is little information about flaviviruses from anopheline mosquitoes, except for a few recent reports from Africa [40, 41]. In addition to *Ae. aegypti*, we also obtained flavivirus sequences from *An. gambiae* s.l. Our phylogenetic data using flavivirus NS5 gene sequences suggest that the sequences from *Ae. aegypti* are related to CFAV and that the sequences from *An. gambiae* s.l. are most closely related to mosquito flaviviruses (KM088037.1 and KM088036.1) from *An. gambiae* s.l. in West Africa and Kenya [40, 41]. Overall, reports of mosquito-specific flaviviruses are increasing.

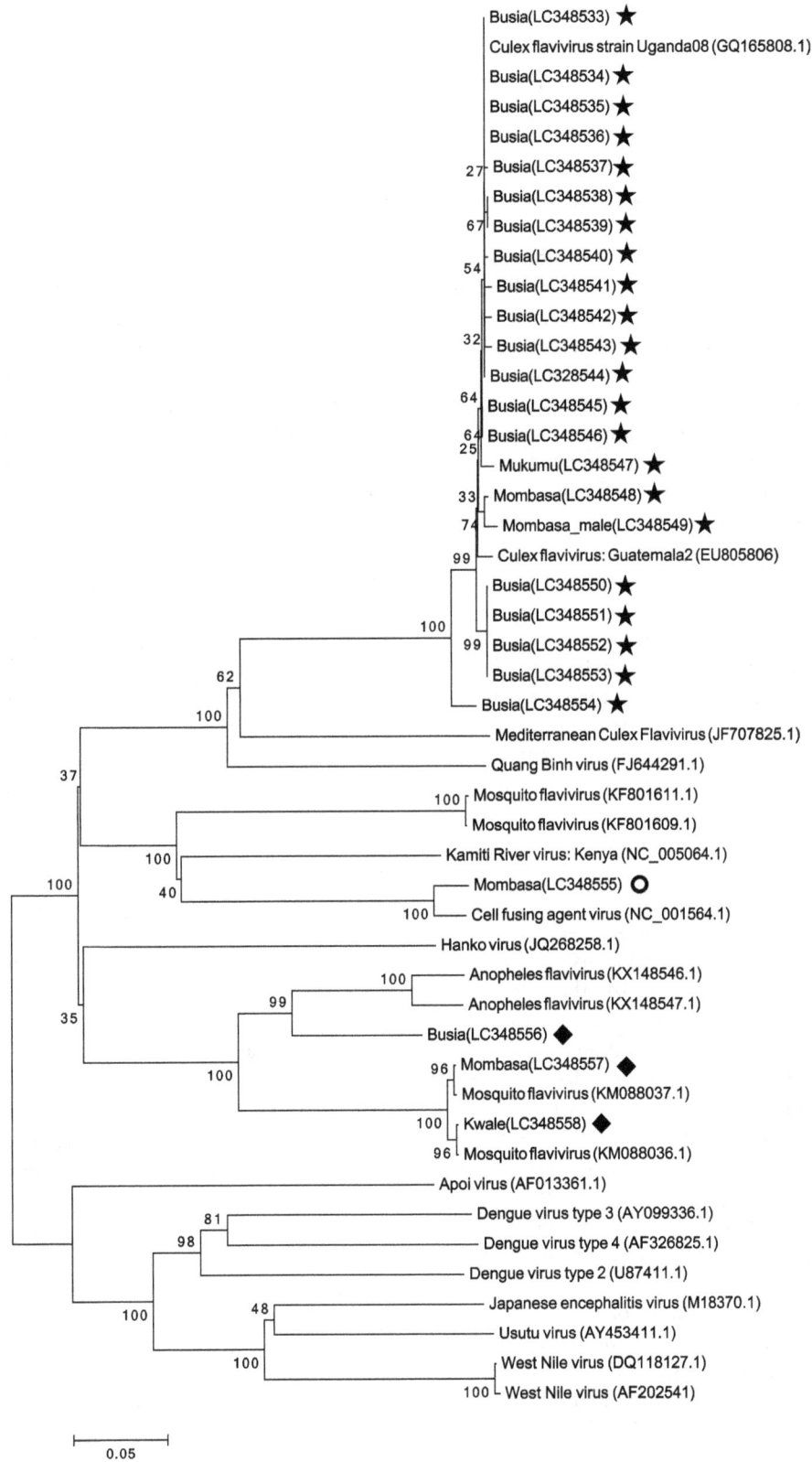

Fig. 2 (See legend on next page.)

(See figure on previous page.)
Fig. 2 Phylogenetic tree of the positive sequences based on the 597 nucleotides of the NS5 gene. The tree was constructed by employing the program MEGA 6, using the neighbor-joining method and distance-p model with 1000 bootstrap replicates. GenBank accession numbers are indicated in the parenthesis in the tree. Numbers on internal branches indicate bootstrap values for 1000 replicates. Our samples are marked with star (*Cx. quinquefasciatus*), with circle (*Ae. aegypti*), and with diamond shape (*An. gambiae*)

Our results are based on partial sequences (NS5) of flaviviruses directly detected in mosquitoes. However, other regions of flavivirus nucleotide sequences (such as a region of NS3) were not determined, and there is a possibility that these sequences differ. Thus, further sequence information might be required, especially for a novel mosquito flavivirus, to establish the detailed taxonomic status of arboviruses. None of the mosquitoes in our samples were infected with human-related flaviviruses, though the detection rate might have been slightly higher if we had performed cell culture. Another limitation is the small sample size, and the number of mosquito species was also small. Larger studies are needed to provide a more accurate view of the prevalence of arboviruses.

Additionally, the abundance of *Ae. aegypti*, one of the most effective arboviral vectors in the human environment, obtained was relatively smaller than we expected. This mosquito is thought to have originated from Africa and to have been introduced to other continents such as Asia and South America through maritime trade [1]. Because this mosquito can easily adapt to urban areas on these continents, DENV transmitted by *Ae. aegypti* has become a major threat to humans. In this study, there were no positive pools of arboviruses, including DEN and CHIK, among 107 female *Ae.* aegypti samples. It is clear that this small sample size is insufficient. Additionally, due to this small sample size, the existence of another important vector, *Aedes albopictus*, cannot be determined, even though the distribution of this Asian-based mosquito has already been extended throughout the world, including West and Central Africa [42, 43]. Currently, this mosquito is not reported in Kenya. However, methods of collecting *Aedes* mosquitoes in Kenya remain an issue. We recognize that the effectiveness of the BG sentinel trap is quite low in certain areas such as Africa [44], though we did not analyze the effectiveness of each trap.

Here, we report the detection of CxFV from *Cx. quinquefasciatus*, CFAV from *Ae. aegypti*, mosquito flavivirus from *An. gambiae* s.l., and a new virus from *An. gambiae* s.l. However, we did not detect any arboviruses that are responsible for human disease. Many individuals might be exposed to a considerable risk of arbovirus infection in Kenya. Muyeku et al. reported the seroprevalence of CHIKV, YFV, and WNV in children at a hospital in Busia. According to their data for 2010, the virus with the highest positive rate was WNV (31% of 296 tested) followed by YFV (17% of 310 tested) and CHIV (11% of 298 tested) [45]. Moreover, there is an anecdotal report that the WNV infection rate might be higher than that reported because many infections are not obvious or are mild among those who live on the border of Kenya and Uganda, where this virus was first isolated in 1937 [46]. Regardless, the detection of human-related arboviruses in mosquitoes is very difficult in the absence of an outbreak. Our results, which indicate relatively high CxFV positivity among *Cx. quinquefasciatus* mosquitoes in Busia, might support risk prediction for future patterns of epidemics of arboviral infection. One previous study reported a positive association between insect-specific flaviviruses and human-related arboviruses, such as WNV [23]. Interestingly, Bolling et al. [47] identified early suppression of WNV infection in *Culex pipiens* naturally infected with CxFV. This suppression is one of the possible explanations for the lack of arbovirus detection, despite the high prevalence of CxFV in *Cx. quinquefasciatus* in our study. Thus, it is important to determine whether mosquitoes infected with mosquito-specific flaviviruses are resistant or susceptible to infection with other human-related flaviviruses. Future research on these viruses and their potential interactions with other flaviviruses in arthropod vectors will provide important new insight into not only virological but also public health aspects.

Conclusions

Insect-specific viruses were detected in various species of mosquitoes. In particular, the abundance of CxFV in *Culex* mosquitoes in Busia is higher than in other areas of Kenya. We suspect that this heterogeneity in various areas of Kenya may reflect the heterogeneity of the abundance of human-related virus vectors. These results, together with the absence of positive pools of human-related arbovirus, can be used as a baseline for future studies of human arboviruses. Future efforts to detect the circulation of arboviruses will help clarify the relationship between human-related arboviruses and various arboviruses, including insect-specific viruses. Detection methods that are more sensitive, such as next-generation sequencing (NGS), will facilitate obtaining real data about the presence of arboviruses.

Abbreviations

CFAV: Cell-fusing agent virus; CHIKV: Chikungunya virus; CxFV: Culex flavivirus; DEN: Dengue; DENV: Dengue virus; MIR: Minimum infection rate; NJ: Neighbor-joining; ONN: O'nyong'nyong; PCR: Polymerase chain reaction; RVF: Rift Valley fever; WNV: West Nile virus; YF: Yellow fever; YFV: Yellow fever virus

Acknowledgements

We are deeply grateful to Dr. Kouichi Morita, Dr. Yoshio Ichinose, Dr. Masaaki Shimada, Dr. Charles Mwandawiro, Dr. Futoshi Hasebe, Dr. Shingo Inoue, Dr. Kazuhiko Moji, Dr. Matilu Mwau, and Mr. Haruki Kazama for technical support and Ms. Yukie Saito and Ms. Junko Sakemoto for providing administrative support. Special thanks go to Mr. Matthew Munyao, Mr. Johnstone Muyodi, Ms. Jecinta Odeo Lumumba, Mr. James Omondi Kongere, Ms. Mercy Syombua Mwania, Ms. Scholastica Achieng Wagalla, and Dr. Yuki Takamatsu, who devoted themselves to the fieldwork and experiments. Finally, we wish to express our gratitude to the residents of Kwale, Mombasa, Busia, and Kakamega who participated in this study.

Funding

This study was supported by a Grant-in-Aid for Scientific Research from the Ministry of Education, Culture, Sports, Science and Technology (MEXT), Japan; Young Researcher Overseas Visits Program for Vitalizing Brain Circulation, MEXT, Japan; the Global COE program, MEXT, Japan; the Japan Initiative for Global Network on Infectious Diseases (J-GRID), MEXT, Japan; and a Grant-in-Aid for Scientific Research from the Ministry of Health, Labour, and Welfare, Japan, Nagasaki University Kenya Research Station NUITM-KEMRI Project.

Authors' contributions

HI, YH, KF, and NM conceived and designed this study. SN helped design and plan the study in Kenya. HI, YH, KF, and PA collected the field data, and HI, YH, and KF organized and conducted the laboratory work. HI and TN performed the data analyses. HI drafted the first manuscript, and HI and NM finalized the manuscript. All authors have read and approved the final manuscript.

Competing interests

The authors declare that they have no competing interests.

Author details

[1]Department of Vector Ecology and Environment, Institute of Tropical Medicine, Nagasaki University, 1-12-4 Sakamoto, Nagasaki 852-8523, Japan. [2]Department of Bacteriology, Graduate School of Medicine, University of the Ryukyus, 207 Uehara, Nishiharacho, Okinawa 903-0125, Japan. [3]NUITM-KEMRI Project, Kenya Medical Research Institute, Nairobi, Kenya. [4]Eastern and Southern Africa Centre of International Parasite Control (ESACIPAC), Kenya Medical Research Institute, Nairobi, Kenya. [5]Department of Virology, Institute of Tropical Medicine, Nagasaki University, Nagasaki, Japan.

References

1. Gubler DJ. The global emergence/resurgence of arboviral diseases as public health problems. Arch Med Res. 2002;33:330–42.

2. Weaver SC, Reisen WK. Present and future arboviral threats. Antivir Res. 2010;85:328–45.

3. Sutherland LJ, Cash AA, Huang YJ, Sang RC, Malhotra I, Moormann AM, et al. Serologic evidence of arboviral infections among humans in Kenya. Am J Trop Med Hyg. 2011;85:158–61.

4. Johnson BK, Ocheng D, Gichogo A, Okiro M, Libondo D, Kinyanjui P, et al. Epidemic dengue fever caused by dengue type 2 virus in Kenya: preliminary results of human virological and serological studies. East Afr Med J. 1982;59:781–4.

5. Sanders EJ, Marfin AA, Tukei PM, Kuria G, Ademba G, Agata NN, et al. First recorded outbreak of yellow fever in Kenya, 1992-1993. I. Epidemiologic investigations. Am J Trop Med Hyg. 1998;59:644–9.

6. Nguku PM, Sharif S, Mutonga D, Amwayi S, Omolo J, Mohammed O, et al. An investigation of a major outbreak of Rift Valley fever in Kenya: 2006–2007. Am J Trop Med Hyg. 2010;83(2 Suppl):05–13.

7. Woods CW, Karpati AM, Grein T, McCarthy N, Gaturuku P, Muchiri E, et al. An outbreak of Rift Valley fever in Northeastern Kenya, 1997-98. Emerg Infect Dis. 2002;8:138–44.

8. Crabtree M, Sang R, Lutomiah J, Richardson J, Miller B. Arbovirus surveillance of mosquitoes collected at sites of active Rift Valley fever virus transmission: Kenya, 2006–2007. J Med Entomol. 2009;46(4):961–4.

9. Sergon K, Njuguna C, Kalani R, Ofula V, Onyango C, Konongoi LS, et al. Seroprevalence of chikungunya virus (CHIKV) infection on Lamu Island, Kenya, October 2004. Am J Trop Med Hyg. 2008;78:333–7.

10. Charrel RN, De Lamballerie X, Raoult D. Chikungunya outbreaks - the globalization of vectorborne diseases. N Engl J Med. 2007;356:769–71.

11. Haddow AJ, Davies CW, Walter AJ. O'nyong-nyong fever: an epidemic virus disease in East Africa - introduction. Trans R Soc TropMed Hyg. 1960;54:517–22.

12. Williams MC, Woodall JP, Corbet PS, Gillett JD. O'nyong-nyong fever: an epidemic virus disease in East Africa. 8. Virus isolations from anopheles mosquitoes. Trans R Soc Trop Med Hyg. 1965;59:300–6. https://doi.org/10.1016/0035-9203(65)90012-X.

13. Geser A, Henderson BE, Christensen S. A multipurpose serological survey in Kenya. 2. Results of arbovirus serological tests. Bull World Health Organ. 1970;43:539–52.

14. Mease LE, Coldren RL, Musila LA, Prosser T, Ogolla F, Ofula VO, et al. Seroprevalence and distribution of arboviral infections among rural Kenyan adults: a cross-sectional study. Virol J. 2011;8:371.

15. Sang RC, Dunster LM. The growing threat of arbovirus transmission and outbreaks in Kenya: a review. East Afr Med J. 2001;78:655–61.

16. Weaver SC, Barrett AD. Transmission cycles, host range, evolution and emergence of arboviral disease. Nat Rev Microbiol. 2004;2:789–801.

17. Lutomiah J, Bast J, Clark J, Richardson J, Yalwala S, Oullo D, et al. Abundance, diversity, and distribution of mosquito vectors in selected ecological regions of Kenya: public health implications. J Vector Ecol. 2013;38:134–42.

18. Labeaud AD, Sutherland LJ, Muiruri S, Muchiri EM, Gray LR, Zimmerman PA, et al. Arbovirus prevalence in mosquitoes, kenya. Emerg Infect Dis. 2011;17:233–41.

19. Gould EA, Higgs S. Impact of climate change and other factors on emerging arbovirus diseases. Trans R Soc Trop Med Hyg. 2009;103(2):109–21.

20. Vazeille M, Moutailler S, Coudrier D, Rousseaux C, Khun H, Huerre M, et al. Two chikungunya isolates from the outbreak of La Reunion (Indian Ocean) exhibit different patterns of infection in the mosquito, *Aedes albopictus*. PLoS One. 2007;2(11):e1168.

21. Hoshino K, Isawa H, Tsuda Y, Sawabe K, Kobayashi M. Isolation and characterization of a new insect flavivirus from Aedes albopictus and Aedes flavopictus mosquitoes in Japan. Virology. 2009;391:119–29.

22. Ciota AT, Kramer LD. Vector-virus interactions and transmission dynamics of West Nile virus. Viruses. 2013;5(12):3021–47. https://doi.org/10.3390/v5123021.

23. Newman CM, Cerutti F, Anderson TK, Hamer GL, Walker ED, Kitron UD, et al. Culex Flavivirus and west Nile virus mosquito coinfection and positive ecological association in Chicago, United States. Vector Borne Zoonotic Dis. 2011;11:1099–105.

24. Gu W, Novak RJ. Short report: detection probability of arbovirus infection in mosquito populations. Am J Trop Med Hyg. 2004;71:636–8.

25. Weaver SC. Urbanization and geographic expansion of zoonotic arboviral diseases: mechanisms and potential strategies for prevention. Trends Microbiol. 2013;21(8):360–3.

26. Hanley KA, Monath TP, Weaver SC, Rossi SL, Richman RL, Vasilakis N. Fever *versus* fever: the role of host and vector susceptibility and interspecific

competition in shaping the current and future distributions of the sylvatic cycles of dengue virus and yellow fever virus. Infect Genet Evol. 2013;19: 292–311.

27. Berens DG, Farwig N, Schaab G, Boehning-Gaese K. Exotic guavas are foci of forest regeneration in Kenyan farmland. Biotropica. 2008;40:104–12.

28. Southwood TRE, ECOLOGICAL METHODS second Edition 1977.

29. Gu W, Unnasch TR, Katholi CR, Lampman R, Novak RJ. Fundamental issues in mosquito surveillance for arboviral transmission. Trans R Soc Trop Med Hyg. 2008;102:817–22.

30. Harbach RE. Pictorial keys to the genera of mosquitoes, subgenera of Culex and the species of Culex (Culex) occurring in southwestern Asia and Egypt, with a note on the subgeneric placement of Culex deserticola (Diptera: Culicidae). Mosq Syst. 1985;17:83–107.

31. Huang YM. A pictorial key to the mosquito genera of the world, including subgenera of Aedes and Ochlerotatus (Diptera: Culicidae). Ins Koreana. 2002; 19:1–130.

32. Reinert JF. Descriptions of Zavortinkius, a new subgenus of Aedes, and the eleven included species from the Afrotropical region (Diptera: Culicidae). Contributions of the American Entomological Institute (Gainesville).1999; 31 (2): 1–105.

33. Rueda LM. Pictorial keys for the identification of mosquitoes (Diptera:Culicidae) associated with dengue virus transmission. Zootaxa. 2004;589:1–60.

34. Biggerstaff BJ. PooledInfRate, version 3.0: a Microsoft excel add-in to compute prevalence estimates from pooled samples. Ft. Collins, CO: Centers for Disease Control and Prevention; 2006.

35. Tamura K, Dudley J, Nei M, Kumar S. MEGA4: molecular evolutionary genetics analysis (MEGA) software version 4.0. Mol Biol Evol. 2007;24(8): 1596–9.

36. Kuno G, Chang GJ, Tsuchiya KR, Karabatsos N, Cropp CB. Phylogeny of the genus Flavivirus. J Virol. 1998;72:73–83.

37. Cook S, Moureau G, Harbach RE, Mukwaya L, Goodger K, Ssenfuka F, et al. Isolation of a novel species of flavivirus and a new strain of Culex flavivirus (Flaviviridae) from a natural mosquito population in Uganda. J Gen Virol. 2009;90:2669–78.

38. Mwangangi JM, Midega J, Kahindi S, Njoroge L, Nzovu J, Githure J, et al. Mosquito species abundance and diversity in Malindi, Kenya and their potential implication in pathogen transmission. Parasitol Res. 2012;110:61–71. https://doi.org/10.1007/s00436-011-2449-6.

39. Kasai S, Komagata O, Tomita T, Sawabe K, Tsuda Y, Kurahashi H, et al. PCR-based identification of Culex pipiens complex collected in Japan. Jpn J Infect Dis. 2008;61:184–91.

40. Fauver JR, Grubaugh ND, Krajacich BJ, Weger-Lucarelli J, Lakin SM, Fakoli LS 3rd, et al. West African Anopheles gambiae mosquitoes harbor a taxonomically diverse virome including new insect-specific flaviviruses, mononegaviruses, and totiviruses. Virology. 2016;498:288e99.

41. Villinger J, Mbaya MK, Ouso D, Kipanga PN, Lutomiah J, Masiga DK. Arbovirus and insect-specific virus discovery in Kenya by novel six genera multiplex high resolution melting analysis. Mol Ecol Resour. 2017;17:466–80. https://doi.org/10.1111/1755-0998.12584.

42. Paupy C, Delatte H, Bagny L, Corbel V, Fontenille D. Aedes albopictus, an arbovirus vector: from the darkness to the light. Microbes Infect. 2009;11: 1177–85.

43. Kraemer MU, Sinka ME, Duda KA, Mylne AQ, Shearer FM, Barker CM, et al. The global distribution of the arbovirus vectors Aedes aegypti and Ae. albopictus. elife. 2015;4:e08347.

44. Sivagnaname N, Gunasekaran K. Need for an efficient adult trap for the surveillance of dengue vectors. Indian J Med Res. 2012;136:739–49.

45. Muyeku MI, Seroprevalence of chikungunya, yellow fever and West Nile viruses in children at the Alupe District Hospital in Western Kenya. http://erepository.uonbi.ac.ke/bitstream/handle/11295/3785/Muyeku_Seropr evalence%20of%20Chikungunya%2c%20Yellow%20fever%20and%20 West%20Nile%20Viruses%20in%20Children.pdf?sequence=1&isAllowed=y (2011). Accessed 5 Dec 2017.

46. Smithburn KC, Hughes TP, Burke AW, Paul JH. A neurotropic virus isolated from the blood of a native of Uganda. Am J Trop Med Hyg. 1940;20:471–3.

47. Bolling BG, Olea-Popelka FJ, Eisen L, Moore CG, Blair CD. Transmission dynamics of an insect-specific flavivirus in a naturally infected Culex pipiens laboratory colony and effects of co-infection on vector competence for West Nile virus. Virology. 2012;427:90–7.

48. Scaramozzino N, Crance JM, Jouan A, DeBriel DA, Stoll F, Garin D. Comparison of flavivirus universal primer pairs and development of a rapid, highly sensitive heminested reverse transcription–PCR assay for detection of flaviviruses targeted to a conserved region of the NS5 gene sequences. J Clin Microbiol. 2001;39:1922–7. https://doi.org/10.1128/JCM.39.5.1922-1927.2001.

49. Ayers M, Adachi D, Johnson G, Andonova M, Drebot M, Tellier R. A single tube RT-PCR assay for the detection of mosquito-borne flaviviruses. J Virol Methods. 2006;135:235–9. https://doi.org/10.1016/j.jviromet.2006.03.009.

50. Tanaka M. Rapid identification of flavivirus using the polymerase chain reaction. J Virol Methods. 1993;41:311–22.

51. Hasebe F, Parquet MC, Pandey BD, Mathenge EG, Morita K, Balasubramaniam V, et al. Combined detection and genotyping of chikungunya virus by a specific reverse transcription-polymerase chain reaction. J Med Virol. 2002;67:370–4. https://doi.org/10.1002/jmv.10085.

52. Jupp PG, Grobbelaar AA, Leman PA, Kemp A, Dunton RF, Burkot TR, et al. Experimental detection of Rift Valley fever by reverse transcription-polymerase chain reaction assay in large samples of mosquitoes. J Med Entomol. 2000;37:467–71. https://doi.org/10.1603/0022-2585(2000)037[0467: EDORVF]2.0.CO;2.

53. Staley M, Dorman KS, Bartholomay LC, Fernández-Salas I, Farfan-Ale JA, Loroño-Pino MA, et al. Universal primers for the amplification and sequence analysis of actin-1 from diverse mosquito species. J Am Mosq Control Assoc. 2010;26:214–8.

54. Higa Y, Toma T, Tsuda Y, Miyagi IA. Multiplex PCR-based molecular identification of five morphologically related, medically important subgenus Stegomyia mosquitoes from the genus Aedes(Diptera: Culicidae) found in the Ryukyu Archipelagon Japan. Jpn J Infect Dis. 2010;63:312–6.

55. Koekemoer LL, Kamau L, Hunt RH, Coetzee M. Cocktail polymerase chain reaction assay to identify members of the Anopheles funestus (Diptera: Culicidae) group. Am J Trop Med Hyg. 2002;66:804–11.

18

Tuberculosis disease burden and attributable risk factors in Nigeria, 1990–2016

Felix Akpojene Ogbo[1,2]* (iD), Pascal Ogeleka[2], Anselm Okoro[3], Bolajoko O. Olusanya[4], Jacob Olusanya[4], Ifegwu K. Ifegwu[2], Akorede O. Awosemo[2], John Eastwood[5,6,7,8,9] and Andrew Page[1]

Abstract

Background: According to the World Health Organization, Nigeria is one of the countries with a high burden of tuberculosis (TB) worldwide. Improving the burden of TB among HIV-negative people would require comprehensive and up-to-date data to inform targeted policy actions in Nigeria. The study aimed to describe the incidence, prevalence, mortality, disability-adjusted life years (DALYs) and risk factors of tuberculosis in Nigeria between 1990 and 2016.

Methods: This study used the most recent data from the global burden of disease study 2016. TB deaths were estimated using the Cause of Death Ensemble model, while TB incidence, prevalence and DALYs, as well as years of life lost and years of life lived with disability were calculated in the DisMod-MR 2.1, a Bayesian meta-regression tool. Using a comparative risk assessment approach, TB burden attributable to risk factors was estimated in a spatial-temporal Gaussian Process Regression tool.

Results: In 2016, the prevalence of TB among HIV-negative people was 27% (95% uncertainty interval [95% UI] 23–31%) in Nigeria. TB incidence rate (new and relapse cases) was 158 per 100,000 people (95% UI; 128-193), while the total number of TB mortality was 39,933 deaths (95% UI; 30,488-55,039) in 2016. Between 2000 and 2016, the age-standardised prevalence and incidence rates of TB-HIV negative decreased by 20.0 and 87.6%, respectively. The age-standardised mortality rate also dropped by 191.6% over the same period. DALYs due to TB among HIV-negative Nigerians was high but varied across the age groups. Of the risk factors studied, alcohol use accounted for the highest number of TB deaths and DALYs, followed by diabetes and smoking in 2016.

Conclusion: The study shows an improving trend in TB disease burden among HIV-negative individuals in Nigeria from 1990 to 2016. Despite this progress, this study suggests that additional efforts are still needed to ensure that Nigeria is not left behind in the current global strategy to end TB disease. Reducing TB disease burden in the country will require a multipronged approach that includes increased funding, health system strengthening and improved TB surveillance, as well as preventive efforts for alcohol use, smoking and diabetes.

Keywords: Tuberculosis, Burden, Nigeria, Mortality, Global burden of disease

* Correspondence: felgbo@yahoo.co.uk
[1]Translational Health Research Institute, School of Medicine, Western Sydney University, Penrith, New South Wales, Australia
[2]Prescot Specialist Medical Centre, Welfare Quarters, Makurdi, Benue State, Nigeria
Full list of author information is available at the end of the article

Background

Tuberculosis (TB) remains a significant public health issue in low-income and middle-income countries and is the leading cause of deaths as a single infectious disease, ranking above human immunodeficiency virus and acquired immune deficiency syndrome (HIV/AIDS) [1]. The World Health Organization's (WHO) Global Tuberculosis Report 2017 reported 6.3 million new cases of TB among HIV-negative people in 2016 [1], compared to 6.1 million in 2015 [2]. Similarly, the Global Burden of Diseases, Injuries and Risk Factors (GBD) Study 2016 estimated 9.0 million TB-HIV-negative incident cases (new and relapse cases) compared to 8.8 million in 2015 [3]. These reports highlighted the considerable burden of TB globally. For example, the WHO African region accounted for 25% of the total number of incident cases (i.e., TB-HIV-negative and TB-HIV infection) globally, where Nigeria accounted for 8% or 407 cases per 100,000 population in 2016 [1], up from 322 cases per 100,000 population in 2015 [2]. These estimates may be lower than the actual number of TB cases in Nigeria because only less than a quarter of TB cases (15%) were notified in 2015 [2].

In the past two decades, the WHO has listed Nigeria as one of the countries with a high burden of TB in order to stimulate targeted interventions and advocacy for funding and policies to improve TB control [4]. This initiative has led to focused and practical actions for TB control worldwide [1]. Recently, the Nigeria National TB Control Programme and its donor partners have commenced the scale-up of availability and accessibility to improved methods for TB diagnosis and effective treatment regimen [5, 6]. While those efforts are needed and well deserved in Nigeria, there are limited pragmatic policy actions to tackle emerging risk factors for TB at the population level, including diabetes [7, 8], alcohol intake [8–11] and tobacco smoking [8, 12]. Country-specific epidemiologic studies which investigate trends in TB disease burden and the attributable risk factors for TB would be useful for public health experts and policy-makers to strengthen TB control and preventive efforts.

Evidence shows that TB mortality among HIV-negative people has declined in many developing countries (including Nigeria); but that TB incidence has remained unchanged in many communities [1, 3]. To ensure a continued reduction in TB disease burden in Nigeria, it is essential to understand not only the trends in TB burden but also the extent to which risk factors contribute to TB disease burden to inform targeted and high-priority TB programmes. We have provided a detailed exposition of TB disease burden in Nigeria from the GBD findings because this is not practicable in the GBD capstone publications due to the huge size and scope of the study, which have also led to further characterisation of the results for other health focus areas and locations [3, 13–16]. Additionally, by distilling the findings for TB burden in Nigeria, we aim to increase awareness and understanding of TB estimates for clinicians, national, and international health experts for TB prevention and control programmes, especially that Nigeria is the largest recipient of developmental assistance for health in Sub-Saharan Africa [17]. The present study aimed to highlight the incidence, prevalence, deaths, disability-adjusted life years (DALYs) and risk factors for tuberculosis in Nigeria from 1990 to 2016 using data from the GBD Study 2016.

Methods

Overview of data sources

The GBD study is a systematic and scientific effort that provides comparable estimates of incidence, prevalence, the cause of death and health loss, and risk factors for diseases and injuries by age, sex, year, location, and over time. In the past two decades, the GBD study has been quantifying health loss from diseases and injuries to inform health programmes and policy decision-making worldwide [18, 19]. The GBD 2016 complied with the Guidelines for Accurate and Transparent Health Estimates Reporting (GATHER) statement, a global agreement that ensures transparency, accurate reporting, interpretation and use of health estimates [20].

For this study, the complete information on data sources, the conceptual framework, and the analytical strategy for the calculation of TB incidence, prevalence, mortality, DALYs and attributable risk factors in Nigeria has been described elsewhere [3, 21–25]. Data used for the TB estimation in Nigeria have been extracted from the Global Health Exchange website (GHDx, http://ghdx.healthdata.org/gbd-2016/data-input-sources). GHDx provides researchers and policy-makers access to the most recent GBD input sources and results, and also creates opportunities for discussing population health based on the best available data, as well as acknowledgment of data owners' contributions [26].

Case definition

TB is an infectious disease caused by the bacterium *Mycobacterium tuberculosis*, an acid-fast bacillus that is spread mainly via the respiratory pathway. The GBD study provides estimates for all forms of TB, including pulmonary and extrapulmonary TB using the International Classification of Diseases (ICD-10) codes [27]. In this study, we have reported estimates for TB (drug-susceptible TB, extensively drug resistance TB, latent TB infection and multidrug-resistant TB, MDR-TB) among HIV-negative people in Nigeria. Information on TB-HIV is provided elsewhere [3, 28].

Overview of the estimation of incidence, prevalence, mortality, disability-adjusted life years and risk factors for tuberculosis

TB mortality was modelled in the GBD Cause of Death Ensemble model (CODEm), a Bayesian, hierarchical, ensemble modelling tool, which has been used to estimate cause-specific mortality for a range of diseases and injuries globally [21, 29]. CODEm modelling strategy used data from the WHO Global Project on Anti-Tuberculosis Drug Resistance Surveillance data (1988–2015) and community-based surveillance data for Nigeria and applied different functional forms (mixed-effects models and spatiotemporal Gaussian process regression models) to mortality rates with varying combinations of predictive models [21].

TB incidence was estimated based on age-specific and sex-specific notification data from the WHO and was defined as new and relapse cases diagnosed within a given calendar year [25]. Categorised notification data (i.e. new pulmonary smear-positive, new pulmonary smear-negative, new extrapulmonary and relapse) were combined to represent all forms of TB [3]. The GBD study estimated point prevalence of TB, defined as the people in the population who at any point within a calendar year with active TB [25].

DALYs are a summary metric of disease or injuries, defined as the number of years lost due to ill-health, disability or premature death, and were computed as the sum of years of life lost (YLLs) and years lived with disability (YLDs) for each year and age in Nigeria [24]. YLLs were calculated by multiplying TB deaths by normative standard life birth (86.9 years), measured as the lowest observed death rates for each 5-year age group in populations higher than five million [30]. In the estimation of YLDs, TB epidemiologic data from the WHO and the Nigeria National Tuberculosis Prevalence Survey 2012 were multiplied by a TB-specific disability weight. The disability weight was obtained from population-based surveys, where respondents rated their health status, from 'perfect health' to 'death' to quantify the severity of the health loss due to a given disease or injury [24].

TB mortality and DALYs attributable to risk factors were computed as the proportion of deaths and DALYs that could be attributed to risk factors (alcohol use, diabetes and tobacco smoking) as a counterfactual relative to the theoretical minimum level of exposure had the population not been exposed to the given risk factor previously. Based on the available evidence on the causal relationship between risk factors and TB, GBD 2016 estimated the attributable burden of diabetes, alcohol use and tobacco smoking for TB in Nigeria using the comparative risk assessment (CRA) strategy developed by Murray and Lopez [31]. Estimates of the attributable number of deaths or DALYs were calculated by multiplying the number of deaths, or DALYs for the outcome by the population attributable fraction (PAF) for the risk-outcome pair for a given age and year in Nigeria [3].

The analyses were conducted in DisMod-MR 2.1, the GBD meta-regression tool that adjusts for variations in epidemiologic data sources and other parameters, including model predictions, as well as propagates uncertainty around the estimates. DisMod-MR 2.1 also estimated 95% corresponding uncertainty intervals for TB incidence, prevalence, deaths and DALYs. A full description of the analytical strategy for the estimation of TB epidemiology in Nigeria is provided in respective GBD study publications [21–25].

Results

Levels and trends of tuberculosis prevalence, incidence, mortality and DALYs

In 2016, age-standardised prevalence rate of TB among HIV-negative people was 31,643.5 per 100,000 population (95% uncertainty interval [95% UI] 27,316-36,249) (Table 1), while the absolute prevalence was 27% (95% UI; 23–31%), highest in people aged 50–69 years and lowest in children under 5 years (Fig. 1). Absolute TB incidence rate (new and relapse cases) was 158 per 100,000 people (95% UI; 128-193) (Table 2).

In the same year, the total number of TB mortality was 39,933 deaths (95% UI; 30,488-55,039), highest in people aged 15–49 years (13,916, 95% UI; 9311-20,530) but lowest in those aged between 5 and 14 years (875, 95% UI; 600-1,211) (Table 3). A similar pattern in the prevalence of TB mortality was observed (Fig. 2). Between 2000 and 2016, the age-standardised prevalence and incidence rates of TB-HIV negative decreased by 20.0 and 87.6%, respectively. The age-standardised mortality rate also dropped by 191.6% over the same period. Drug-susceptible TB was the most common variant, followed by multidrug- resistance TB in 2016 (Table 1).

In Nigeria, the burden of TB among HIV-negative people was highest in those aged 15–49 years (660,942 DALYs [477,430-921,111]), followed by people aged 50–69 years (312,294, 95% UI; 227,215-440,406) (Table 4).

In 2016, YLLs were highest among people aged 15–49 years (623,955, 95% UI; 442,103-888,510), followed by those aged 50–69 years (301,086, 95% UI; 216,478-428,083) (Additional file 1: Table S1). YLDs were highest in those aged 15–49 years (36,987, 95% UI; 22,578-55,926) and adults between 50 and 69 years (11,208, 95% UI; 6263-17,761]) (Additional file 1: Table S2). Between 1990 and 2016, DALYs and YLLs decreased in all age group over time, while there were variations in the YLDs across the age groups.

Table 1 Age-standardised cases of tuberculosis, drug-susceptible tuberculosis, multidrug-resistant tuberculosis and extensively drug-resistant tuberculosis among HIV-negative individuals in Nigeria, 2000–2016

	Prevalence			Incidence		
	2000 Rate/100,000 (95% UI)	2016 Rate/100,000 (95% UI)	% change, 2000–2016	2000 Rate/100,000 (95% UI)	2016 Rate/100,000 (95% UI)	% change, 2000–2016
Tuberculosis	37,964.1 (32,963.3–43,057.0)	31,643.5 (27,316.3–36,249.3)	−20.0%	373.9 (300.2–455.4)	199.2 (162.0–238.5)	−87.6%
Drug-susceptible tuberculosis	269.9 (217.2–329.6)	147.3 (119.4–180.2)	−83.3%	362.8 (292.3–442.1)	192.9 (157.3–231.8)	−88.0%
Multidrug-resistant tuberculosis	8.2 (2.7–18.5)	4.8 (2.0–9.5)	−72.5%	11.1 (3.8–25.2)	6.3 (2.7–12.8)	−76.6%
Latent tuberculosis infection	37,685.9 (32,701.1–42,774.3)	31,491.4 (27,161.1–36,074.3)	−19.7%	–	–	–
	Deaths			DALYs		
Tuberculosis	131.3 (101.7–177.9)	45.0 (35.2–59.3)	−191.6%	3524.8 (2696.8–4867.8)	1159.3 (897.4–1557.6)	−204.1%
Drug-susceptible tuberculosis	120.0 (92.0–163.4)	40.9 (31.6–54.2)	−193.2%	3228.3 (2414.1–4569.2)	1056.5 (808.5–1427.6)	−205.6%
Multidrug-resistant tuberculosis	11.3 (3.8–25.0)	4.0 (1.7–7.9)	−179.1%	295.7 (98.2–640.7)	101.1 (43.0–199.7)	−192.5%
Extensively drug-resistant tuberculosis	–	–	–	0.9 (0.3–1.9)	1.7 (0.7–3.4)	48.1%

- indicate less than one per 100,000 population

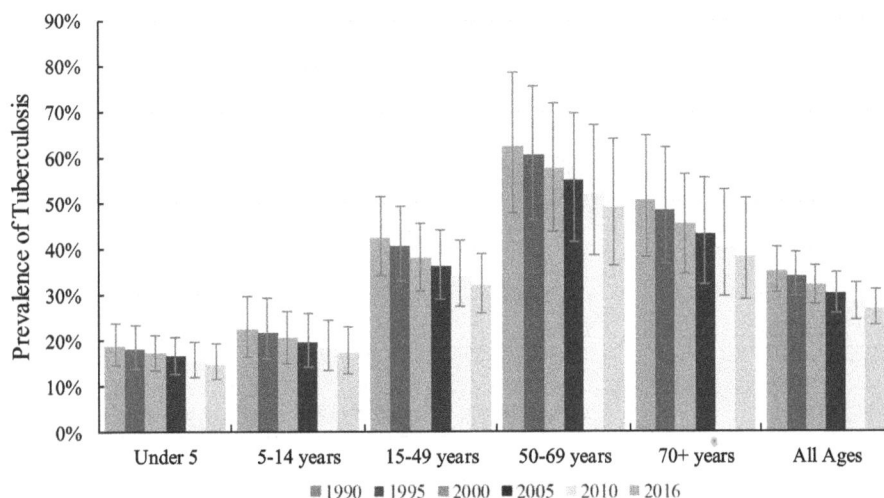

Fig. 1 Prevalence of tuberculosis in Nigeria by age, 1990–2016

TB mortality and DALYs attributable to individual risk factors

In Nigeria, alcohol use accounted for 13,196 (95% UI; 7277-20,605) TB deaths among HIV-negative people in 2016, followed by diabetes (1486 deaths [818–2493]) and smoking (942 deaths [349–1756]) (Additional file 1: Table S3). Proportionally, TB deaths that could be attributed to alcohol use was 38%, (95% UI; 23–52%), diabetes (4%, 95% UI; 3–6%) and smoking (3%, 95% UI; 1–5%) in 2016. The number of DALYs from TB due to alcohol use was 496,147 (95% UI; 283,342-777,331), followed by diabetes at 45,926 (95% UI; 26,297-75,452) and smoking at 32,369 (95% UI; 11,417-60,737) in 2016 (Additional file 1: Table S3).

Discussion

In Nigeria, the prevalence of TB among HIV-negative people was 27%, the TB incidence rate was 158 per 100,000 population, and the total number of TB mortality was 39,933 in 2016. From 2000 to 2016, the age-standardised prevalence, incidence and mortality rates dropped considerably, with variations across the age groups. The number DALYs due to TB among HIV-negative Nigerians varied

across the age groups; highest in those aged 15–49 years, followed by people aged 50–69 years and children under 5 years in 2016. Alcohol use accounted for the highest number of deaths and DALYs that could be attributed to TB in 2016, followed by diabetes and smoking, probably reflecting the high burden of TB among older adults.

Consistent with previous studies [1, 32, 33], this study showed that the prevalence and incidence of TB among HIV-negative people were higher in adults compared to children in Nigeria. Evidence has shown that not all individuals who are exposed to the *Mycobacterium tuberculosis* progress to having active TB infections. Studies from high burden TB environments suggest that approximately 20% of people maintain negative tuberculin skin tests throughout their lifespan despite repeated exposure to the mycobacteria [34]. In young children, active TB disease usually results from the haematogenous spread of the mycobacterium after primary infection, associated with subsequent pulmonary and extrapulmonary infections in some cases. In adults, however, TB infection is usually pulmonary and may reflect the reactivation of the latent TB infection (LTBI) from a

Table 2 Incidence rate of tuberculosis (with 95% uncertainty interval, UI) by age in Nigeria, 1990–2016 (per 100,000 population)

Age	1990	1995	2000	2005	2010	2016	% change (1990–2016)
	N (95% UI)	N (95% UI)	N (95% UI)	N (95% UI)	N (95% UI)	N (95% UI)	
Under 5 years	218 (153–306)	226 (156–323)	220 (150–317)	179 (122–264)	136 (91–199)	102 (71–148)	− 53.3
5–14 years	68 (43–100)	71 (45–106)	78 (48–117)	77 (47–117)	65 (38–102)	56 (34–85)	− 16.9
15–49 years	356 (273–461)	377 (273–497)	358 (254–487)	290 (201–400)	228 (161–312)	210 (155–274)	− 41.1
50–69 years	536 (399–699)	558 (398–742)	557 (377–773)	474 (321–669)	354 (235–506)	276 (182–396)	− 48.6
70+ years	799 (591–1045)	807 (601–1073)	759 (543–1007)	607 (428–821)	425 (304–574)	342 (244–464)	− 57.2
All ages	277 (233–329)	292 (240–356)	285 (228–352)	236 (188–293)	182 (146–231)	158 (128–193)	− 42.9

Table 3 Number of deaths from tuberculosis (with 95% uncertainty interval, UI) by age in Nigeria, 1990–2016

Age	1990 N (95% UI)	1995 N (95% UI)	2000 N (95% UI)	2005 N (95% UI)	2010 N (95% UI)	2016 N (95% UI)	% change (1990–2016)
Under 5 years	9313 (5939–13,651)	9557 (6136–14,356)	8577 (5421–13,213)	5868 (3733–8747)	3519 (2148–5743)	4720 (3030–7196)	− 49.3
5–14 years	1382 (964–1926)	1517 (1055–2095)	1447 (981–1975)	1113 (756–1572)	746 (503–1060)	875 (600–1211)	− 36.7
15–49 years	21,542 (16,162–31,474)	24,437 (17,214–34,397)	25,107 (16,951–37,381)	20,300 (13,190–30,585)	12,187 (8543–17,420)	13,916 (9311–20,530)	− 35.4
50–69 years	18,723 (14,227–27,847)	21,405 (15,544–31,463)	22,178 (15,703–32,747)	17,871 (12,701–26,285)	10,573 (7688–1,4845)	12,357 (8797–17,817)	− 34
70+ years	11,553 (9091–15,539)	13,613 (10,740–17,887)	14,034 (10,930–18,725)	11,274 (8711–14,819)	7377 (5655–9722)	8065 (6129–10,550)	− 30.2
All ages	62,513 (50,969–85,245)	70,530 (54664–94,278)	71,343 (54,497–98,715)	56,427 (42,423–77,678)	34,403 (26,533–46,550)	39,933 (30,488–55,039	− 36.1

primary site, which may partly be responsible for the increased prevalence and incidence observed in adults [35]. While only a limited number of individuals with LTBI progress to active TB disease, it is worth noting that one untreated infected person can transmit the disease to many healthy people, with broader implications for population health and TB control programmes [36, 37]. Early treatment of advanced LTBI in high TB-endemic countries like Nigeria is been advocated [38], and if the intervention is well implemented, it would reduce TB incidence and improve survival and productivity.

The present study showed that the number of deaths from TB mortality had dropped substantially over time in Nigeria, consistent with other reports [1, 2]. Similarly, between 2000 and 2016, this study indicated that TB incidence has declined. This improvement could be attributed to the scale-up of strategic policies and interventions, socioeconomic growth and a stable political environment [33, 39, 40], as well as increased

developmental assistance for health and impact of the Millennium Development Goal agenda [17]. However, the WHO Tuberculosis Report 2017 indicated that TB incident cases have remained stagnant in Nigeria since the year 2000 [1]. The variation in the findings may be due to the data sources and methodological approach used wherein the WHO estimated TB incidence based on WHO notification [1]. The GBD study, however, employed a statistical triangulation method that utilised all data sources (including data from the WHO global TB database and surveillance data) in Nigeria for TB estimation [3, 41]. A recent systemic review conducted in Nigeria reported higher levels of MDR-TB compared to the WHO estimate [42]. Despite the differences in data sources and methodology, both the WHO and GBD study reported similar estimates for global TB incidence and mortality in 2016 [1, 28].

Globally, delayed TB diagnosis and treatment has been shown to increase the transmission of the mycobacterium, exacerbate the disease, increase the likelihood of

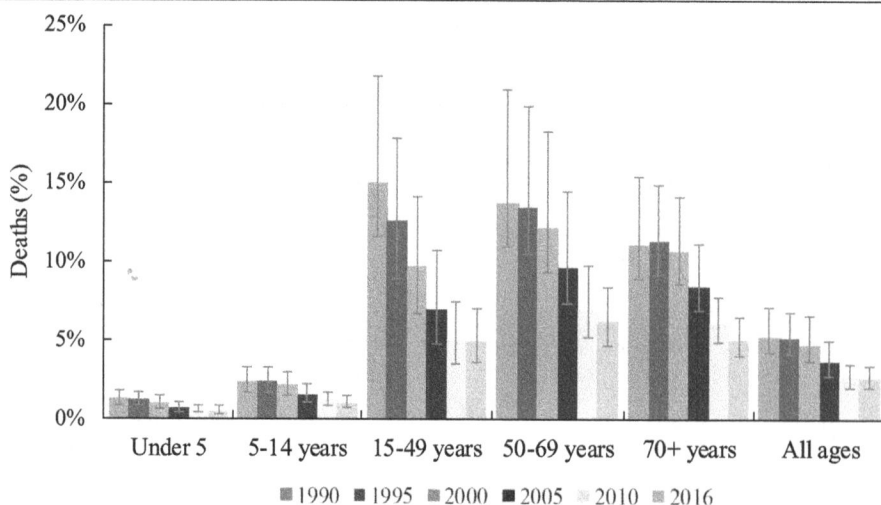

Fig. 2 Prevalence of deaths from tuberculosis in Nigeria by age, 1990–2016

Table 4 Numbers of disability-adjusted life years (with 95% uncertainty interval, UI) due to tuberculosis in Nigeria, 1990–2016

Age	1990 N (95% UI)	1995 N (95% UI)	2000 N (95% UI)	2005 N (95% UI)	2010 N (95% UI)	2016 N (95% UI)	% change (1990–2016)
Under 5 years	796,326 (509,536–1,167,425)	818,094 (526,989–1,225,994)	735,514 (466,850–1,131,697)	504,739 (325,725–750,223)	406,505 (263,324–617,181)	303,628 (186,059–490,830)	−61.9
5–14 years	109,450 (77,440–151,691)	120,172 (84,493–165,691)	115,521 (78,775–155,780)	90,261 (62,470–125,194)	71,786 (50,534–99,023)	61,720 (43,117–86,028)	−43.6
15–49 years	1,144,635 (872,156–1,633,936)	1,308,897 (930,238–1,818,531)	1,349,558 (922,957–1,973,510)	1,089,776 (723,744–1,636,032)	755,490 (520,518–1,080,864)	660,942 (477,430–921,111)	−42.3
50–69 years	541,198 (411,353–813,917)	619,595 (449,209–901,830)	643,310 (455,098–948,833)	519,960 (372,897–763,299)	363,631 (259,050–524,544)	312,294 (227,215–440,406)	−42.3
70+ years	162,936 (127,597–221,855)	191,308 (149,138–256,179)	196,198 (150,260–266,630)	156,696 (119,232–207,194)	111,538 (84,317–148,261)	101,646 (77,262–134,947)	−37.6
All ages	2,754,545 (2,222,630–3,625,684)	3,058,066 (2,396,218–3,929,792)	3,040,101 (2,347,459–4,075,851)	2,361,431 (1,801,039–3,192,772)	1,708,950 (1,321,347–2,300,534)	1,440,229 (1,127,285–1,921,654)	−47.7

mortality [43–45] and may be a reason for why TB incident cases have not reduced considerably compared to TB mortality [1, 3]. Evidence from regional areas of Nigeria found that delayed diagnosis and treatment of TB was due to factors such as a lack of awareness of TB symptoms by primary health professionals, older age, distance to the public health facility, male gender, and first clinic visit to a non-tuberculosis control programme providers [43, 46–48]. Additional studies have suggested that a lack of knowledge about TB in the community and patients preference for private health practitioners are the major reasons for why patients delay TB treatment [44, 45]. However, Lambert and Van der Stuyft argued that the failed health care system should be blamed and not the patient because there is limited evidence to indicate that health education about TB could reduce treatment delays [49]. Improving timely diagnosis and treatment of TB in Nigeria will require improved human resources, better coordination and decentralisation of TB control programmes [6], as well as increased and monitoring of public health financing [50].

The estimation of the population attributable risk for a specific disease or injury is crucial for health and other relevant agencies to identify opportunities for preventive efforts and policy priorities [22, 51, 52]. In the current study, we found that alcohol use, tobacco smoking and diabetes were essential contributors to the burden of TB in Nigeria. Studies have shown that the association between alcohol use [53, 54], smoking [55] and tuberculosis is due to impairment of the host immune system (innate and adaptive response), which increases vulnerability to TB infection, or reactivation of latent TB infection. Diabetes leads to increased susceptibility to tuberculosis through direct effects of hyperglycaemia and inadequate secretion of insulin at the cellular level, as well as indirect effects on specialised anti-TB immune cells (macrophages and lymphocytes), where chemotaxis, phagocytosis, activation and antigen presentation by macrophages are impaired [7, 56].

Evidence from regional areas of Nigeria has suggested that the lifetime prevalence of alcohol use was 57.9% [57], while the overall prevalence of current alcohol use ranged from 15 to 24% [57–60]. In Nigeria, there are some policy initiatives (excise tax on beer, wine and spirits, the national legal minimum age for on/off-premise sales of alcoholic beverages and regulations on alcohol advertising) to limit alcohol use. However, there is currently no written national action plan, nor is there a national monitoring system or enforcement of relevant policies to reduce alcohol use [61]. For tobacco smoking, an estimated 5.6% Nigerian adults aged over 15 years smoked tobacco products in 2017 [62]. Similar to alcohol use initiatives, strategic policies to support Nigerians to quit smoking [62], as well as efforts to prevent diabetes, are weak [63, 64]. Our finding implies that efforts

must not only be made to strengthen the health system and its human resources for TB control but also calls for collaborative, targeted and measurable socioeconomic reforms that address issues of alcohol use, tobacco, smoking and vulnerabilities, galvanised with strong political support to reduce TB burden in Nigeria.

The current study has policy implications for national health agencies and development partners aiming to reduce the high burden of TB and improve the quality of life in Nigeria because it provides relevant country-specific epidemiologic data for TB disease. The World Health Organization End TB Strategy highlights priority areas for attention to end the global TB epidemic, with targets to reduce TB deaths by 95% and to cut incidence by 90% between 2015 and 2035 [65, 66]. The WHO domains include integrated, patient-centred TB care and prevention; bold policies and supportive systems; and intensified research and innovation. For Nigeria to achieve the WHO goal of ending TB, a multipronged approach will be needed. Those strategic measures will include closing the funding gaps for TB control programmes and reducing the reliance on international donors; scaling up the national immunisation schedule (including the anti-TB vaccine, bacillus calmette–guérin) in underserved areas; improving the political commitment at all levels of government; and strengthening the healthcare system and TB diagnosis and surveillance [3, 42], including improving coordination, integration and consistency in the primary health care structure through the National Primary Care Health Development Agency [6]. Additional measures to reduce the high burden of TB in Nigeria should also include initiatives to limit alcohol use and prevent tobacco smoking and diabetes [3].

The study has several methodological limitations, and they have been described in detail elsewhere [3, 21, 22]. Briefly, caution should be exercised when interpreting the study findings especially that vital registration and other high-quality data for TB are sparse at the subnational and national levels in Nigeria. Importantly, the availability of high-quality TB data at the subnational level is essential given differences in the socioeconomic and political situation in Nigeria which have been shown to influence healthcare and social policies [67, 68]. In the present study, the assessment of TB mortality was based on various modelling strategies of WHO notification and other published data. Consequently, the TB estimates for Nigeria with limited high-quality data are reflected in the wide uncertainty intervals. Efforts at improving both subnational and national research, surveys and vital statistics on TB disease burden are warranted in Nigeria to guide strategic policy interventions. While there is biological plausibility for the association between malnutrition and TB, the attributable burden of malnutrition due to TB was not examined in GBD 2016 because of limited evidence of a casual association. The limitations related to the estimation of TB incidence, YLLs, YLDs and DALYs using the GBD Bayesian meta-regression tool also applied to this study [24, 25]. Publication bias relating to the use of the GBD data may also be a limitation. Despite these limitations, this study provides comprehensive country-level epidemiologic data on TB disease burden and attributable risk factors to inform better TB prevention and control programmes in Nigeria, a country with Africa's largest population of over 186 million people [40]. Future studies which investigate the rate of decline of TB incidence and mortality at the subnational level and whether those declines are fast enough to meet the WHO End TB Strategy may be warranted.

Conclusion

Between 1990 and 2016, the present study showed a decreasing trend in TB disease burden among HIV-negative people in Nigeria. Despite this progress, TB disease remains a significant public health issue in the country. Efforts to ensure a further reduction in TB disease burden, as well as improve the health and well-being of Nigerians, will require a multipronged approach that includes increased funding and appropriate monitoring, health system strengthening and enhanced national and subnational surveillance for TB disease.

Abbreviations
CRA: Comparative risk assessment; DALYs: Disability-adjusted life years; GBD: Global burden of disease; LTBI: Latent tuberculosis infection; MDR-TB: Multidrug-resistant TB; TB: Tuberculosis; UI: Uncertainty intervals; WHO: World Health Organization; YLDs: Years lived with disability; YLLs: Years of life lost

Acknowledgements
The authors are grateful to the Institute for Health Metrics and Evaluation for providing the data.

Funding
This study received no specific grant from any funding agency in the public, commercial or not-for-profit sectors.

Authors' contributions
FAO conceptualised the study, contributed to the data preparation and interpreted the results, drafted the original manuscript and critically revised the manuscript. PO prepared the data, interpreted results and critically revised the manuscript. AO, BOO, JO, IKI, AOA, JE and AP provided advice on data preparation and interpretation and critically revised the manuscript. All authors read and approved the final manuscript as submitted.

Competing interests
The authors declare that they have no competing interests.

Author details
[1]Translational Health Research Institute, School of Medicine, Western Sydney University, Penrith, New South Wales, Australia. [2]Prescot Specialist Medical Centre, Welfare Quarters, Makurdi, Benue State, Nigeria. [3]Society for Family Health, Justice Ifeyinwa Nzeako House, 8 Port Harcourt Crescent Area 11, Garki, Abuja, Nigeria. [4]Centre for Healthy Start Initiative, 286A Corporation Drive, Dolphin Estate, Ikoyi, Lagos, Nigeria. [5]Ingham Institute for Applied Medical Research, 1 Campbell Street, Liverpool, New South Wales 2170, Australia. [6]School of Women's and Children's Health, The University of New South Wales, Kensington, Sydney, New South Wales 2052, Australia. [7]School of Public Health, The University of Sydney, Sydney, New South Wales 2006, Australia. [8]School of Public Health, Griffith University, Queensland, Gold Coast 4222, Australia. [9]Department of Community Paediatrics, Sydney Local Health District, Croydon Community Health Centre, 24 Liverpool Rd, Croydon, New South Wales 2132, Australia.

References
1. World Health Organization. Global tuberculosis report 2017. Geneva: World Health Organization; 2017. Licence: CC BY-NCSA 3.0 IGO
2. World Health Organization. Global tuberculosis report 2016. Geneva: World Health Organization; 2016.
3. GBD Tuberculosis Collaborators. The global burden of tuberculosis: results from the Global Burden of Disease Study 2015. Lancet Infect Dis. 2017; 3099(17):30692–8. https://doi.org/10.1016/S1473-3099(17)30703-X.
4. World Health Organization. Use of high burden country lists for TB by WHO in the post-2015 era. Geneva: World Health Organization; 2015. Contract No.: WHO/HTM/TB/2015.29
5. Owoseye A. Nigeria adopts shorter treatment for drug-resistant tuberculosis. Online: Premuim Times 2017 [cited 2018 11 January]. Available from: https://www.premiumtimesng.com/news/more-news/235781-nigeria-adopts-shorter-treatment-drug-resistant-tuberculosis.html.
6. Federal Ministry of Health - Nigeria. The National Strategic Plan for Tuberculosis Control - Towards Universal Access to Prevention, Diagnosis and Treatment 2015-2020. Abuja: Federal Ministry of Health; 2015.
7. Dooley KE, Chaisson RE. Tuberculosis and diabetes mellitus: convergence of two epidemics. Lancet Infect Dis. 2009;9(12):737–46.
8. Patra J, Jha P, Rehm J, Suraweera W. Tobacco smoking, alcohol drinking, diabetes, low body mass index and the risk of self-reported symptoms of active tuberculosis: individual participant data (IPD) meta-analyses of 72,684 individuals in 14 high tuberculosis burden countries. PLoS One. 2014;9(5):e96433.
9. Rehm J, Samokhvalov AV, Neuman MG, Room R, Parry C, Lönnroth K, et al. The association between alcohol use, alcohol use disorders and tuberculosis (TB). A systematic review. BMC Public Health. 2009;9(1):450.
10. Nelson S, Zhang P, Bagby GJ, Happel KI, Raasch CE. Alcohol abuse, immunosuppression, and pulmonary infection. Curr Drug Abus Rev. 2008; 1(1):56–67.
11. Volkmann T, Moonan P, Miramontes R, Oeltmann J. Tuberculosis and excess alcohol use in the United States, 1997–2012. Int J Tuberc Lung Dis. 2015; 19(1):111–9.
12. Leung CC, Yew WW, Chan CK, Chang KC, Law WS, Lee SN, et al. Smoking adversely affects treatment response, outcome and relapse in tuberculosis. Eur Respir J. 2015;45(3):738–45.
13. Akinyemiju T, Abera S, Ahmed M, Alam N, Alemayohu MA, Allen C, et al. The burden of primary liver cancer and underlying etiologies from 1990 to 2015 at the global, regional, and national level: results from the Global Burden of Disease Study 2015. JAMA Oncol. 2017;3(12):1683–91.
14. Melaku YA, Appleton SL, Gill TK, Ogbo FA, Buckley E, Shi Z, et al. Incidence, prevalence, mortality, disability-adjusted life years and risk factors of cancer in Australia and comparison with OECD countries, 1990–2015: findings from the Global Burden of Disease Study 2015. Cancer Epidemiol. 2018;52:43–54.
15. Charara R, Bcheraoui EC, Mokdad HA, Khalil I, Moradi-Lakeh M, Afshin A, et al. The burden of mental disorders in the Eastern Mediterranean region, 1990–2015: findings from the global burden of disease 2015 study. Int J Public Health. 2017:1–13.

16. Fitzmaurice C, Allen C, Barber RM, Barregard L, Bhutta ZA, Brenner H, Fleming T. Global, regional, and national cancer incidence, mortality, years of life lost, years lived with disability, and disability-adjusted life-years for 32 cancer groups, 1990 to 2015: a systematic analysis for the global burden of disease study. JAMA oncology. 2017;3(4):524–548.

17. Institute for Health Metrics and Evaluation (IHME). Financing Global Health 2016: development assistance, public and private health spending for the pursuit of universal health coverage. Seattle: IHME; 2017.

18. Murray CJ, Lopez AD. Alternative projections of mortality and disability by cause 1990–2020: Global Burden of Disease Study. Lancet. 1997;349(9064): 1498–504.

19. Murray CJ, Lopez AD. Measuring global health: motivation and evolution of the Global Burden of Disease Study. Lancet. 2017;390(10100):1460–4.

20. Stevens GA, Alkema L, Black RE, Boerma JT, Collins GS, Ezzati M, et al. Guidelines for accurate and transparent health estimates reporting: the GATHER statement. PLoS Med. 2016;13(6):e1002056.

21. Naghavi M, Abajobir AA, Abbafati C, Abbas KM, Abd-Allah F, Abera SF, et al. Global, regional, and national age-sex specific mortality for 264 causes of death, 1980–2016: a systematic analysis for the Global Burden of Disease Study 2016. Lancet. 2017;390(10100):1151–210.

22. Gakidou E, Afshin A, Abajobir AA, Abate K, Hassen AC, Abbas MK, et al. Global, regional, and national comparative risk assessment of 84 behavioural, environmental and occupational, and metabolic risks or clusters of risks, 1990–2016: a systematic analysis for the Global Burden of Disease Study 2016. Lancet. 2017;390:1345–422.

23. Haidong W, Amanuel AA, Kalkidan HA, Cristiana A, Kaja MA, Foad A-A, et al. Global, regional, and national under-5 mortality, adult mortality, age-specific mortality, and life expectancy, 1970–2016: a systematic analysis for the Global Burden of Disease Study 2016. Lancet. 2017;390:1084–150.

24. Hay IS, Abajobir AA, Abate KH, Abbafati C, Abbas KM, Abd-Allah F, et al. Global, regional, and national disability-adjusted life-years (DALYs) for 333 diseases and injuries and healthy life expectancy (HALE) for 195 countries and territories, 1990–2016: a systematic analysis for the Global Burden of Disease Study 2016. Lancet. 2017;390(10100):1260–344.

25. Vos T, Abajobir AA, Abbafati C, Abbas MK, Abate KH, Abd-Allah F, et al. Global, regional, and national incidence, prevalence, and years lived with disability for 328 diseases and injuries for 195 countries, 1990–2016: a systematic analysis for the Global Burden of Disease Study 2016. Lancet. 2017;390:1211–59.

26. Institute for Health Metrics and Evaluation (IHME). Global Burden of Disease Study 2016 (GBD 2016) Data Input Sources Tool Online: IHME; 2018 [cited 2018 29 March]. Available from: http://ghdx.healthdata.org/gbd-2016/data-input-sources.

27. World Health Organization. The ICD-10 classification of mental and behavioural disorders: clinical descriptions and diagnostic guidelines. Geneva: World Health Organization; 1992.

28. Institute for Health Metrics and Evaluation. GBD Compare Online2018 [cited 2018 14 January]. Available from: https://vizhub.healthdata.org/gbd-compare/.

29. Wang H, Naghavi M, Allen C, Barber RM, Bhutta ZA, Carter A, et al. Global, regional, and national life expectancy, all-cause mortality, and cause-specific mortality for 249 causes of death, 1980–2015: a systematic analysis for the Global Burden of Disease Study 2015. Lancet. 2016;388(10053):1459–544.

30. Murray CJ, Barber RM, Foreman KJ, Ozgoren AA, Abd-Allah F, Abera SF, et al. Global, regional, and national disability-adjusted life years (DALYs) for 306 diseases and injuries and healthy life expectancy (HALE) for 188 countries, 1990–2013: quantifying the epidemiological transition. Lancet. 2015; 386(10009):2145–91.

31. Murray CJ, Lopez AD. On the comparable quantification of health risks: lessons from the Global Burden of Disease Study. Epidemiology-Baltimore. 1999;10(5):594–605.

32. Dim CC, Dim NR. Trends of tuberculosis prevalence and treatment outcome in an under-resourced setting: the case of Enugu state, South East Nigeria. Niger Med J. 2013;54(6):392.

33. Federal Ministry of Health - Nigeria. Report first national TB prevalence survey 2012, Nigeria. Abuja: Federal Ministry of Health; 2012.

34. Kassim S, Zuber P, Wiktor S, Diomande F, Coulibaly I, Coulibaly D, et al. Tuberculin skin testing to assess the occupational risk of Mycobacterium tuberculosis infection among health care workers in Abidjan, Cote d'Ivoire. Int J Tuberc Lung Dis. 2000;4(4):321–6.

35. Alcaïs A, Fieschi C, Abel L, Casanova J-L. Tuberculosis in children and adults: two distinct genetic diseases. J Exp Med. 2005;202(12):1617–21.

36. Flynn JL, Chan J. Tuberculosis: latency and reactivation. Infect Immun. 2001; 69(7):4195–201.

37. Getahun H, Matteelli A, Chaisson RE, Raviglione M. Latent mycobacterium tuberculosis infection. N Engl J Med. 2015;372(22):2127–35.

38. World Health Organization. Guidelines on the management of latent tuberculosis infection. Geneva: World Health Organization; 2015.

39. Kana MA, Doctor HV, Peleteiro B, Lunet N, Barros H. Maternal and child health interventions in Nigeria: a systematic review of published studies from 1990 to 2014. BMC Public Health. 2015;15(1):334.

40. The World Bank. Nigeria: The World Bank; 2017 [cited 2018 22 January]. Available from: https://data.worldbank.org/country/nigeria.

41. Institute for Health Metrics and Evaluation. Global Burden of Disease Study 2016 (GBD 2016) Data Input Sources Tool Online2018 [cited 2017 14 December]. Available from: http://ghdx.healthdata.org/gbd-2016/data-input-sources.

42. Onyedum CC, Alobu I, Ukwaja KN. Prevalence of drug-resistant tuberculosis in Nigeria: a systematic review and meta-analysis. PLoS One. 2017;12(7):e0180996.

43. Sullivan BJ, Esmaili BE, Cunningham CK. Barriers to initiating tuberculosis treatment in sub-Saharan Africa: a systematic review focused on children and youth. Glob Health Action. 2017;10(1):1290317.

44. Sreeramareddy CT, Qin ZZ, Satyanarayana S, Subbaraman R, Pai M. Delays in diagnosis and treatment of pulmonary tuberculosis in India: a systematic review. Int J Tuberc Lung Dis. 2014;18(3):255–66.

45. Takarinda KC, Harries AD, Nyathi B, Ngwenya M, Mutasa-Apollo T, Sandy C. Tuberculosis treatment delays and associated factors within the Zimbabwe national tuberculosis programme. BMC Public Health. 2015;15(1):29.

46. Ukwaja KN, Alobu I, Nweke CO, Onyenwe EC. Healthcare-seeking behavior, treatment delays and its determinants among pulmonary tuberculosis patients in rural Nigeria: a cross-sectional study. BMC Health Serv Res. 2013; 13(1):25.

47. Odusanya OO, Babafemi JO. Patterns of delays amongst pulmonary tuberculosis patients in Lagos, Nigeria. BMC Public Health. 2004;4(1):18.

48. Babatunde OI, Bismark EC, Amaechi NE, Gabriel EI, Olanike A-UR. Determinants of treatment delays among pulmonary tuberculosis patients in Enugu Metropolis, South-East, Nigeria. Health. 2015;7(11).

49. Lambert M, Van Der Stuyft P. Delays to tuberculosis treatment: shall we continue to blame the victim? Tropical Med Int Health. 2005;10(10):945–6.

50. Ogbo FA, Page A, Idoko J, Claudio F, Agho KE. Have policy responses in Nigeria resulted in improvements in infant and young child feeding practices in Nigeria? Int Breastfeed J. 2017;12:9.

51. Forouzanfar MH, Afshin A, Alexander LT, Aasvang GM, Bjertness E, Htet AS, et al. Global, regional, and national comparative risk assessment of 79 behavioural, environmental and occupational, and metabolic risks or clusters of risks, 1990-2015: a systematic analysis for the Global Burden of Disease Study 2015. Lancet. 2016;388:1659–724.

52. Ogbo FA, Page A, Idoko J, Agho KE. Population attributable risk of key modifiable risk factors associated with non-exclusive breastfeeding in Nigeria. BMC Public Health. 2018;18:247. https://doi.org/10.1186/s12889-018-5145-y.

53. Lönnroth K, Williams BG, Stadlin S, Jaramillo E, Dye C. Alcohol use as a risk factor for tuberculosis—a systematic review. BMC Public Health. 2008;8(1):289.

54. Imtiaz S, Shield KD, Roerecke M, Samokhvalov AV, Lönnroth K, Rehm J. Alcohol consumption as a risk factor for tuberculosis: meta-analyses and burden of disease. Eur Respir J. 2017;50(1):1700216.

55. Feldman C, Anderson R. Cigarette smoking and mechanisms of susceptibility to infections of the respiratory tract and other organ systems. J Infect. 2013;67(3):169–84.

56. Moutschen M, Scheen A, Lefebvre P. Impaired immune responses in diabetes mellitus: analysis of the factors and mechanisms involved. Relevance to the increased susceptibility of diabetic patients to specific infections. Diabete Metab. 1992;18(3):187–201.

57. Lasebikan VO, Ola BA. Prevalence and correlates of alcohol use among a sample of Nigerian semirural community dwellers in Nigeria. J Addict. 2016;2016. https://doi.org/10.1155/2016/2831594.

58. Okonoda KM, Mwoltu G, Yakubu K, James B. Alcohol use disorders among participants of a community outreach in Jos, Nigeria: prevalence, correlates and ease of acceptance of brief intervention. J Med Sci Clin Res. 2017;5(5): 22049–56.

59. Awosusi A, Adegboyega J. Alcohol consumption and tobacco use among secondary school students in Ekiti State, Nigeria. Int J Educ Res. 2015;3(5): 11–20.

60. Adelekan M, Ndom R, Makanjuola A, Parakoyi D, Osagbemi G, Fagbemi O, et al. Trend analysis of substance use among undergraduates of university of Ilorin, Nigeria, 1988–1998. African J Drug Alcohol Studies. 2000;1(1):39–52.

61. World Health Organization. Global status report on alcohol and health, 2014. World Health Organization Management of Substance Abuse Unit, editor. Geneva: World Health Organization; 2014.

62. World Health Organization. WHO report on the global tobacco epidemic, 2017; Country profile: Nigeria. Geneva: World Health Organzation.

63. Fasanmade OA, Dagogo-Jack S. Diabetes care in Nigeria. Ann Glob Health. 2015;81(6):821–9.

64. Adeloye D, Ige JO, Aderemi AV, Adeleye N, Amoo EO, Auta A, et al. Estimating the prevalence, hospitalisation and mortality from type 2 diabetes mellitus in Nigeria: a systematic review and meta-analysis. BMJ Open. 2017;7(5):e015424.

65. Uplekar M, Weil D, Lonnroth K, Jaramillo E, Lienhardt C, Dias HM, et al. WHO's new End TB Strategy. Lancet. 2015;385(9979):1799–801.

66. World Health Organization. The End TB Strategy. Geneva, Switzerland: World Health Organization; 2015. Contract No.: WHO/HTM/TB/2015.19

67. Ogbo FA, Agho KE, Page A. Determinants of suboptimal breastfeeding practices in Nigeria: evidence from the 2008 demographic and health survey. BMC Public Health. 2015;15:259.

68. The Federal Government of Nigeria. The millenium development goals performance tracking survey 2015 report. Abuja, Nigeria: National Bureau of Statistics; 2015.

19

Pneumonia mortality and healthcare utilization in young children in rural Bangladesh: a prospective verbal autopsy study

Farzana Ferdous[1], Shahnawaz Ahmed[2], Sumon Kumar Das[2,3], Mohammod Jobayer Chisti[2], Dilruba Nasrin[4], Karen L. Kotloff[5], Myron M. Levine[5], James P. Nataro[5,6], Enbo Ma[7,9], Khitam Muhsen[8], Yukiko Wagatsuma[9], Tahmeed Ahmed[2] and Abu Syed Golam Faruque[2,10*]

Abstract

Background: The present study aimed to examine the risk factors for death due to pneumonia in young children and healthcare behaviors of the guardians for children in rural Bangladesh. A prospective autopsy study was conducted among guardians of children aged 4 weeks to 59 months in Mirzapur, Bangladesh, from 2008 to 2012.

Results: Pneumonia was the primary cause of death, accounting for 26.4% ($n = 81$) of all 307 deaths. Of the pneumonia deaths, 58% ($n = 47$) deaths occurred in younger infants (aged 4 weeks to < 6 months) and 24.7% ($n = 20$) in older infants (aged 6–11 months). The median duration of illness before pneumonia death was 8 days (interquartile range [IQR] 3–20 days). Prior to death, 91.4% ($n = 74$) children with pneumonia sought treatment, and of those who sought treatment, 52.7% ($n = 39$) sought treatment ≥ 2 days after the onset of disease. Younger infants of 4 weeks to < 6 months old were at 5.5-time (95% confidence interval [CI] 2.5, 12.0) and older infants aged 6–11 months were at 3-time (1.2, 7.5) greater risk of dying from pneumonia than older children aged 12–59 months. Children with a prolonged duration of illness (2–10 days) prior to death were at more risk for death by pneumonia than those who died from other causes (5.8 [2.1, 16.1]). Children who died from pneumonia sought treatment 3.4-time more than children who died from other causes. Delayed treatment seeking (≥ 2 days) behavior was 4.9-time more common in children who died from pneumonia than those who died from other causes. Children who died from pneumonia more often had access to care from multiple sources (5.7-time) than children who died from other causes.

Conclusions: Delay in seeking appropriate care and access to multiple sources for treatment are the underlying risk factors for pneumonia death in young children in Bangladesh. These results indicate the perplexity in guardians' decisions to secure appropriate treatment for children with pneumonia. Therefore, it further underscores the importance of focusing on mass media coverage that can outline the benefits of seeking care early in the progression of pneumonia and the potential negative consequences of seeking care late.

Keywords: Death, Infant, Health care, Health facilities, Pneumonia

* Correspondence: gfaruque@icddrb.org
[2]International Centre for Diarrhoeal Disease Research, Bangladesh (icddr,b), Dhaka, Bangladesh
[10]Nutrition and Clinical Services Division, icddr,b, 68 Shaheed Tajuddin Ahmed Sarani, Mohakhali, Dhaka 1212, Bangladesh
Full list of author information is available at the end of the article

Background

Pneumonia is the leading cause of childhood death, accounting for 16% of 5.6 million deaths of children aged less than 5 years globally, more than 95% of which occur in developing countries [1]. In Bangladesh, pneumonia accounts for 15% of the 119,000 total deaths of children aged less than 5 years in 2015 [2].

Numerous pathogens can cause pneumonia. The respiratory syncytial virus, *Streptococcus pneumoniae*, and *Haemophilus influenzae* are the leading causes of childhood pneumonia, with the latter two being preventable through vaccination [3]. These vaccines are currently included in the immunization programs of numerous countries. The main risk factors for pediatric pneumonia include not being breastfed, undernutrition, indoor air pollution, household crowding, low birth weight, incomplete immunization, HIV, and pre-existing illnesses such as underlying heart disease [4, 5]. Muscle weakness, soft rib abnormalities, chest wall deformities, and impaired immune function may increase the severity of the disease [6–8]. Cyanosis [9], inability to feed, malnutrition [9, 10], prolonged duration of illness [11], altered mental state [10], and the presence of underlying chronic illness (such as heart disease) [12] are related with increased pneumonia-associated mortality in young children.

In 2010, 48 million deaths, 7 million of which were children, occurred in low- and middle-income countries (LMICs), and most of these deaths occurred without medical attention, at homes in rural areas [13, 14]. It is commonly believed that child mortality is higher in rural rather than in urban areas [15]. It has been also reported that the post-discharge mortality due to pneumonia is as high as in-hospital mortality even after receiving successful treatment at hospital [16]. Parents living in remote areas have a lack of adequate knowledge about clinical features of pneumonia and do not perceive the illness as serious or life-threatening [17]. Although Bangladesh has achieved 80% immunization coverage, only 22% of children receive postnatal checkups for immunizations and only 37% receive facility treatment for acute respiratory infections (ARI) [18]. However, 12% of children do not receive any kind of treatment for ARI and a larger portion of ARI children do not receive facility treatment; their treatment forms do not yet reveal, where routine checkups have the potential to detect health problems and provide optimal health care [18]. Previous studies have highlighted prompt identification of symptoms or risk markers of pneumonia, and subsequent interventions may prevent complications and child deaths [19, 20]. Even with these suggestions and solutions, there are some underlying risks that have not yet come to light that require understanding and consideration to reduce the risk of death by pneumonia in children. Verbal autopsy is a technique of growing importance used to estimate the distribution of the cause of death in populations lacking vital registries or other medical death certificates [21]. The technique focuses on the child or maternal deaths to elicit information on the signs, symptoms, and sequence of events during the final illness leading to death, which has been increasingly used in LMICs [14, 22]. Therefore, this study aimed to examine the risk factors for deaths due to pneumonia in children less than 5 years of age in rural Bangladesh and describe patterns of healthcare utilization that preceded death.

Methods

Study design and study population

This prospective post-mortem verbal autopsy study was conducted from January 2008 to December 2012 within the framework of the Global Enteric Multicenter Study (GEMS). The present study comprised a secondary data analysis of risk factors of pneumonia mortality. The GEMS was conducted in four sites in sub-Saharan Africa (Gambia, Mali, Mozambique, and Kenya) and three sites in South Asia (India, Bangladesh, and Pakistan) and a rural sub-district (Mirzapur) which was the field site of the GEMS in Bangladesh [23, 24].

Mirzapur is a sub-district of the Tangail district located about 60 km north of Dhaka, the capital city of Bangladesh, and has a geographical area of 374 km^2. The GEMS established a demographic surveillance system (DSS) in Mirzapur in January 2007 that covered eight out of 13 unions (the minimum administrative unit in rural Bangladesh). The DSS of GEMS regularly updated vital events including deaths in the study populations. In 2007, the mid-year population in the surveillance area was 238,463. The crude birth and death rates were 20.7 and 5.6 per thousand populations, respectively. The total fertility rate was 2388 per thousand women aged 15–49 years. The rate of neonatal mortality was 28.7 per thousand live births [25].

Data collection—verbal autopsy

Verbal autopsies were conducted in case of any deaths of a child aged less than 5 years in the DSS area. The DSS of Mirzapur collected information on demographic vital events three times a year (every 4 months). The total area was divided into 15 clusters; one data collector was responsible for each cluster, and each cluster was further divided into 80 blocks. Each data collector visited a block (40–50 households) each day and covered 80 blocks within 16 weeks. Additionally, four data collectors were assigned to collect the most recent information on pregnancy outcomes. The database was updated on a weekly basis, and a list of recent deaths of children less than 5 years old, including neonatal deaths, was generated to conduct verbal autopsies. Eventually, an overall list of total deaths of children aged less than 5 years was obtained and the information was cross-checked with the weekly list generated on all deaths to detect any mismatches and/or to complete information that was not provided in the weekly list.

The causes of death were classified according to International Classification of Disease 10th edition (ICD-10) codes [26]. Information on the causes of death was collected in a standardized manner from the medical chart or healthcare providers and, if available, death certificate. The caretaker, typically the mother, was interviewed by a trained research assistant using a World Health Organization (WHO) standard verbal autopsy questionnaire 3 or 4 weeks after the child's death [27]. Anonymous forms were reviewed by two clinicians independently to determine both the primary and antecedent causes of death of the child. In case of disagreement between the two clinicians, that was resolved through discussions with a third clinician. Detailed information on clinical signs and symptoms around the time of the child's death, as well as care-seeking practices, were obtained. The questionnaire included both closed and open-ended questions.

Inclusion and exclusion criteria

The present study only focused on data collected by the WHO verbal autopsy questionnaire for children aged 4 weeks to 59 months. Two different WHO verbal autopsy questionnaires were used for data collection from two different age groups of children (0–28 days and 4 weeks to 59 months). Given the difficulty in matching data obtained from these two age groups for analysis, data collected from another WHO verbal autopsy questionnaire for neonates aged 0–28 days were excluded from present study analysis. We further excluded sepsis from the pneumonia risk factor analysis as severe cases of pneumonia can eventually lead to sepsis if not properly treated [28].

Definitions

According to WHO classification, pneumonia was defined as the "presence of a cough and/or respiratory difficulty with any of the following symptoms reported by caregivers, such as first breathing, chest wall indrawing, noisy breathing, or flaring of nostril" [9].

In this study, the term "infant" denotes a child who was 4 weeks to 11 months old with children aged 4 weeks to < 6 months defined as "younger infants", and children 6 to 11 months old are defined as "older infants." The term "treatment" refers to any type of care including home remedies or other medical attention as reported by caregivers that were administered to the child with an illness that led to death. The term "indigenous healer" implies a person who is authorized by a particular culture or subculture to provide "indigenous treatment" even though

he/she has not been so trained according to acceptable professional standards. The term, therefore, includes a whole range of individuals from *religious shamans*, *witch doctors*, and *medicine men* (*homeopathic*) within a community. The term "delay in treatment" represents a child who did not seek treatment within days of disease onset [29]. The term, therefore, considers a child with a delay of two and more days to seek treatment (median 1 day) for an illness that leads to death. "Malnutrition" denotes a child who had inadequate growth and thinness according to caregiver's perception.

Statistical analysis

Descriptive statistics were employed to describe the study sample and distribution of causes of death. The normality of the distribution was checked, and in case of a skewed distribution, median and interquartile range (IQR) values were given. Differences in the proportions of pneumonia death and other causes of death according to independent categorical variables were examined using the chi-square test. Crude and adjusted odds ratios (OR) and 95% confidence intervals (CI) were calculated for each independent variable. Age of the children was categorized into three groups considering younger infants at higher risk of death: (i) 4 weeks to < 6 months, (ii) 6 to 11 months, and (iii) 12 to 59 months (12–59 months was not further categorized due to insufficient frequency). Based on the median number of days to begin treatment after the disease onset, children were classified into three groups: (i) delayed in seeking treatment for ≥ 2 days, (ii) sought treatment within 0–1 day, and (iii) did not seek any treatment. The duration of disease that leads to death was categorized into three groups denoting prolonged duration of illness (> 10 days) at a higher risk of death: (i) 11 days and more, (ii) 2–10 days, and (iii) 0–1 day. Diagnosed medical conditions were classified into two groups based on presence or absence of any previous disease before the final illness that leads to death (yes/no). Before classifying diagnosed medical conditions into two groups, a cumulative frequency for all pre-existing diseases (congenital heart disease, malnutrition, kidney or liver diseases, cancer, asthma, and diarrhea) was estimated based on the presence or absence of the symptoms (yes/no). Symptoms noted during the final illness that leads to death were classified into two groups based on the presence or absence of any symptoms (yes/no). Before classification of symptoms into two groups, a cumulative frequency for all symptoms (diarrhea, vomiting, abdominal pain, no passage of stool, headache, presence of any mass, pain in neck, unconsciousness, convulsion, paralysis of lower limb, any change in urine flow, skin rash, red color of eyes, nasal bleeding, yellow color of urine, weight loss, thinness or wasting, and a change in hair color) was estimated based on the presence or absence of the symptoms (yes/no). Data from each source accessed for the treatment were collected separately. Responses from sources were merged into a separate variable, where government hospitals and government clinics were considered a single source, and as private hospitals, and private clinics were also considered as another single source of treatment.

Correlations between the independent variables were assessed using Spearman's correlation coefficient. Highly correlated variables such as variables measuring health-care utilization (correlation coefficients > 0.70) were ana-lyzed in separate models to avoid multicollinearity among predictor variables. $P < 0.10$ in bivariate analysis was set as an inclusion criterion of variables in the mul-tivariable models along with known predisposing factors such as age at death, previous illness diagnosed of the child, and symptoms noted during illness (any symptoms reported by mother) before death. Several multivariable logistic regressions were performed to identify the risk factors for pneumonia (ICD-10-CM code J18.8) as the primary cause, whereas other causes of death were used as a comparison group. In model 1, we included the following variables: seeking treatment before death (yes or no), age at death, preexisting diagnosed illness, symp-toms, and duration of illness before death (symptoms which were likely to lead to death). An additional two models included variables relating to healthcare utilization and the interval between receiving treatment and death due to pneumonia. In model 2, all variables from model 1 were included except the variable "seeking treatment before death" which was replaced by another variable "sought care a number of days after onset of the disease." In model 3, similar variables of model 2 were included, except "sought care a number of days after onset of the disease" variable was replaced by a variable denoting the "number of sources accessed to seek treat-ment." $P < 0.05$ was considered as statistically significant. IBM SPSS (version 23.0; New York, USA) was used for data entry and analysis. Chi-square for linear trend was calculated by EpiInfo software (version 7.2).

Results

From January 2008 to December 2012, a total of 24,561 children were born in the DSS area of the Mirzapur and 307 (23.5/10,000) children aged 4 weeks to 59 months died during the study period. The cause-specific death rate for pneumonia (6.2/10,000) did not change during the study period (Table 1). The mean age at death was 14.6 months [standard deviation (SD) 15.3] (median 9.0 months). Approximately, 40.7% ($n = 125$) of all deaths occurred in younger infants (4 weeks to < 6 months), 16.9% ($n = 52$) occurred in older infants aged 6 to 11 months, and 42.3% ($n = 130$) in children 12 to 59 months old. Overall, 26.4% ($n = 81$) of all deaths were accounted for pneumonia. Other primary causes of deaths were sepsis (ICD-10-CM code A41.9) (20.2%; $n = 62$), drowning (18.9%; $n = 58$) (ICD-10-CM code V92), diar-rhea/dysentery (9.4%; $n = 29$), congenital heart disease (4.6%; $n = 14$), and illness suggestive of central nervous system (CNS) disorders (3.9%; $n = 12$) (Fig. 1).

To avoid overlapping clinical features, sepsis deaths (ICD-10-CM code A41.9) ($n = 62$) were excluded from the analysis of risk factors for death from pneumonia (Fig. 1). Of the children enrolled in the study ($n = 245$), 11.4% ($n = 28$) had a previous diagnosis of heart disease; 11% ($n = 27$) suffered from liver or kidney diseases, cancer, asthma, and diarrhea, etc.; and 4.9% ($n = 12$) had malnutrition. During the final illness that leads to death, fever was noted among 40% ($n = 122$) of the children and one third of them reported a cold and cough ($n = 84$), difficulty in breathing ($n = 98$), and chest indrawing ($n = 75$). The median duration of illness before child death was 4 days (interquartile range [IQR] 1–15 days) for all children, and for pneumonia deaths, the median duration of illness before death was 8 days (IQR 3–20 days). The median duration before seeking treatment after disease onset was 1 day (IQR 0–60 days [median 1.5 days for pneumonia]). For 66.5% ($n = 163$) of the children, treatment was sought before death, and of those who sought treatment, 67.5% ($n = 110$) children were admitted to a hospital or health facility for treat-ment and, for 43.6% ($n = 71$) children, treatment was

Table 1 Fertility and mortality indicators of rural Mirzapur DSS, 2008–2012

Indicators	2008	2009	2010	2011	2012	Overall	p value
Total population	239,233	244,754	258,061	263,085	264,998	239,233	
Total under-5 population	26,103	26,143	26,090	26,161	25,912	130,409	
Number of live births (CBR)	5176 (21.6)	4844 (19.8)	5040 (19.5)	5156 (19.6)	4345 (16.4)	24,561 (19.7)	0.0
Childhood deaths (4 weeks–59 months; CMR)	62 (23.8)	62 (23.7)	61 (23.4)	59 (22.6)	63 (24.3)	307 (23.5)	0.9
Childhood pneumonia deaths (4 weeks–59 months; CPMR) by under-5 population	21 (8.0)	11 (4.2)	16 (6.1)	16 (6.1)	17 (6.6)	81 (6.2)	0.8

Childhood death rate was measured as number of deaths per 10,000 total under-5 populations by each year period. Childhood pneumonia death rate was measured as number of pneumonia deaths per 10,000 under-5 population per year
CBR crude birth rate, *CMR* child mortality rate, *CPMR* childhood pneumonia mortality rate, *DSS* demographic surveillance system

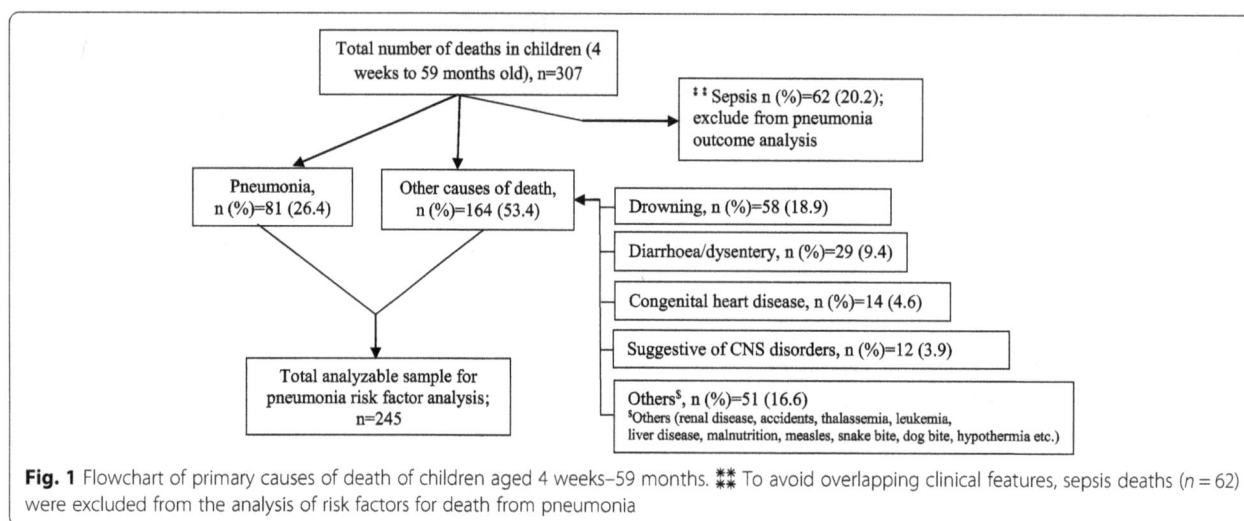

Fig. 1 Flowchart of primary causes of death of children aged 4 weeks–59 months. ✚✚ To avoid overlapping clinical features, sepsis deaths ($n = 62$) were excluded from the analysis of risk factors for death from pneumonia

sought ≥ 2 days after disease onset. Of those who sought treatment before death ($n = 163$), treatment was sought largely from private clinics/hospitals (79.7%; $n = 130$), followed by government facilities (28.2%; $n = 46$), pharmacies/drug stores (28.2%; $n = 46$), indigenous healers (16.6%; $n = 27$), and home treatment (6.1%; $n = 10$) (note: guardians accessed multiple sources for their child's treatment; therefore, the figures do not add up to 100%).

Risk factors for pneumonia deaths

Children aged 4 weeks to < 6 months, and those aged 6 to 11 months, when compared with older children 12 to 59 months old, were at increased risk to die from pneumonia than children who died from other causes. Children who died from pneumonia were ill for a longer period before death than those who died from other causes (53.2 vs. 21.4% were ill for 2–10 days, and 38 vs. 28.3% were ill for 11 days or more, respectively; $p < 0.05$). Children who died from pneumonia received treatment for their illnesses more often than those who died from other causes. Children who died from pneumonia were more likely to seek treatment ≥ 2 days after the onset of the illness than children who died from other causes (Table 2). Of the children with pneumonia who had visited three and more sources for treatment ($n = 14$), 71.4% ($n = 10$) of them delayed in seeking treatment until ≥ 2 days after the onset of disease and 75.0% ($n = 11$) of them had a duration of illness ≥11 days before death. Of those children with pneumonia who visited two sources for treatment ($n = 24$), 41.7% ($n = 10$) of them were delayed in seeking treatment ≥ 2 days after onset of disease and 58.3% ($n = 14$) of them had a duration of illness of 2–10 days before death (data not shown in the table).

Highly significant correlations ($r > 0.7$, $p < 0.05$) were found between three variables: seeking treatment, time

elapsed (in days) between disease onset and seeking care, and the number of sources accessed for treatment ($r = 0.869$, 0.854, and 0.764, respectively) (Additional file 1: Table S1). As a result, these variables were not included in the same multivariable model.

Multivariable model 1 showed that younger infants aged 4 weeks to < 6 months were 5-time and older infants 6–11 months old were 3-time at increased risk of death for pneumonia than the older children 12–59 months old. Children with pneumonia had a prolonged duration of illness (6-fold more), particularly with duration of illness of 2–10 days than children who died from other causes. Children with pneumonia were more likely to seek treatment (3-fold more) than children who died from other causes (Table 2). The present study performed additional analyses (multivariable analyses) to identify knowledge gaps between care-seeking behavior and deaths from pneumonia. Multivariable model 2 showed that, in addition to age and duration of illness, children with pneumonia, who delayed ≥ 2 days from the onset of disease to seek care, were at more risk of death than the children who died from other causes. Multivariable model 3 showed that children with pneumonia were more likely to visit multiple sources (3 or more) to seek treatment than children who died due to other causes (Additional file 2: Table S2).

Discussion

We assessed the risk factors for death due to pneumonia in children aged less than 5 years old in rural Bangladesh. Pneumonia was the leading cause of death found in 81/307 of all deaths of children aged 4 weeks to 59 months. Children who died from pneumonia were predominantly infants, with those aged less than 6 months being particularly at a higher risk. The present study revealed some important findings relating to death

Table 2 Correlates of pneumonia deaths compared to other causes of deaths in children aged 4 weeks to 59 months in rural Bangladesh (n = 245)

Variables	Pneumonia, n = 81 (%)	Other causes of death, n = 164 (%)	Unadjusted OR (95% CI)	Adjusted OR (95% CI)***
Age				
4 weeks–5 months	47 (58.0)	38 (23.2)	8.9 (4.4–18.0)*	5.5 (2.5–12.0)*
6–11 months	20 (24.7)	25 (15.2)	5.1 (2.6–13.0)*	3.0 (1.2–7.5)*
12–59 months	14 (17.3)	101 (61.6)	1	1
Sex				
Male	41 (50.6)	85 (51.8)	0.5 (0.6–1.6)	NA
Female	40 (49.4)	79 (48.2)	1	1
History of medical condition (multiple frequency)				
Heart disease	14 (17.3)	14 (8.5)	2.2 (1.0–5.0)*	1.4 (0.6–3.0)
Malnutrition	5 (6.2)	7 (4.3)	1.5 (0.5–4.8)	
Others (liver disease, kidney disease, cancer, asthma, diarrhea, etc.)	10 (12.3)	17 (10.4)	1.2 (0.4–2.8)	
None	52 (64.1)	126 (76.8)	1	1
Small at birth (< 1 year), n = 131[†]	21/67 (31.3)	16/64 (25.0)	1.4 (0.6–3.0)	NA
Premature (< 37 weeks) (< 1 year), n = 131[†]	15/67 (22.4)	4/64 (6.3)	4.3 (1.4–13.9)*	NA
Symptoms noted during last illness (multiple frequency)				
Fever	44 (54.3)	54 (32.3)	2.5 (1.4–4.3)*	0.9 (0.4–2.2)
Vomiting	13 (16.0)	34 (20.7)	0.7 (0.4–1.5)	
Not passed stool	5 (6.2)	22 (13.4)	0.4 (0.2–1.2)	
Unconscious	6 (7.4)	15 (9.1)	0.8 (0.3–2.1)	
Convulsion	9 (11.1)	17 (10.4)	1.1 (0.5–2.5)	
Others	39 (48.1)	67 (40.9)	1.3 (0.8–2.3)	
None	35 (43.2)	73 (44.5)	1	1
Duration of illness that leads to death (days), n = 238				
≥ 11	30 (38.0)	45 (28.3)	7.6 (3.1–18.7)*	2.5 (0.8–7.4)
2–10	42 (53.2)	34 (21.4)	14.1 (5.8–34.6)*	5.8 (2.1–16.1)*
0–1	7 (8.9)	80 (50.3)	1	1
Sought care for illness that leads to death				
Yes	74 (91.4)	89 (54.3)	8.9 (3.9–20.5)*	3.4 (1.1–10.1)*
No	7 (8.6)	75 (45.7)	1	1
Sought care a number of days after onset of the disease (days)				
≥ 2	39 (48.1)	32 (19.5)	12.4 (5.0–30.7)*	NA
0–1	35 (43.2)	57 (34.8)	7.0 (2.9–16.7)*	
Did not seek treatment for illness	7 (8.6)	75 (45.7)	1	
Admission to a hospital/health facility, n = 163‡				
Yes	54 (73.0)	56 (62.2)	1.6 (0.8–3.2)	NA
No	20 (27.0)	34 (37.8)	1	
Sources of treatment (multiple frequency), n = 163‡				
Home	5 (6.8)	4 (4.5)	1.5 (0.4–5.9)	NA
Indigenous healer	12 (16.2)	15 (16.9)	0.9 (0.4–2.2)	
Government clinic/hospital	17 (23.0)	29 (32.6)	0.6 (0.3–1.2)	
Private clinic/hospital	62 (83.8)	68 (76.4)	1.6 (0.7–3.5)	
Pharmacies/drug stores	22 (29.7)	24 (27.0)	1.1 (0.6–2.3)	
Number of sources accessed to seek treatment				

Table 2 Correlates of pneumonia deaths compared to other causes of deaths in children aged 4 weeks to 59 months in rural Bangladesh ($n = 245$) *(Continued)*

Variables	Pneumonia, $n = 81$ (%)	Other causes of death, $n = 164$ (%)	Unadjusted OR (95% CI)	Adjusted OR (95% CI)***
≥ 3	14 (17.3)	15 (9.1)	10.0 (3.5–29.0)*	NA
2	24 (29.6)	30 (18.3)	8.6 (3.3–22.0)*	
1	36 (44.4)	44 (26.8)	8.8 (3.6–21.4)*	
0 (not sought treatment)	7 (8.6)	75 (45.7)	1	1
Place of death				
Hospital	33 (40.7)	29 (17.7)	3.2 (1.8–5.8)*	NA
Home	48 (59.3)	135 (82.3)	1	

Children who died from sepsis were exlcuded from the analysis

OR odds ratio, *CI* confidence interval, *NA* not applicable (those variables not included in the mutivariable model)

*$p < 0.05$

†Only available sample, $n = 131$

‡Only available sample, $n = 238$

‡Only available sample, $n = 163$

***Model 1: dependent variable; causes of death (1 = pneumonia, 0 = other causes); variables included in the model were age at death, previous diagnosed illness (used as binominal variable—yes or no), symptoms noted during final illness (used as binominal variable—yes or no), duration of illness that leads to death, and sought care for illness that leads to death

due to pneumonia in children and knowledge gaps in healthcare utilization by guardians of ill children in a rural community of Bangladesh. Firstly, only two thirds of these study children received treatment. Secondly, we noted that children who died from pneumonia had a prolonged duration of illness (median of 8 days) before death. Thirdly, a trend of delayed care seeking (≥ 2 days) after the onset of disease was noted in children who died from pneumonia rather than other causes. Lastly, children who died from pneumonia sought treatment from multiple sources more often before death than children who died from other causes. Altogether, these findings suggest that children who died from pneumonia had a time window between onset of symptoms and death, in which appropriate treatment could have been delivered to reduce the risk of death. However, in most cases, appropriate action was not taken during this critical timing. To our knowledge, this is the first study that posits delay in seeking care and access to multiple sources for treatment, as key factors for delaying appropriate care for pneumonia in children.

In seeking treatment, one single child was witnessed to utilize a maximum of four sources, including treatment at home (home remedy). This clearly indicates the reasons for delayed care seeking behavior for illness, which may be associated with families' socioeconomic context and additional determining factors such as inadequate parental knowledge about the disease [17, 30]. The present study findings are consistent in some respects with previous studies as well as a WHO report which revealed the reasons for delayed seeking care (median 7 days) are treatment of children at home by the informal sector or indigenous healers, and such practices were important key barriers to prompt treatment and reduction of unnecessary childhood deaths

due to pneumonia [20, 29]. In the present study, half of the children suffered at least 4 days due to the illness (for pneumonia, 8 days) and delayed at least 1 day (for pneumonia, 1.5 days) to seek treatment for the illness that leads to death. This lag time in between disease onset, treatment, and death of the children can be explained by the treatment sources those had been accessed by the guardians of ill children. Of those who sought treatment, one fourth (28.2%; 29.7% for pneumonia) of them attempted to seek treatment from pharmacies/drug stores, or 16.6% from indigenous healers (16.2% for pneumonia), or 6.1% received remedies at home (6.8% for pneumonia); additionally, 33.5% children never received any treatment for illnesses that lead to death (9% for pneumonia), suggesting inappropriate healthcare utilization patterns by guardians of sick children in this rural community of Bangladesh. It could be possible that guardians of pneumonia children accessed many different facilities, and due to the inappropriate or inadequate quality of care, their children could not recover and, subsequently, died. The present WHO verbal autopsy questionnaire for 4 weeks to 59 months old children could not reveal much meaningful information such as treatment quality at the facility and the places where the child was taken first to seek treatment.

According to UNICEF 2016 report, children younger than 2 years were at higher risk of death from pneumonia [31]; however, in the present study, infants (< 1 year old), especially less than 6 months old, were at a higher risk of death due to pneumonia than the older group. It has been reported that the immune system of children less than 6 months or 1 year old may be weakened if they are malnourished or if have not exclusively breastfed [32], though present study was unable to reveal those associations due to lack of those specific data. Former studies have indicated that guardians from rural as well as urban communities are unable to recognize the signs and symptoms of pneumonia, particularly the danger signs of pneumonia; thus, there is a delay in seeking care [17, 33]. In the present study, children with pneumonia often were reported as having symptoms such as fever, cough, and common cold. Diagnosis based on difficulty in breathing, chest indrawing, and noisy breathing (grunting or wheezing) can be easily performed to identify cases of childhood pneumonia or to measure the severity of disease. However, the present study findings indicate that caregivers were found not to pay careful attention to these symptoms at the time critical for ensuring appropriate treatment. Like other developing countries, the severity of a disease was not given due attention in rural Bangladesh at the initial stage, and parents tried to seek treatment from drug stores or local unlicensed healthcare providers [17, 20, 34]. These practices may have also occurred to the present study children. The advanced stage of the disease characterized by high fever, cough, difficulty in breathing, and first breathing may have influenced family members in the present study to take their children to the health facility, yet it appears guardians did not access them at the appropriate time. It has been also observed that 40% of children with pneumonia died at the hospital; however, 74% of children who died from pneumonia were admitted to hospitals to receive treatment for their illnesses. This gap between death and admission of children with pneumonia has been explained by Chisti et al. who reported that even after a successful treatment at a hospital, post-discharge mortality has been reported to be as high as in-hospital mortality [16] which suggests the possible existence of persistent subclinical infection even after recovery or the survivor of premature microbiota in these children.

Previous studies have reported that inadequate education, lack of decision-making in the family, poor household socioeconomic status, longer distance from healthcare facility, and inadequate knowledge about disease severity are the key barriers to accessing health care [17, 34–36]. Moreover, overall factors such as quality of care, costs, geographic barrier, and existing social network influence families to rely on community-level healthcare providers for their care [37]. Access to qualified healthcare providers to receive care is often impeded due to a lack of household income and the location of the family in a remote area, which is often accentuated by physical geographic barriers or the lack of transportation to reach the health facility in a timely manner [17, 37, 38].

Guardians of children living in areas similar to this study should be knowledgeable about child health and the advance signs and symptoms of common morbidities and further be aware of the appropriate measures necessary for prevention and early treatment. Moreover, programs, such as community-based treatment of childhood pneumonia, should consider the referral of children with complications

to larger facilities for better treatment. A previous study in Zambia suggested health education in the rural community can help community members recognize clinically severe pneumonia and understand the importance of early and appropriate care seeking [39]. This study also proposes training and retraining of personnel in different levels of health care with an emphasis on case definition and case management, where management includes preventive measures and appropriate means of referral. Such training should prioritize the use of available protocols for health workers who play a key role in maternal and child health clinics, especially in the rural settings. By promoting appropriate care for young children, the mortality rate of children less than 5 years old would be reduced in Bangladesh, especially in the case of infants.

Limitations of the study

In the present study, all the information was collected on the basis of recall method (usually 3 to 4 weeks after death); to overcome this recall bias, trained research assistants carefully interviewed respondents which were again reviewed by research physicians. It is often accepted that details pertaining to stressful events like death are not easily forgotten; thus, authors believe these recalls as likely to be accurate [40]. Additionally, verbal autopsy questionnaires that were developed by WHO have some generic limitations due to lacking information on parent's education, family income, the number of antenatal care (ANC) visits made by pregnant women, breastfeeding history, rate of breathing/minute, and the places where the first attempts to seek care were made. However, the likelihood of missing of data after conducting interviews was avoided by regular checks by the DSS personnel. Any mismatch or confusion on diagnosis was also avoided through quality training and reviewing of questionnaires by a group of trained and experienced physicians.

Conclusions

Pneumonia is the number one killer in children less than 5 years of age in rural Bangladesh based on post-mortem verbal autopsies, and deaths mostly occur in infants. This study addresses important knowledge gaps by identifying factors such as caregivers' delay in seeking appropriate care and access to multiple sources of treatment as the underlying risk factors for death due to pneumonia in young children in Bangladesh. The study findings suggest a time window between onset of symptoms and death for pneumonia, in which appropriate treatment can be delivered to reduce the risk of death. Prompt identification and treatment of less severe cases of pneumonia at the beginning may prevent their progression to severe pneumonia and death. A mass media program at the community level aimed at educating caregivers about the simple clinical features of pneumonia and intelligent utilization of health services might reduce childhood pneumonia deaths in

Bangladesh. The government of Bangladesh should consider setting priorities and formulating appropriate strategies to educate the population to ensure improved healthcare behaviors which may address the basic need to improve health care in a resource-constraint setting like Bangladesh. Such an effort would achieve better results if both the public and the private sectors are involved in service delivery in rural Bangladesh.

Abbreviations
ANC: Antenatal care; CI: Confidence intervals; CNS: Central nervous system; DSS: Demographic surveillance systems; GEMS: Global Enteric Multicénter Study; ICD-10: International Classification of Disease 10th edition codes; IQR: Interquartile range; LMICs: Low- and middle-income countries; OR: Odds ratios; SD: Standard deviation; UNICEF: The United Nations Children's Fund; WHO: World Health Organization

Acknowledgements
The icddr,b acknowledges with gratitude the commitment of The Bill & Melinda Gates Foundation (BMGF) to its research efforts. We acknowledge the following donors for providing unrestricted support to icddr,b's effort and advancement to its strategic plan: the Government of the People's Republic of Bangladesh and Canada (Global Affairs, Canada-GAC), Sweden (Sida), and the United Kingdom (DFID). The authors would lastly like to thank Joshua Gallagher (Department of Health Services Research, University of Tsukuba) for his contribution in English language editing to finalize the paper.

Funding
This research protocol was funded by The Bill & Melinda Gates Foundation (BMGF), grant number GR-00505 (OPP 1033572).

Authors' contributions
FF, EM, KM, and ASGF performed, analyzed, and interpreted the present study and played the major roles in writing the manuscript. FF, SKD, KM, EM, YW, and ASGF analyzed and interpreted all the data produced and contributed to the writing of the manuscript. All authors read and approved the final manuscript.

Competing interests
The authors declare that they have no competing interests.

Author details
[1]Graduate School of Comprehensive Human Sciences, University of Tsukuba, Tsukuba, Japan. [2]International Centre for Diarrhoeal Disease Research, Bangladesh (icddr,b), Dhaka, Bangladesh. [3]School of Public Health, The University of Queensland, Brisbane, Australia. [4]Center for Vaccine Development and Department of Medicine, University of Maryland School of Medicine, Baltimore, MD, USA. [5]Center for Vaccine Development, Department of Pediatrics and Medicine, University of Maryland School of Medicine, Baltimore, MD, USA. [6]Department of Pediatrics, University of Virginia School of Medicine, Charlottesville, VA, USA. [7]Health Promotion Center, Fukushima Medical University, Fukushima, Japan. [8]Department of Epidemiology and Prevention Medicine, School of Public Health, Sackler Faculty of Medicine, Tel Aviv, Israel. [9]Department of Clinical Trial and Clinical Epidemiology, Faculty of Medicine, University of Tsukuba, Tsukuba, Japan. [10]Nutrition and Clinical Services Division, icddr,b, 68 Shaheed Tajuddin Ahmed Sarani, Mohakhali, Dhaka 1212, Bangladesh.

References
1. UNICEF, Levels & trends in child mortality. Report 2017. New York: the United Nations Children's fund; 2017.
2. UNICEF, Committing to child survival. A promise renewed. Progress report 2015. In: New York: the United Nations Children's fund; 2015.
3. Leung DT, Chisti MJ, Pavia AT. Prevention and control of childhood pneumonia and diarrhea. Pediatr Clin N Am. 2016;63:67–79.
4. Rudan I, Boschi-Pinto C, Biloglav Z, Mulholland K, Campbell H. Epidemiology and etiology of childhood pneumonia. Bull World Health Organ. 2008;86:408–16.
5. Jackson S, Mathews KH, Pulanic D, et al. Risk factors for severe acute lower respiratory infections in children: a systematic review and meta-analysis. Croat Med J. 2013;54:110–21.
6. Spooner V, Barker J, Tulloch S, et al. Clinical signs and risk factors associated with pneumonia in children admitted to Goroka hospital, Papua New Guinea. J Trop Pediatr. 1989;35:295–300.
7. Suwanjutha S, Ruangkanchanasetr S, Chantarojanasiri T, Hotrakitya S. Risk factors associated with morbidity and mortality of pneumonia in Thai children under 5 years. Southeast Asian J Trop Med Public Health. 1994;25:60–6. 7825027.
8. Banajeh SM, al-Sunbali NN, al-Sanahani SH. Clinical characteristics and outcome of children aged under 5 years hospitalized with severe pneumonia in Yemen. Ann Trop Paediatr. 1997;17:321–6.
9. WHO, Pocket book of hospital care for children. Guidelines for the management of common childhood illnesses. In: Geneva: WHO; 2013.
10. Subhi R, Adamson M, Campbell H, et al. The prevalence of hypoxaemia among ill children in developing countries: a systematic review. Lancet Infect Dis. 2009;9:219–27.
11. Shann F, Barker J, Poore P. Clinical signs that predict death in children with severe pneumonia. Pediatr Infect Dis J. 1989;8:852–5.
12. Nascimento-Carvalho CM, Rocha H, Santos-Jesus R, Benguigui Y. Childhood pneumonia: clinical aspects associated with hospitalization or death. Braz J Infect Dis. 2002;6:22–8.
13. Jha P. Reliable direct measurement of causes of death in low- and middle-income countries. BMC Med. 2014;12:19.
14. Leitao J, Desai N, Aleksandrowicz L, et al. Comparison of physician-certified verbal autopsy with computer-coded verbal autopsy for cause of death assignment in hospitalized patients in low- and middle-income countries: systematic review. BMC Med. 2014;12:22.
15. Susuman AS. Child mortality rate in Ethiopia. Iran J Public Health. 2012; 41:9–19. 23113145.
16. Chisti MJ, Salam MA, Bardhan PK, et al. Treatment failure and mortality amongst children with severe acute malnutrition presenting with cough or respiratory difficulty and radiological pneumonia. PLoS One. 2015;10:e0140327.
17. Ferdous F, Dil Farzana F, Ahmed S, et al. Mothers' perception and healthcare seeking behavior of pneumonia children in rural Bangladesh. ISRN family med. 2014;2014:690315. https://doi.org/10.1155/2014/690315.
18. Sayem AM, Nury AT, Hossain MD. Achieving the millennium development goal for under-five mortality in Bangladesh: current status and lessons for issues and challenges for further improvements. J Health Popul Nutr. 2011;29:92–102.
19. Graham SM, English M, Hazir T, Enarson P, Duke T. Challenges to improving case management of childhood pneumonia at health facilities in resource-limited settings. Bull World Health Organ. 2008;86:349–55.
20. WHO/UNICE, WHO/UNICEF joint statement: management of pneumonia in community settings. 2004.
21. Sibai AM, Fletcher A, Hills M, Campbell O. Non-communicable disease mortality rates using the verbal autopsy in a cohort of middle aged and older populations in Beirut during wartime, 1983-93. J Epidemiol Community Health. 2001;55:271–6.
22. Hill K, Lopez AD, Shibuya K, Jha P. Monitoring of Vital E. Interim measures for meeting needs for health sector data: births, deaths, and causes of death. Lancet. 2007;370:1726–35.
23. Kotloff KL, Blackwelder WC, Nasrin D, et al. The global enteric multicenter study (GEMS) of diarrheal disease in infants and young children in developing countries: epidemiologic and clinical methods of the case/control study. Clin Infect Dis. 2012;55(Suppl 4):S232–45.
24. Levine MM, Kotloff KL, Breiman RF, Preface ZAK. Am J Trop Med Hyg. 2013;
25. Darmstadt GL, Choi Y, Arifeen SE, et al. Evaluation of a cluster-randomized controlled trial of a package of community-based maternal and newborn interventions in Mirzapur, Bangladesh. PLoS One. 2010;5:e9696.

26. Engmann C, Jehan I, Ditekemena J, et al. An alternative strategy for perinatal verbal autopsy coding: single versus multiple coders. Tropical Med Int Health. 2011;16:18–29.

27. Perry HB, Ross AG, Fernand F. Assessing the causes of under-five mortality in the Albert Schweitzer hospital service area of rural Haiti. Rev Panam Salud Publica. 2005;18:178–86.

28. Florescu DF, Kalil AC. The complex link between influenza and severe sepsis. Virulence. 2014;5:137–42.

29. Kallander K, Hildenwall H, Waiswa P, Galiwango E, Peterson S, Pariyo G. Delayed care seeking for fatal pneumonia in children aged under five years in Uganda: a case-series study. Bull World Health Organ. 2008;86:332–8.

30. Chisti MJ, Duke T, Robertson CF, et al. Co-morbidity: exploring the clinical overlap between pneumonia and diarrhoea in a hospital in Dhaka, Bangladesh. Ann Trop Paediatr. 2011;31:311–9.

31. UNICEF, One is too many: ending child deaths from pneumonia and diarrhea. New York: UNICEF; 2016.

32. Lamberti LM, Zakarija-Grkovic I, Fischer Walker CL, et al. Breastfeeding for reducing the risk of pneumonia morbidity and mortality in children under two: a systematic literature review and meta-analysis. BMC Public Health. 2013;13(Suppl 3):S18.

33. Hildenwall H, Nantanda R, Tumwine JK, et al. Care-seeking in the development of severe community acquired pneumonia in Ugandan children. Ann Trop Paediatr. 2009;29:281–9.

34. Das SK, Nasrin D, Ahmed S, et al. Health care-seeking behavior for childhood diarrhea in Mirzapur, rural Bangladesh. Am J Trop Med Hyg. 2013;89:62–8.

35. Ferdous F, Das SK, Ahmed S, et al. The impact of socio-economic conditions and clinical characteristics on improving childhood care seeking behaviors for families living far from the health facility. Science Journal of Public Health. 2013;1:69–76. https://doi.org/10.11648/j.sjph.20130102.14.

36. Sonego M, Pellegrin MC, Becker G, Lazzerini M. Risk factors for mortality from acute lower respiratory infections (alri) in children under five years of age in low and middle-income countries: a systematic review and meta-analysis of observational studies. PLoS One. 2015;10:e0116380.

37. Sack DA. Achieving the millennium development goals for health and nutrition in Bangladesh: key issues and interventions—an introduction. J Health Popul Nutr. 2008;26:253–60. 18831222

38. Shah R, Mullany LC, Darmstadt GL, et al. Determinants and pattern of care seeking for preterm newborns in a rural Bangladeshi cohort. BMC Health Serv Res. 2014;14:417.

39. Stekelenburg J, Kashumba E, Wolffers I. Factors contributing to high mortality due to pneumonia among under-fives in Kalabo district, Zambia. Tropical Med Int Health. 2002;7:886–93.

40. Lacy JW, Stark CEL. The neuroscience of memory: implications for the courtroom. Nat Rev Neurosci. 2013;14:649–58.

20

Spatial, temporal, and spatiotemporal analysis of under-five diarrhea in Southern Ethiopia

Hunachew Beyene[1,2*], Wakgari Deressa[2], Abera Kumie[2] and Delia Grace[3]

Abstract

Background: Despite improvements in prevention efforts, childhood diarrhea remains a public health concern. However, there may be substantial variation influenced by place, time, and season. Description of diarrheal clusters in time and space and understanding seasonal patterns can improve surveillance and management. The present study investigated the spatial and seasonal distribution and purely spatial, purely temporal, and space-time clusters of childhood diarrhea in Southern Ethiopia.

Methods: The study was a retrospective analysis of data from the Health Management Information System (HMIS) under-five diarrheal morbidity reports from July 2011 to June 2017 in Sidama Zone. Annual diarrhea incidence at district level was calculated. Incidence rate calculation and seasonal trend analysis were performed. The Kulldorff SaTScan software with a discrete Poisson model was used to identify statistically significant special, temporal, and space-time diarrhea clusters. ArcGIS 10.1 was used to plot the maps.

Results: A total of 202,406 under-five diarrheal cases with an annual case of 5822 per 100,000 under-five population were reported. An increasing trend of diarrhea incidence was observed over the 6 years with seasonal variation picking between February and May. The highest incidence rate (135.8/1000) was observed in the year 2016/17 in Boricha district. One statistically significant most likely spatial cluster (Boricha district) and six secondary clusters (Malga, Hulla, Aleta Wondo, Shebedino, Loka Abaya, Dale, and Wondogenet) were identified. One statistically significant temporal cluster (LLR = 2109.93, $p < 0.001$) during December 2013 to May 2015 was observed in all districts. Statistically significant spatiotemporal primary hotspot was observed in December 2012 to January 2015 in Malga district with a likelihood ratio of 1214.67 and a relative risk of 2.03. First, second, third, and fourth secondary hotspots occurred from January 2012 to May 2012 in Loka Abaya, December 2011 in Bursa, from March to April 2014 in Gorchie, and March 2012 in Wonsho districts.

Conclusion: Childhood diarrhea was not distributed randomly over space and time and showed an overall increasing trend of seasonal variation peaking between February and May. The health department and other stakeholders at various levels need to plan targeted interventional activities at hotspot seasons and areas to reduce morbidity and mortality.

Keywords: Southern Ethiopia, Under-five diarrhea, SatScan, Cluster, Spatial, Temporal

* Correspondence: hunachew@gmail.com
[1]College of Health Sciences, Hawassa University, P.O. Box 1560, Hawassa, Ethiopia
[2]School of Public Health, Addis Ababa University, P.O. Box 1176, Addis Ababa, Ethiopia
Full list of author information is available at the end of the article

Background

Globally, diarrheal disease is the second leading cause of death in children under 5 years of age, and there are nearly 1.7 billion cases of childhood diarrheal disease every year [1]. In 2015, diarrhea was a leading cause of disability-adjusted life years (DALYs) on young children [2]. If not properly treated, diarrhea will be responsible for dehydration and death in children [2–4]. Despite a decrease in the proportions of diarrheal morbidity among under-five children, a growing trend of inequalities among neighborhoods and villages of countries has been observed [2, 5, 6].

Based on the 2016 Ethiopian Demographic and Health Survey (DHS) report, access to improved water supply and sanitation facilities have shown improvements. The percentage of children aged between 12 and 23 months, who received all basic vaccinations, also increased from 14% in 2000 to 20% in 2005, 24% in 2011, and 39% in 2016. In addition, the 2 weeks under-five diarrheal morbidity prevalence reduced from 24% in 2000 to 18% in 2005, 13% in 2011, and 12% in 2016 [7]. Studies which were conducted in different times and places in Ethiopia, however, indicated that diarrhea remains a public health problem with morbidity prevalence ranging from 18 to 30.5% [8–12]. In the study area, high rate of reversion to open defecation was reported [13].

Several studies indicated that morbidity patterns of childhood diarrhea showed spatial variation, with the occurrence of clusters [14–16]. However, studies indicated that under-five diarrhea disease did not differ significantly across different study locations [17, 18]. Seasonal patterns of childhood diarrheal morbidity have been reported from different countries with different seasonal features [14, 18–21]. Diarrheal morbidity has also been observed to be influenced by metrological parameters such as precipitation and temperature anomalies in different parts of the world including Ethiopia [14, 22–25].

Analysis of disease trends in space and time provides context which can be linked to possible risk factors in a research environment [26]. Scan statistics has been used widely in the field of epidemiology for investigation of spatial, temporal, and space-time clusters of infectious disease such as hemorrhagic fever [27], *Clostridium difficile* infection clusters [28], healthcare-associated infections or colonizations with *Pseudomonas aeruginosa* [29], visceral leishmaniasis [30], typhoid fever [31], cholera [32], malaria [33], and diarrhea [14, 15].

Description of diarrheal clusters in time and space and understanding seasonal patterns is important for informed decision-making at various levels of the health department and may lead to improvements in disease surveillance. However, studies in Ethiopia which assessed the seasonal trend, spatial, temporal, and space-time clusters of diarrhea are lacking. The very few available

studies used different data sources and did not include the current study area. Acute watery diarrhea (AWD) has been a public health threat since 2006 in the study area and caused the morbidity of thousands of people. These outbreaks were linked to lack of basic sanitation and safe water supply, as well as to the high sensitivity of the pathogens to variations in climatic variability [34]. In addition to this, the effect of climate change is reported in parts of the study area [35]. The present study, therefore, was conducted to investigate the seasonal distribution, purely spatial, purely temporal, and space-time clusters of childhood diarrhea in Sidama Zone, Southern Ethiopia. The study adds to the already existing knowledge, and identifying the risk areas would help in designing effective intervention mechanisms to reduce childhood diarrhea in these areas.

Methods
Description of the study area
The study was conducted in Sidama Administration Zone, Southern Ethiopia (Fig. 1). It consists of 19 rural districts and two administrative towns.

Its geographic location lies between 6°14′ and 7°18′ North latitude and 37°92′ and 39°14′ East longitude. The total area of the Sidama Administrative Zone is about 6981.8 km². The administrative zone is bounded by Oromiya in North, East, and South East, with Gedieo Zone in the South and Wolayta Zone in the West. The altitude ranges between the highest peak of Garamba mountains 3500 m above sea level (masl) to low lands (1190 m) around Bilate River in Loka-Abaya and Borcha districts. The climatic condition can be described as wet moist highland (27.7%), wet moist midland (45.4%), dry midland (14.5%), dry lowland (8.6%), and wet moist lowland (3.8%) [36]. In 2017, the administrative zone had a total population of 3,668,304 with 1,849,128 male and 1,819,176 female [37].

Study design and population
This is a retrospective longitudinal study design using the Sidama Zone HMIS under-five diarrheal morbidity report from July 2011 to June 2017. In the study area, the annual morbidity report is compiled based on the Ethiopian fiscal year which spans from July to June. The study population was all under-five children of the 19 districts who lived during the study period. Each district was represented by a geographical point location by the geographic coordinates taken from a representative location in the district. Coordinates were specified using the standard Cartesian coordinate system.

Population projection for the years 2011 to 2017 was made based on the 2007 census report as a referee population, using the population projection formula: $P = Po(1 + r)^t$, where P is the projected total

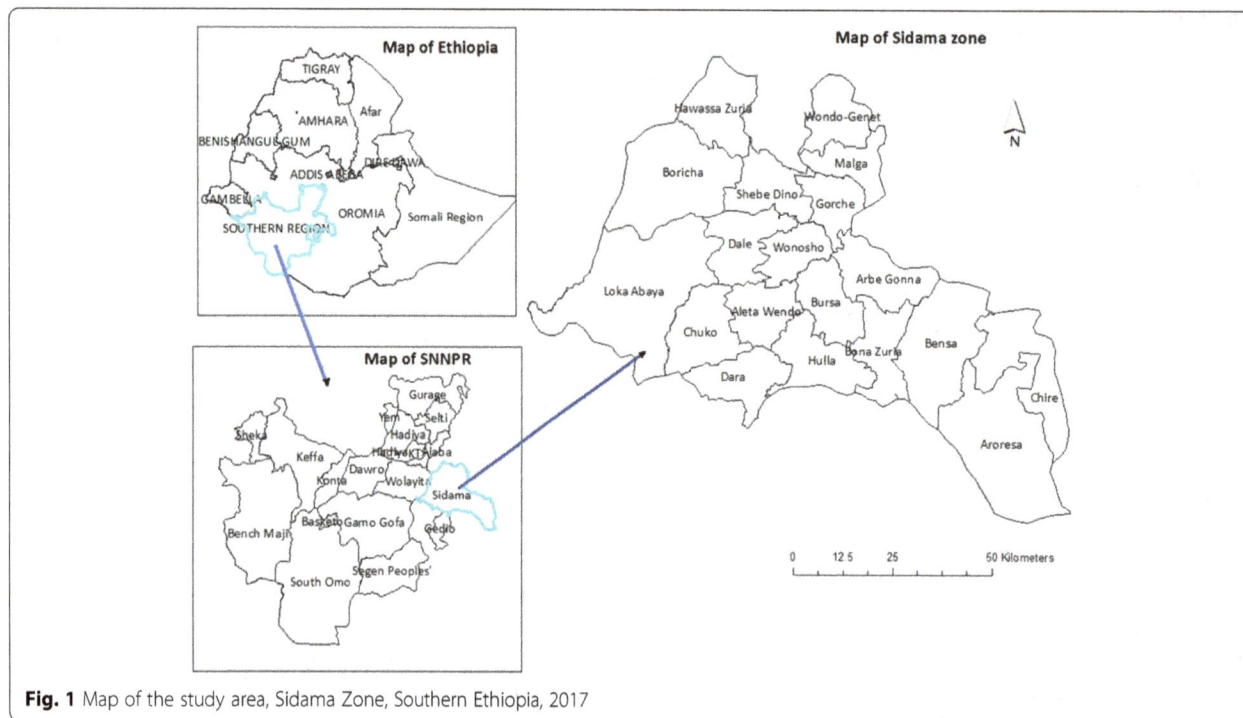

Fig. 1 Map of the study area, Sidama Zone, Southern Ethiopia, 2017

population, *Po* the reference population, *r* the regional annual population growth rate (2.9), and *t* the time of the year when the projection was made. The under-five population was calculated to be 15.6% of the total population in Southern Nations, Nationalities, and Peoples' Region (SNNPR) [38]. The projected under-five population data of each district was specified continuously over each month for the 6 years from July 2011 to June 2017 and matched with its location ID, monthly under-five diarrheal morbidity data, and *XY* coordinate of each study location.

Cases were defined as the number of under-five children who were diagnosed to have diarrhea in each health facility of the study districts. Since July 2011, the SNNPR Health Bureau has adopted electronic Health Management Information System (HMIS), where diarrheal cases have been compiled electronically at health facility level. The compiled data are reported monthly to the Zonal Health Department and Regional Health Bureau. For this study, a 6-year monthly under-five diarrheal morbidity data from July 2011 to June 2017 was collected from the e-HMIS database. The data was collected by using a checklist. Data were collected by trained health professionals who had knowledge of the HMIS data management.

Data analysis

The 30 years (1983–1984) average monthly rainfall, the maximum temperature, and the minimum temperature of the administrative zone were calculated from the National Meteorology Agency (NMA) Climate Analysis and Application (map room) [39]. The annual under-five diarrhea incidence per 1000 individuals in each district for the years between July 2011 and June 2017 and seasonal trend were calculated using Excel'. Smoothing of the data was done by calculating the 12 months (1 year) moving average followed by calculating the centered moving average (CMA). The trend of the monthly morbidity data of the 6 years was calculated by using the deseasonalized data and time. The incidence rate per 1000 under-five children, the CMA, and the trend component of the data were plotted to observe seasonal variations and trend of childhood diarrhea in the study areas (Additional file 1).

The excess hazard (the ratio of observed to expected cases greater than one) for each district was calculated by dividing the observed cases by the expected cases and plotted using the geographic information system (GIS). The expected number of cases in each area under the null hypothesis was calculated using the following formula: $E[c] = p*C/P$, where *c* is the observed number of cases and *p* the population in the location of interest, while *C* and *P* are the total number of cases and population respectively [40].

Cluster analysis

The Kulldorff scan statistic, implemented in SaTScan software (SaTSCan v9.4.4), was used to detect if diarrhea was randomly distributed over space, time, or space and time and to evaluate the statistical significance of disease clusters [41]. SaTScan was preferred among software programs capable of space-time disease surveillance analysis, as it was found to be the best-equipped package for use in surveillance system [26].

The scan statistic technique detects and evaluates the statistical significance of spatial or space-time clusters that cannot be explained by the assumption of spatial or space-time randomness, noting the number of observed and expected observations inside the window at each location. In the SaTScan software, the scanning window is an interval (in time), a circle or an ellipse (in space), or a cylinder with a circular or elliptic base (in space-time). The discrete Poisson-based model was used assuming that the reported monthly diarrheal cases are Poisson-distributed in the study area with the projected under-five underlying population at risk. The statistical principles behind the spatial and space-time scan statistics used in the SaTScan software for our specific analysis have been described in detail by Martin Kulldorff [42].

Purely spatial clusters

In this study, the maximum spatial cluster size of the population at risk was set to 50%. The observed diarrheal cases were compared with expected cases inside and outside of each window, and the risk ratios were estimates on the basis of Poisson distribution. The null hypothesis of the spatial scan statistic states that childhood diarrhea is randomly distributed throughout the districts of the administrative zone and that the expected event count is proportional to the population at risk. For any circular window, if the null hypothesis is statistically rejected, then the geographic area defined by the scan window can be considered as a spatial cluster. For each circle, rejection of the null hypothesis is based on a likelihood ratio statistic. The p value was calculated through Monte Carlo hypothesis testing, by comparing the rank of the maximum likelihood from the real data set with the maximum likelihoods from random data sets. To evaluate the statistical significance of the primary cluster, the 999 random replications of the data set are generated under the null hypothesis.

For each location and size of the scanning window, SaTScan uses a Monte Carlo simulation to test the null hypothesis, that is, there is no an elevated risk within the window as compared to outside. Under the Poisson assumption, the likelihood function for a specific window is proportional to:

$$\left[\frac{c}{E(c)}\right]^c \left[\frac{C-c}{C-E(c)}\right]^{C-c} I()$$

where C is the total number of cases, c is the observed number of cases within the window and $E[c]$ is the covariate-adjusted expected number of cases within the window under the null-hypothesis, $C-E(c)$ is the expected number of cases outside the window, and $I()$ is an indicator function. In this study, since SaTScan is set to scan only for clusters with high rates, $I()$ is equal to 1 when the window has more cases than expected under the null hypothesis, and 0 otherwise.

Purely temporal cluster

A purely temporal cluster analysis scanning was performed to detect the temporal clusters of childhood diarrheal cases with high rates, representing the whole geographic area but a 1-month time aggregation length. The maximum time was specified to be the default 50% within the study period. To identify clusters, a likelihood function was maximized across all locations and times. The maximum likelihood indicates the cluster least likely to have occurred by chance (primary cluster). The p value is obtained through Monte Carlo hypothesis testing. Secondary clusters are those that are in rank order after primary cluster by their likelihood ratio test statistic.

Space-time clusters

The space-time scan statistic was defined by a cylindrical window with a circular (or elliptic) geographic base and with a height corresponding to time. The base is defined exactly as for the purely spatial scan statistic, while the height reflects the time period of potential clusters. The cylindrical window is then moved in space and time so that for each possible geographical location and size, it also visits each possible time period, where each cylinder reflects a possible cluster. A likelihood ratio was calculated for each space-time window to indicate to what extent the rate of cases inside the area is higher than expected. Monte Carlo hypothesis testing is then used to indicate the significance level of specific space-time windows.

Results

Monthly diarrheal morbidity data were collected from all the 19 study districts from the 6 years HMIS data. There was no missing data from each district during the study period. A total of 202,406 under-five diarrheal cases were reported, with an annual childhood diarrheal case of 5822 per 100,000 under-five population. The incidence rate varies from place to place and year to year, and an overall increasing trend of childhood diarrhea with seasonal variation peaking between February and May was observed. The highest incidence rate (135.8/1000) was observed in Boricha district in the year 2016/17, and the lowest incidence rate (17.3 per 1000 under-five children) was observed in Bensa district in 2016/17 and Chirie district in 2015/16 (Table 1).

Table 1 Yearly diarrheal incidence rate under-five children of each district, Sidama Zone, Southern Ethiopia, 2017

SN	District name	Yearly incidence rate per 1000 under-five population					
		2011/12	2012/13	2013/14	2014/15	2015/16	2016/17
1	Aleta Chuko	56.0	44.9	57.9	56.6	61.2	54.7
2	Aleta Wondo	56.0	64.0	84.7	95.4	60.2	70.6
3	Arbegona	52.4	42.5	63.9	68.3	43.9	52.0
4	Aroresa	31.6	35.5	43.8	27.7	22.4	31.2
5	Bensa	24.5	18.3	26.1	27.9	17.5	17.3
6	Bona	26.1	49.1	51.2	48.1	40.2	65.2
7	Boricha	88.3	62.0	85.1	121.8	95.7	135.8
8	Bursa	50.7	31.4	33.9	26.7	24.2	17.5
9	Chirie	18.6	91.3	82.7	37.4	17.3	27.2
10	Dale	115.2	38.5	50.7	59.6	53.4	58.1
11	Dara	59.7	48.0	53.0	64.2	52.8	44.4
12	Gorchie	45.9	42.0	65.8	63.8	46.3	32.1
13	Hawassa Zuria	40.2	37.8	30.3	59.8	41.2	51.3
14	Hulla	35.9	39.9	94.4	129.2	111.1	107.1
15	Loka Abaya	94.7	61.2	55.8	64.9	40.3	63.7
16	Malga	71.4	99.2	115.7	106.7	76.3	85.9
17	Shebedino	55.3	60.9	77.3	90.6	62.6	79.3
18	Wonsho	44.2	20.8	55.6	52.9	50.1	60.9
19	Wondogenet	32.0	40.9	56.1	63.8	79.9	75.8
Average		52.6	48.9	62.3	66.6	52.5	58.6

The 6 years seasonal trend of the smoothed and deseasonalized incidence rate of childhood diarrhea showed an increasing trend, with an equation of $Yt = 0.015t + 4.27$, which starts to increase in January and reaches its peak in February. The incidence rate starts to slowly decline through time to reach its lowest peaks in the months of July to November (Fig. 2).

The 30 years average monthly precipitation, maximum temperature, and minimum temperature of the study area are indicated in Fig. 3. The minimum average monthly rainfall was registered in the months of

November, December, January, and February, between 20 and 60 mm. The precipitation starts to increase in March (nearly 95 mm) and reaches its peak in the months of April and May (170–190 mm). A slight reduction is observed in the months of July to August (100–120 mm), then increase in September (145 mm) and October (140 mm). A significant reduction of precipitation was observed in November (nearly 60 mm) (Fig. 3). The 30 years monthly average maximum temperature of the study area showed that November, December, January, February, and March had a higher temperature, where its peak reaches in the months of February and March. It starts to drop in April and reaches its lowest in July and August and then starts to slowly increase again.

The distribution of excess risk, which was defined as the ratio of the number of observed over the number of expected cases was indicated in Table 2 and Fig. 4. Eight districts (Boricha, Malga, Hulla, Aleta Wondo, Shebedion, Dale, Loka Abaya, and Wondogenet) had standard mortality ration (SMR) greater than one.

Purely spatial cluster

The purely spatial cluster analysis result indicated a non-random distribution of under-five diarrhea incidence in Sidama Zone during July 2011–June 2017

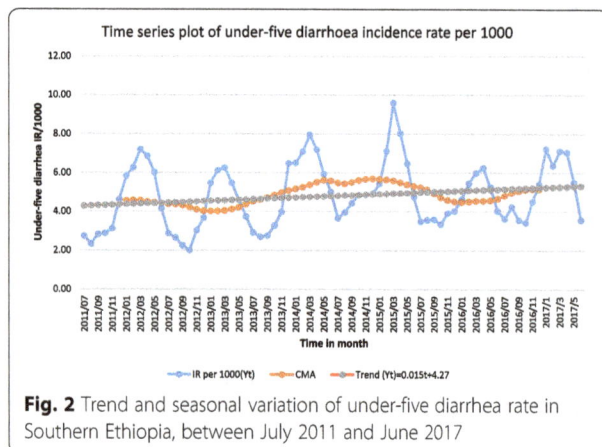

Fig. 2 Trend and seasonal variation of under-five diarrhea rate in Southern Ethiopia, between July 2011 and June 2017

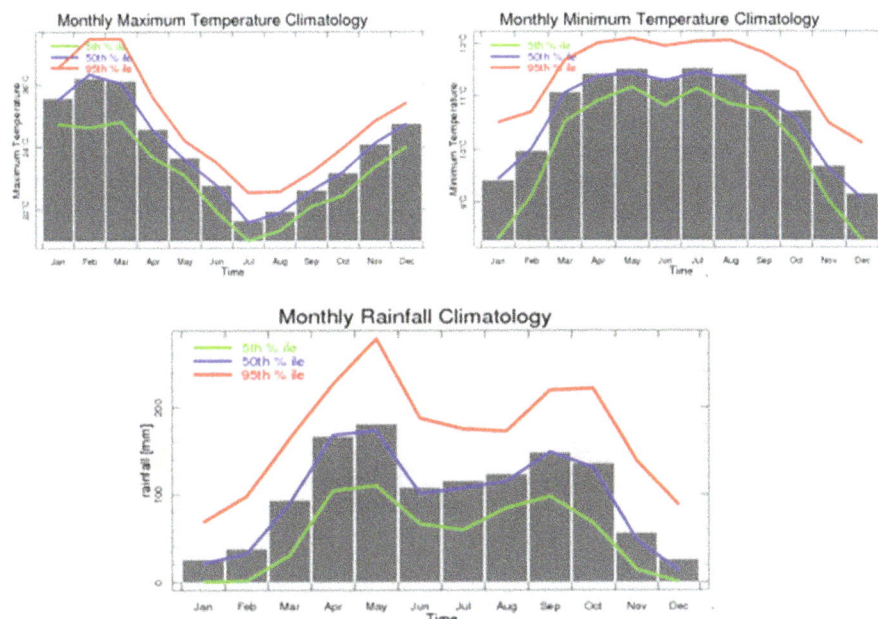

Fig. 3 Thirty years historical (1983–2014) monthly data of precipitation, maximum temperature, and minimum temperature calculated from the National Meteorology Agency (NMA) Climate Analysis and Application (map room)

Table 2 Values of excess risk and relative risk of diarrhea, July 2011 to June 2017, Southern Ethiopia, 2017

SN	District	Obs.*	Exp¥	Obs./exp.	RR
1	Boricha	29,153	17,146.87	1.70	1.82
2	Malga	11,952	7522.60	1.59	1.63
3	Hulla	13,335	8856.59	1.51	1.54
4	Aleta Wondo	16,005	12,947.92	1.24	1.26
5	Shebedino	19,636	16,027.43	1.23	1.25
6	Loka Abaya	7351	6799.06	1.08	1.08
7	Dale	17,713	16,626	1.07	1.07
8	Wondogenet	10,792	10,668.99	1.01	1.01
9	Aleta Chuko	10,883	11,462.75	0.95	0.95
10	Arbegona	8606	9308.74	0.92	0.92
11	Dara	9786	10,638.18	0.92	0.92
12	Gorchie	6102	7226.53	0.84	0.84
13	Wensho	5045	6143.31	0.82	0.82
14	Bona	6713	8306.62	0.81	0.80
15	Chirie	6407	8252.70	0.78	0.77
16	Hawassa Zuria	6391	8528.34	0.75	0.74
17	Aroresa	6393	11,664.18	0.55	0.53
18	Bursa	3691	7100.39	0.52	0.51
19	Bensa	6452	17,178.83	0.38	0.36

RR relative risk, *SN* serial number
*Number of observed cases in a cluster
¥Number of expected cases in a cluster

(Table 3 and Fig. 5). Out of the 19 districts, eight of them (Boricha, Malga, Hulla, Aleta Wondo, Shebedino, Loka Abaya, Dale, and Wondogenet) had significantly higher cases than expected (log likelihood ratio greater than 1). Using the maximum spatial cluster size of ≤ 50% of the total population, one most likely cluster and six secondary clusters were identified. The most likely cluster had a relative risk (RR) of 1.82 ($p < 0.001$), with an observed number of cases of 29,153 and expected cases of 17,146.87. The RR of secondary clusters within a non-random distribution pattern was also significant ($p < 0.001$).

Purely temporal cluster

The purely temporal cluster analysis indicated that one most likely cluster was identified in all districts (LLR = 2109.93, $p < 0.001$) during December 2013 to May 2015 (01/12/2013 to 31/5/2015). The overall RR within the cluster was 1.37 ($p < 0.001$) with an observed number of cases of 63,683 and 50,695.23 expected cases. There was no secondary cluster identified.

Spatiotemporal clusters of childhood diarrhea

The space-time cluster analysis of cases of under-five diarrhea from July 2011 to June 2017 in Sidama Zone showed that diarrhea was not distributed randomly in space-time. Using the maximum spatial cluster size of 50% of the total population, and the maximum temporal cluster size of 50% of the total population, one most likely cluster and four secondary clusters were identified

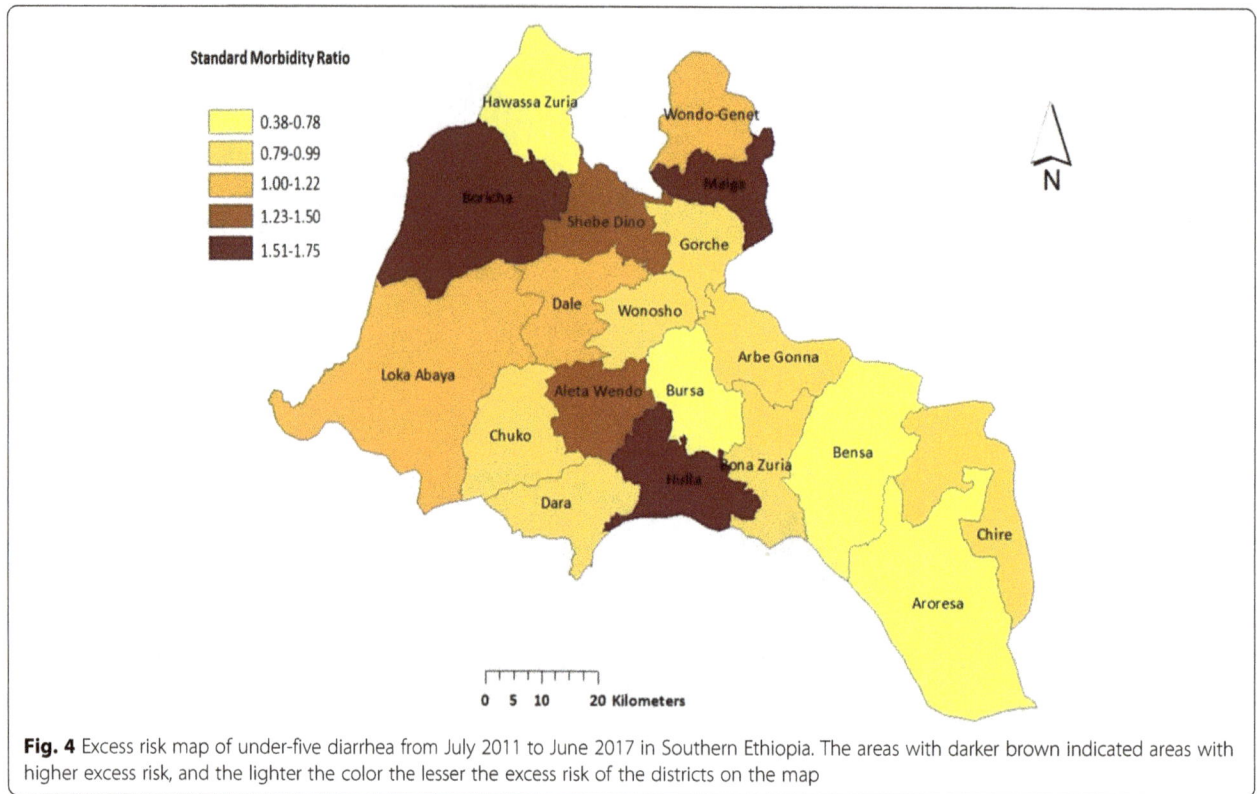

Fig. 4 Excess risk map of under-five diarrhea from July 2011 to June 2017 in Southern Ethiopia. The areas with darker brown indicated areas with higher excess risk, and the lighter the color the lesser the excess risk of the districts on the map

(Table 4). The overall RR within the most likely cluster was 2.03 ($p < 0.001$) with an observed number of cases of 6186 compared with expected cases of 3097.21. The RR of secondary clusters, within a non-random distribution pattern, was also significant ($p < 0.001$).

Discussion

In this study, seasonal variation and hotspots of under-five diarrhea are indicated. The 6-year monthly under-five diarrhea report shows an overall increasing trend and seasonal variation in the study area. The highest incidence rate peaked in Boricha district in the year 2016/17. Spatial, temporal, and space-time hotspots of diarrhea were also observed in Boricha, Malga, Hulla, Loka Abaya, Bursa, Gorchie, and Wonsho districts of Southern Ethiopia.

The current study showed that childhood diarrhea occurred in a cyclical pattern over the months of the

Table 3 Spatial clusters of under-five diarrhea in Southern Ethiopia between July 2011 and June 2017

Cluster number	District	Population	Coordinates	Obs.*	Exp¥	Annual cases/100,000	Obs./exp	RR	LLR	P value
Primary cluster	Boricha	49,076	6.939005 N, 38.253064 E	29,153	17,146.87	9898.2	1.70	1.82	3864.33	< 0.001
1st secondary cluster	Malga	21,530	6.933700 N, 38.562860 E	11,952	7522.60	9249.8	1.59	1.65	1154.94	< 0.001
2nd secondary cluster	Hulla	25,348	6.487117 N, 38.522366 E	13,335	8856.59	8765.7	1.51	1.54	1030.89	< 0.001
3rd secondary cluster	Shebedino	45,872	6.874400 N, 38.441810 E	19,636	16,027.43	7132.6	1.23	1.25	413.94	< 0.001
4th secondary cluster	Aleta Wondo	37,058	6.596820 N, 38.422840 E	16,005	12,947.92	7196.4	1.24	1.26	360.24	< 0.001
5th secondary cluster	Dale	47,585	6.745428 N, 38.409888 E)	17,713	16,626.00	6202.4	1.07	1.07	37.97	< 0.001
6th secondary cluster	Loka Abaya	19,459	6.694306 N, 38.202427 E	7351	6799.06	6294.4	1.08	1.08	22.60	< 0.001

RR relative risk, *LLR* log-likelihood ratio
*Number of observed cases in a cluster
¥Number of expected cases in a cluster

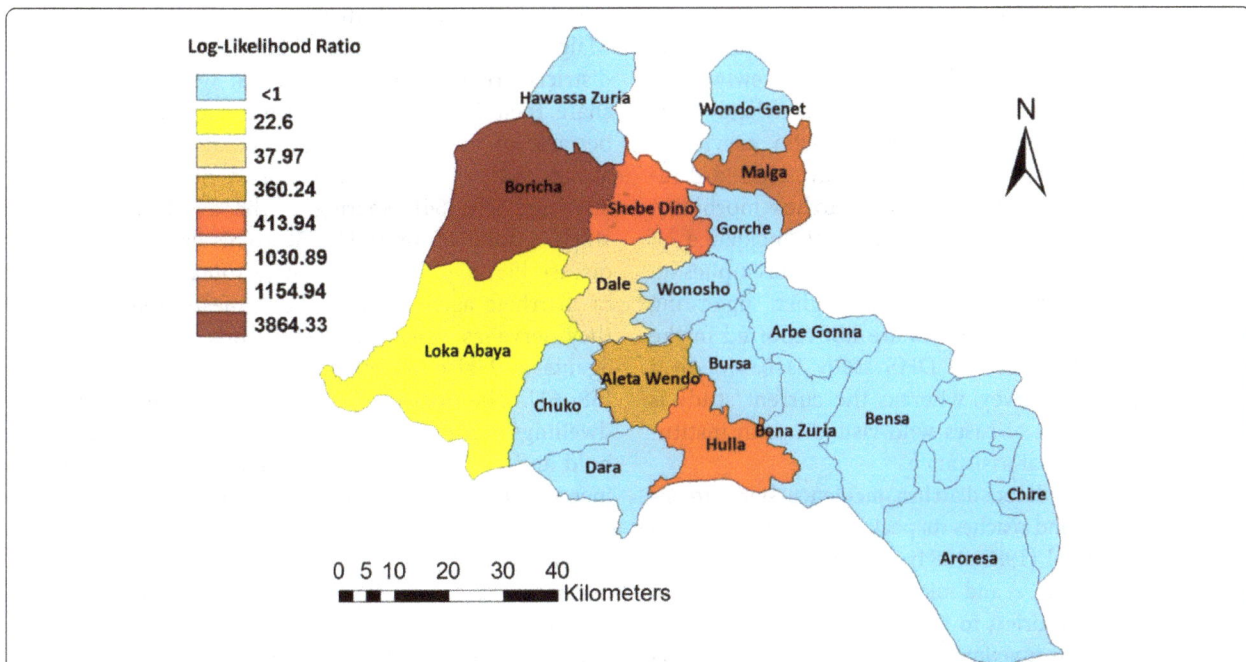

Fig. 5 Most likely spatial cluster and secondary clusters of under-five diarrhea in Southern Ethiopia between July 2011 and June 2017. The primary cluster is found in Boricha district, and the secondary clusters were identified in Malga, Hulla, Shebedino, Aleta Wondo, Dale, and Loka Abaya districts. The order of the names of the districts is based on their likelihood ratio with decreasing order. Numerical identification of the clusters are in order of their likelihood ratio. Tuscan red color indicates the cluster with the likelihood ratio and labeled cluster 1 (most likely cluster or primary cluster), while cluster 2 (flame red), cluster 3 (fire red), cluster 4 (mars red), cluster 5 (seville orange), and cluster 6 (mango) are secondary clusters from the highest to lowest likelihood ratio. Olive color indicates no cluster districts (Table 3)

6 years study period. Previous reports found this. For example, in Brazil, hospitalization rate caused by acute diarrhea in children under the age of one showed annual seasonal and 6-monthly patterns [20]. A study in Northwest Ethiopia also showed that peak childhood diarrheal cases showed a seasonal trend [14]. In China, diarrhea in children under 5 years showed a bimodal distribution, where it showed its peak in fall-winter seasons [43].

Despite reported improvements in water, sanitation, hygiene, and vaccination coverage in the study area

over the years, the annual number of reported childhood diarrheal cases showed an increasing trend. Our finding contradicts the previous report in Gojam, Northwest Ethiopia, where childhood diarrhea showed a decreasing trend [14]. The previous four DHS reports of Ethiopia also showed a decreasing trend in childhood diarrhea in [44]. Another study based on DHS data in Burkina Faso, Mali, Nigeria, and Niger during the period between 1990 and 2013 identified a decrease in the proportions of diarrheal morbidity

Table 4 Spatiotemporal clusters of under-five diarrhea in Southern Ethiopia between July 2011 and June 2017

Cluster number	District	Population	Coordinates	Time frame	Obs.*	Exp[¥]	Annual cases/100,000	Observed/ expected	RR	LLR	P value
1	Malga	21,530	6.933700 N, 38.562860 E	2012/12/1 to 2015/5/31	6186	3097.21	11,627.8	2.00	2.03	1214.67	< 0.001
2	Loka Abaya	19,459	6.694306 N, 38.202427 E	2012/1/1 to 2012/5/31	900	441.07	11,879.4	2.04	2.05	183.47	< 0.001
3	Bursa	20,322	6.590160 N, 38.606330 E	2011/12/1 to 2011/12/31	327	93.27	20,410.6	3.51	3.51	176.61	< 0.001
4	Gorchie	20,683	6.876740 N, 38.584650 E	2014/3/1 to 2014/4/30	479	199.43	13,983.0	2.40	2.41	140.34	< 0.001
5	Wensho	17,583	6.749010 N, 38.517450 E	2012/3/1 to 2012/3/31	216	81.28	15,471.9	2.66	2.66	76.44	< 0.001

RR relative risk, *LLR* log-likelihood ratio
*Number of observed cases in a cluster
[¥]Number of expected cases in a cluster

among under-five children [45]. The fact that the childhood diarrhea morbidity showed an increasing trend over the years might be because newly built health facilities started reporting the diarrheal morbidity and health extension workers, who previously did not diagnose and treat diarrhea, have started diagnosing, treating, and reporting of diarrhea morbidity. Our data suggest an annual diarrheal incidence of around six cases per 100 while the DHS data implies an annual incidence order of magnitude higher, suggesting that the great majority of cases are not reported in the HMIS. This is because the DHS study is based on a community-based survey, whereas the current study is based on the report of cases who visited health institutions seeking medical assistance.

The 6 years childhood diarrhea incidence starts to increase in January and reaches its peak in February. According to the historical (1983–1984) monthly data of rainfall, maximum temperature, and minimum temperature, this is the transition from driest to the rainy season. During this time, the average maximum temperature reaches its highest [39]. Similar studies also showed that increase in temperature was positively associated with diarrhea incidence [46, 47]. The incidence rate starts to slowly decline through time to reach its lowest peaks in the months of July to November. Shortage of water in the dry season has been associated with increased prevalence of diarrhea [22]. This may be due to less availability of fresh water or concentration of contaminants in smaller volumes of water [48] or longer water storage [49]. A large outbreak of diarrhea occurred following severe droughts due to decreased water availability and worsened personal hygiene [50]. Extreme rainfall days and associated flooding were also strongly related to diarrhea-associated morbidity [51, 52]. This is because flooding could result in the breakdown of sanitary conditions and contamination of drinking water sources by washing nutrients, pathogens, and toxins into water bodies [53].

The study also showed the existence of substantial variation in the spatial distribution of diarrhea within the study area. The finding was in agreement with another national study [15]. However, there is the difference in the nature of the data sources between the studies in that the later used cross-sectional DHS data. The highest risk of diarrhea was found in Boricha district. This might be due to the fact that most of the residents of the district relied heavily on pond water, which is open for both human and animal. In addition, the population is agro-pastoralist, where they move from place to place in search of food and water for their animals. These types of people would not have the chance to construct and use their own latrines. It can also be due to other factors such as differing levels of poverty, education, and lifestyle.

Spatial hotspots of diarrhea were also observed in Malga and Hulla districts. This might be because these districts are located in Highlands, where most people share their home with their domestic animals at night because of fear of cold and theft. It is estimated that around 90% of rural households in Ethiopia own some farm animals [54]. Sharing of the dwellings with livestock is quite common [55, 56]. This has been linked to disease [55, 57]. One of the main routes of transmission of diarrheic agents is through domesticated animals as they serve as reservoirs for various zoonotic diseases agents and also to other domestic and wild animals [58–61]. The presence of domestic animals around the dwellings can compromise the sanitation of the household and their neighborhood environment, and thus, it increases the chance of the dwellers come in contact with animal droppings; thereby, there are chances of vertical transmission of the microbes to the owners [62, 63]. Zoonotic diseases such as *Campylobacter* diarrhea, *Cryptosporidium* diarrhea, and *E. coli* O157 infection have been reported following exposure to unhygienic environments as a result of domestic animals living in and around the human dwellings [61, 64, 65].

The findings showed temporal variation in the overall risk of diarrhea, which indicated that childhood diarrhea was not distributed randomly in time. This might be due to the influence of socio-economical, environmental, or climate-related factors. Statistically significant space-time hotspots ($p < 0.001$) were also observed (Table 4). This consisted of a primary hotspot and four secondary hotspots. The primary hotspot was observed in December 2012 to January 2015 in Malga district with a likelihood ratio of 1214.67 and relative risk of 2.03. The first, second, third, and fourth secondary hotspots occurred from January 2012 to May 2012 in Loka Abaya, December 2011 in Bursa, from March to April 2014 in Gorchie, and March 2012 in Wonsho districts. The primary hotspot spanned for slightly more than 2 years, and the other secondary clusters existed from 1 to 5 months only. This might be due to the occurrence of risk factors specific to the local areas and time periods.

This study has strengths and limitations. The fact that complete monthly morbidity data were obtained from all districts throughout the study period was a strength. The other strength was the existence of historical 30 years precipitation, maximum temperature, and minimum temperature data which were compared with the seasonal variation of childhood diarrhea that could have been influenced by metrological parameters. The use of the SaTScan software allowed us to both detect the location of clusters and evaluate their statistical significance without problems with multiple testing. A limitation is under-reporting of childhood diarrhea as the data reflects only those who sought healthcare setup level treatment. As a result, the study might not be indicative of the true picture of diarrheal morbidity of the study area. However, this limitation might be minimal as the problem is assumed to be uniform across all districts over the study period.

Conclusions

This study assessed the seasonal variation and spatial, temporal, and space-time clusters of under-five diarrhea using 6 years HMIS morbidity data (July 2011 to June 2017) in Southern Ethiopia. An increasing trend with a seasonal variation of childhood diarrhea which peaks in the transition period from driest to the rainy season occurred. An excess risk of diarrhea was also observed in Boricha, Malga, and Hulla districts. Statistically significant space-time hotspots were also observed in five districts from December 2012 to January 2015 in Malga district, from January 2012 to May 2012 in Loka Abaya, December 2011 in Bursa, from March to April 2014 in Gorchie, and March 2012 in Wonsho districts.

The spatial, temporal, and space-time clusters, generated in this research, can be used by the various stakeholders to prioritize places of intervention. In addition, season-specific interventional strategies can be developed with efficient resource use to reduce the childhood morbidity, mortality, and financial losses related to visiting health instructions as a result of diarrhea morbidity. Further studies are required to clarify the effect of weather variabilities on under-five diarrhea incidence and to investigate the specific risk factors of childhood diarrhea in hotspot areas.

Acknowledgements
The authors would like to thank the funding organizations, the SNNPR Health Bureau, and the Sidama Zone Health Department people for providing access to the HMIS data, the Central Statistical Agency of Ethiopia Hawassa Branch Office, the SNNPR Finance and Economy Bureau, and the Sidama Zone Finance and Economy Department for providing relevant information about the study area.

Funding
Financial support for this study was obtained from the German Academic Exchange Program (DAAD), through the International Livestock Research Institute, and from Addis Ababa and Hawassa Universities.

Authors' contributions
HB, WD, DG, and AK participated from the conception to the final write up of the study. DG also revised the English language. All authors read and approved the manuscript.

Authors' information
HB is a lecturer of Environmental and Public Health at Hawassa University, Ethiopia. WD is the associate professor and dean of the School of Public Health, College of Health Sciences, Addis Ababa University. He has been teaching several courses including biostatistics, epidemiology, and research methodology. He has had supervised many masters and doctoral students. He also has more than 60 publications in the national and international journals. AK is an associate professor, head of Environmental Health Unit, and PhD program coordinator at the School of Public Health, Addis Ababa University, Ethiopia. He has been teaching environmental health courses for various groups of health science students. He also has supervised several masters and doctoral students. He has more than 60 publications in the peer-reviewed journals. DG is an epidemiologist and veterinarian with nearly 20 years of experience in developing countries. She is a senior researcher at the International Livestock Research Institute in Kenya and program manager of agriculture-associated diseases in the new CGIAR Research Program on Agriculture for Human Nutrition and Health. She is a prolific and effective author in a wide variety of media, including over 70 peer-reviewed journal articles, numerous book chapters, presentations, posters, policy briefs, films, manuals, farmer diagnostic aids, and articles.

Competing interests
The authors declare that they have no competing interest.

Author details
[1]College of Health Sciences, Hawassa University, P.O. Box 1560, Hawassa, Ethiopia. [2]School of Public Health, Addis Ababa University, P.O. Box 1176, Addis Ababa, Ethiopia. [3]International Livestock Research Institute, Box 30709, Nairobi, Kenya.

References
1. World Health Organization (WHO). Diarrhoeal disease. 2017. Available from: http://www.who.int/en/news-room/fact-sheets/detail/diarrhoeal-disease. updated 2 May 2017; cited 2017, November 7.
2. Troeger C, Forouzanfar M, Rao PC, Khalil I, Brown A, Reiner RC Jr, et al. Estimates of global, regional, and national morbidity, mortality, and aetiologies of diarrhoeal diseases: a systematic analysis for the Global Burden of Disease Study 2015. Lancet Infect Dis. 2017;17(9):909–48.
3. Ahmed M, Abedin J, Alam KF, Al Mamun A, Paul RC, Rahman M, et al. Incidence of acute diarrhea-associated death among children <5 years of age in Bangladesh, 2010-12. Am J Trop Med Hyg. 2018;98(1):281–6.
4. van der Westhuizen FP, Slogrove AL, Kunneke HM, Kruger M. Factors associated with severe dehydrating diarrhoea in the rural western cape, South Africa. J Trop Pediatr. 2018. https://doi.org/10.1093/tropej/fmy002. [Epub ahead of print].
5. Bado AR, Susuman AS, Nebie EI. Trends and risk factors for childhood diarrhea in sub-Saharan countries (1990–2013): assessing the neighborhood inequalities. Glob Health Action. 2016;9(1):30166.
6. Stella S, Ajayi A. Viral causes of diarrhea in children in Africa: a literature review. J Mole Biol Tech. 2017;1(1):1042.
7. Central Statistical Agency-CSA/Ethiopia, ICF. Ethiopia demographic and health survey 2016. Addis Ababa: CSA and ICF; 2017.
8. Dessalegn M, Kumie A, Tefera W. Predictors of under-five childhood diarrhea: Mecha District, West Gojam. Ethiopia Ethiop J Health Dev. 2011; 25(3):192–200.
9. Eshete WB. A stepwise regression analysis on under-five diarrhoeal morbidity prevalence in Nekemte town, western Ethiopia: maternal care giving and hygiene behavioral determinants. East African J Public Health. 2008;5(3):193–8.
10. Mengistie B, Berhane Y, Worku A. Household water chlorination reduces incidence of diarrhea among under-five children in rural Ethiopia: a cluster randomized controlled trial. PLoS One. 2013;8(10):e77887.
11. Mengistie B, Berhane Y, Worku A. Prevalence of diarrhea and associated risk factors among children under-five years of age in eastern Ethiopia: a cross-sectional study. Open J Prev Med. 2013;3(7):446–53.
12. Tamiso A, Yitayal M, Awoke A. Prevalence and determinants of childhood diarrhoea among graduated households, in rural area of Shebedino district, southern Ethiopia, 2013. Sci J Public Healtht. 2014;2(3):243–51.

13. Beyene H. Sanitation infrastructure sustainability challenges case study: Ethiopia. In: Bongartz P, Vernon N, Fox J, editors. Sustainable sanitation for all: experiences, challenges, and innovations. Rugby: Practical Action Publishing Ltd; 2016.

14. Azage M, Kumie A, Worku A, Bagtzoglou AC. Childhood diarrhea exhibits spatiotemporal variation in Northwest Ethiopia: a SaTScan spatial statistical analysis. PLoS One. 2015;10(12):e0144690.

15. Bogale GG, Gelaye KA, Degefie DT, Gelaw YA. Spatial patterns of childhood diarrhea in Ethiopia: data from Ethiopian demographic and health surveys (2000, 2005, and 2011). BMC Infect Dis. 2017;17(1):426.

16. Osei FB, Duker AA. Spatial dependency of V. cholera prevalence on open space refuse dumps in Kumasi, Ghana: a spatial statistical modelling. Int J Health Geogr. 2008;7(62). https://doi.org/10.1186/1476-072X-7-62.

17. Thiam S, Diène AN, Fuhrimann S, Winkler MS, Sy I, Ndione JA, et al. Prevalence of diarrhoea and risk factors among children under five years old in Mbour, Senegal: a cross-sectional study. Infectious Dis Poverty. 2017;6:109.

18. Ahmed SF, Farheen A, Muzaffar A, Mattoo GM. Prevalence of diarrhoeal disease, its seasonal and age variation in under-fives in Kashmir, India. Int J Health Sci. 2008;2(2):126–33.

19. Anyorikeya M, Ameme DK, Nyarko KM, Sackey SO, Afari E. Trends of diarrhoeal diseases in children under five years in the war memorial hospital-Navrongo, Ghana: 2010-2013. Pan African Med J. 2016;25(Suppl 1):8.

20. Masukawa MLT, EMd S, Gimenes E, Uchimura NS, Moriwaki AM, Uchimura TT. Time series investigation of changes in seasonality of acute diarrhea hospitalizations before and after rotavirus vaccine in Southern Brazil. Cadernos de Saúde Pública; 2016;32(10):e00080515.

21. Phung D, Huang C, Rutherford S, Chu C, Wang X, Nguyen M, et al. Temporal and spatial patterns of diarrhoea in the Mekong Delta area, Vietnam. Epidemiol Infect. 2015;143(16):3488–97.

22. Bandyopadhyay S, Kanji S, Wang L. The impact of rainfall and temperature variation on diarrheal prevalence in sub-Saharan Africa. Appl Geogr. 2012; 33(Supplement C):63–72.

23. Kulinkina AV, Mohan VR, Francis MR, Kattula D, Sarkar R, Plummer JD, et al. Seasonality of water quality and diarrheal disease counts in urban and rural settings in South India. Sci Rep. 2016;6:20521.

24. Omore R, Tate JE, O'Reilly CE, Ayers T, Williamson J, Moke F, et al. Epidemiology, seasonality and factors associated with rotavirus infection among children with moderate-to-severe diarrhea in rural western Kenya, 2008–2012: the Global Enteric Multicenter Study (GEMS). PLoS One. 2016; 11(8):e0160060.

25. Tornheim JA, Manya AS, Oyando N, Kabaka S, O'Reilly CE, Breiman RF, et al. The epidemiology of hospitalization with diarrhea in rural Kenya: the utility of existing health facility data in developing countries. Int J Infect Dis. 2010; 14(6):e499–505.

26. Robertson C, Nelson TA. Review of software for space-time disease surveillance. Int J Health Geogr. 2010;9(16).

27. Wu W, Guo J, Guan P, Sun Y, Zhou B. Clusters of spatial, temporal, and space-time distribution of hemorrhagic fever with renal syndrome in Liaoning Province, Northeastern China. BMC Infect Dis. 2011;11:229.

28. Faires MC, Pearl DL, Ciccotelli WA, Berke O, Reid-Smith RJ, Weese JS. Detection of Clostridium difficile infection clusters, using the temporal scan statistic, in a community hospital in southern Ontario, Canada, 2006–2011. BMC Infect Dis. 2014;14(1):254.

29. Lefebvre A, Bertrand X, Vanhems P, Lucet JC, Chavanet P, Astruc K, et al. Detection of temporal clusters of healthcare-associated infections or colonizations with Pseudomonas aeruginosa in two hospitals: comparison of SaTScan and WHONET software packages. PLoS One. 2015;10(10):e0139920.

30. Dewan A, Abdullah AYM, Shogib MRI, Karim R, Rahman MM. Exploring spatial and temporal patterns of visceral leishmaniasis in endemic areas of Bangladesh. Trop Med Health. 2017;45(1):29.

31. Dewan AM, Corner R, Hashizume M, Ongee ET. Typhoid fever and its association with environmental factors in the Dhaka metropolitan area of Bangladesh: a spatial and time-series approach. PLoS Negl Trop Dis. 2013;7(1):e1998.

32. Osei FB, Stein A. Spatial variation and hot-spots of district level diarrhea incidences in Ghana: 2010–2014. BMC Public Health. 2017;17(1):617.

33. Hundessa SH, Williams G, Li S, Guo J, Chen L, Zhang W, et al. Spatial and space–time distribution of Plasmodium vivax and Plasmodium falciparum malaria in China, 2005–2014. Malar J. 2016;15(1):595.

34. FMoH. Acute Watery Diarrhea (AWD) prevention and control strategy. Addis Ababa: Federal Minstry of Health; 2011. Report No

35. Hameso SY. Development challenges in the age of climate change: the case of Sidama. Economy of Southern Ethiopia, Ethiopian Economics Association, its Chapter at Hawassa University, Department of Economics; 1 March 2012. Ethiopia: Hawassa University; 2012.

36. Deqamo Y. In: Department SZFaE, editor. Socio-economical and environmental characteristics of Sidama Zone. Hawassa: Sidama Zone Finance & Economic Development Department, Ethiopia; 2011. p. 98.

37. Central Statistical Agency (CSA). Population projection of Ethiopia for all regions at Wereda level from 2014–2017. Addis Ababa: Federal Democratic Republic of Ethiopia, Central Statistical Agency; 2013. p. 118.

38. Central Statistical Agency (CSA). National Census Report of Ethiopia. Addis Ababa: Central Statistical Agency of Ethiopia; 2007.

39. National Meteorology Agency (NMA). Climate Analysis and Application Addis Ababa, Ethiopia: National Metrological Agency of Ethiopia; 2017. Available from: http://www.ethiometmaprooms.gov.et/. cited 2017 November 28.

40. Kulldorff M. SaTScanTM user guide. In: Boston; 2006.

41. Kulldorff M and Information Management Services, Inc. SaTScanTM v9.4.4: Software for the spatial and space-time scan statistics. 2016. http://www.satscan.org/. August 2016.

42. Kulldorff M. A spatial scan statistic. Commun Stat Theory Methods. 1997;26: 1481–96.

43. Xu Z, Hu W, Zhang Y, Wang X, Zhou M, Su H, et al. Exploration of diarrhoea seasonality and its drivers in China. Sci Rep. 2015;5:8241.

44. CSA. Central Statistical Agency (CSA) [Ethiopia] and ICF. Ethiopia Demographic and Health Survey 2016. Addis Ababa, Ethiopia, and Rockville, Maryland: CSA and ICF; 2017.

45. Bado AR, Susuman AS, Nebie EI. Trends and risk factors for childhood diarrhea in sub-Saharan countries (1990–2013): assessing the neighborhood inequalities. Glob Health Action. 2016;9 https://doi.org/10.3402/gha.v9.30166.

46. Checkley W, Epstein LD, Gilman RH, Figueroa D, Cama RI, Patz JA, et al. Effect of El Nino and ambient temperature on hospital admissions for diarrhoeal diseases in Peruvian children. Lancet. 2000;355(9202):442–50.

47. Hashizume M, Armstrong B, Hajat S, Wagatsuma Y, Faruque AS, Hayashi T, et al. Association between climate variability and hospital visits for non-cholera diarrhea in Bangladesh: effects and vulnerable groups. Int J Epidemiol. 2007;36(5):1030–7.

48. Leder K, Sinclair MI, McNeil JJ. Water and the environment: a natural resource or a limited luxury? Med J Aust. 2002;177:609–13.

49. Boelee E, McCartney M, Yohannes M, Hagos F, Lautze J, Kibret S. Climate change, water resource development and malaria in Ethiopia. Water and Health: Where Science Meets Policy; October 25-26, 2010. The University of North Carolina at Chapel Hill, USA; 2010.

50. Jordan E. Drought as a climatic driver of an outbreak of diarrhea in Tuvalu, South Pacific: Public Health Theses; 2015. p. 1079. http://elischolar.library.yale.edu/ysphtdl/1079. Accessed on 26 Aug 2016

51. Chou W, Wu J, Wang Y, Huang H, Sung F, Chuang C. Modelling the impact of climate variability on diarrhea-associated diseases in Taiwan (1996–2007). Sci Total Environ. 2010;409(43–51):43–51.

52. Hashizume M, Armstrong B, Wagatsuma Y, Faruque AS, Hayashi T, Sack DA. Rotavirus infections and climate variability in Dhaka, Bangladesh: a time-series analysis. Epidemiol Infect. 2008;136(9):1281–9.

53. Thomas MK, Charron DF, Waltner-Toews D, Schuster C, Maarouf AR, Holt JD. A role of high impact weather events in waterborne disease outbreaks in Canada, 1975–2001. Int J Environ Health Res. 2006;16:167–80.

54. EDHS. Central Statistical Agency [Ethiopia] and ICF International. Ethiopia Demographic and Health Survey (EDHS). Addis Ababa, Ethiopia and Calverton: Central statistical agency and ICF international; 2012.

55. Ayele WY, Neill SD, Zinsstag J, Weiss MG, Pavlik I. Bovine tuberculosis: an old disease but a new threat to Africa. Int J Tuberc Lung Dis. 2004;8(8):924–37.

56. Haile AA. Assessment of the impact of latrine utilization on idarrhoeal diseases in the rural community of Hulet Ejju Enessie District, Amhara Regional State. Addis Ababa: Addis Ababa University, Ethiopia; 2007.

57. Mulugeta T. Socio-economic, environmental, and behavioural factors associated with the occurrence of diarrhoeal disease among under-five children, Meskanena Mareko Woreda, southern Ethiopia. Addis Ababa: Addis Ababa University, Ethiopia; 2003.

58. Doorduyn Y, Van Den Brandhof WE, Van Duynhoven YT, Breukink BJ, Wagenaar JA, Van Pelt W. Risk factors for indigenous Campylobacter jejuni and Campylobacter coli infections in the Netherlands: a case-control study. Epidemiol Infect. 2010;138(10):1391–404.

59. Mahdi NK, Ali NH. Cryptosporidiosis among animal handlers and their livestock in Basrah, Iraq. East Afr Med J. 2002;79(10):550–3.

60. Moher D, Liberati A, Tetzlaff J, Altman DG. Preferred reporting items for systematic reviews and meta-analyses: the PRISMA statement. Ann Intern Med. 2009;151(4):264–9. w64

61. Rao MR, Naficy AB, Savarino SJ, Abu-Elyazeed R, Wierzba TF, Peruski LF, et al. Pathogenicity and convalescent excretion of campylobacter in rural Egyptian children. Am J Epidemiol. 2001;154(2):166–73.

62. Fayehun OA. Household environmental health hazards and child survival in sub-Saharan Africa. DHS Working Papers No. 74. Calverton: ICF Macro; 2010. Contract No.: 74

63. Ramani SV, Frühauf T, Dutta A, Meijers H. Determinants of the prevalence of diarrhoea in adolescents attending school: a case study of an Indian village school. UNU-MERIT Working Papers. 2012;059:2012.

64. Locking ME, SJ O'BRIEN, Reilly WJ, Wright EM, Campbell DM, Coia JE, et al. Risk factors for sporadic cases of Escherichia coli O157 infection: the importance of contact with animal excreta. Epidemiol Infect. 2001;127:215–20.

65. Molbak K, Jensen H, Ingholt L, Aaby P. Risk factors for diarrheal disease incidence in early childhood: a community cohort study from Guinea-Bissau. Am J Epidemiol. 1997;146(3):273–82.

21

Bottom-up approach to strengthen community-based malaria control strategy from community health workers' perceptions of their past, present, and future: a qualitative study in Palawan, Philippines

Emilie Louise Akiko Matsumoto-Takahashi[1,2], Pilarita Tongol-Rivera[3], Elena Andino Villacorte[3], Ray Uyaan Angluben[4], Masamine Jimba[2] and Shigeyuki Kano[1*]

Abstract

Background: Microscopists have active roles in bringing malaria diagnosis and treatment closer to households in Palawan, the highest malaria-endemic province in the Philippines. To accelerate the elimination of malaria in Palawan, we performed a study based on the bottom-up approach to provide profound data to strengthen this community-based malaria control from the microscopists' point of view.

Methods: We performed a qualitative cross-sectional study in Palawan. Four focus group discussions with 50 microscopists were conducted in Palawan from November 2010 to February 2011. During the discussions, the following open-ended questions were addressed: motivation for applying to be microscopists in the "Past" category; job satisfaction, role, problems, and saddest and happiest experiences working as microscopists in the "Present" category; and willingness towards task shifting in the "Future" category. Data were transcribed and analyzed by framework analysis using the NVivo software program.

Results: The present study innovatively proposed the following strategies: reinforcement strategy (adequate supplies and settings), highly prioritized additional strategies (improving social status of microscopists, issuing a travel budget, and including indigenous populations), regional additional strategies (additional malaria control in the southern region and task shifting in the northern region), and less prioritized additional strategies (employment policy and health checkup).

Conclusion: A bottom-up approach using microscopists' perceptions would be a valuable method to propose practical and effective additional strategies for strengthening community-based malaria control.

Keywords: Malaria, Microscopist, Community health workers, Program development, Program evaluation

* Correspondence: kano@ri.ncgm.go.jp
[1]Department of Tropical Medicine and Malaria, Research Institute, National Center for Global Health and Medicine, 1-21-1 Toyama, Shinjuku-ku, Tokyo 162-8655, Japan
Full list of author information is available at the end of the article

Background

Palawan has the highest incidence/prevalence of malaria among the endemic provinces of the Philippines, where microscopists, as community health workers (CHWs), have active roles in bringing malaria diagnosis and treatment closer to households to support the limited health care services [1, 2]. In many malaria-endemic countries, CHWs have now important roles in malaria intervention including malaria case management, prevention including health surveillance, and health promotion specific to malaria [3]. Microscopists in Palawan prepare Giemsa-stained blood smears, identify malaria infection and species, give anti-malaria drugs if necessary, and conduct community awareness-raising activities for malaria prevention [2].

This community-based malaria control, *Kilusan Ligtas Malaria* (KLM, Tagalog: Movement Against Malaria), was launched in 1999, and since then, early diagnosis and prompt treatment have been implemented and scaled-up throughout Palawan. Consequently, the morbidity and mortality decreased year by year to reach an annual parasite index (API) in 2010 of 13.0 [1]. However, if we analyze the decrease in the API closely, it has actually remained unchanged since 2006. Now, additional strategies to further strengthen the KLM are earnestly desired in Palawan.

In this regard, we conducted three quantitative studies and suggested a new approach to accelerate the universal access of malaria patients to diagnosis, treatment, and prevention [4–6], namely the studies suggested that community awareness-raising activities of the microscopists would strengthen the effective prevention practices of the residents by increasing the likelihood of their seeking appropriate treatment. These activities could be also enhanced by additional follow-up interventions to improve service quality of the microscopists and their usage ability. However, these findings were still raising the question of how to effectively address the recent plateau in malaria incidence in the province.

Thus, in the present study, we performed a qualitative study based on the bottom-up approach to provide more profound data to strengthen this community-based malaria control from the microscopists' points of view. The bottom-up approach could bridge the gap between proposer and practitioner by not relying on central guidance but by using the creativity and will of the people working in the community [7, 8]. Some studies have obtained findings to develop and/or evaluate strategies using qualitative data on specific CHWs' perceptions (such as issues, barriers, or motivations), but no intervention design was discussed by applying the perceptions [9–12]. The present study explained the methods of extracting findings from qualitative data on the CHWs' perceptions that were relevant to intervention design. We gleaned such spatiotemporal and multilateral perceptions of the CHWs as motivation for applying to be microscopists in the "Past" category; job satisfaction, role, problems, and saddest and happiest experiences working as microscopists in the "Present" category; and willingness towards task shifting in the "Future" category, and then tried to provide a path to promote a better strategy in an articulate manner.

Methods

Participants

The present study was a qualitative study conducted in the province of Palawan, Philippines. The population comprises various ethnicities, and the registered population was estimated to be 1,025,800 in 2010 [13]. The southern region has a much higher incidence of malaria than the northern region (Table 1).

Focus group discussions (FGDs) employing a total number of 50 microscopists were successfully conducted in two municipalities (Taytay and San Vicente) from the northern region in February 2011 and in two municipalities (Bataraza and Brooke's Point) from the southern region in November 2010 (Table 2). Not only the variation in localities along the island of Palawan but also the incidence of malaria and the socio-economic status of each region were taken into consideration when choosing the municipalities to be representative study sites.

FGDs

The FGD method was chosen because it could stimulate group dynamics of the participants by providing the facilitator with rich data, which would not have

Table 1 Distribution of confirmed malaria cases, API, and microscopists/region (year 2011)

Region	Confirmed malaria cases (*P. falciparum*)	API	Microscopists	
			Registered	Participants
Total	4984 (76.3%)	5.71	290	50 (17.2%)
Northern region	200 (57.0%)	0.60*	115	28 (24.3%)
Puerto Princesa City	795 (71.2%)	3.84	30	0 (0%)
Southern region	3989 (78.3%)	12.1*	145	22 (15.2%)

API annual parasite index
*Chi-square test between the northern region and southern region ($p < 0.0001$)

Table 2 Socio-demographic status of participants with respect to place of assignment

Socio-demographic status	Total ($N = 50$)	Northern region ($n = 28$)	Southern region ($n = 22$)	p value
Age				
Mean (SD)	38.6 (6.8)	39.2 (6.4)	37.7 (7.4)	0.451[a]
Gender				
Men	8	3	5	0.223[b]
Women	41	24	17	
Marital status				
Never married	5	2	3	0.177[b]
Married	42	26	16	
Divorced	1	0	1	
Widowed	2	0	2	
Education				
No grade completed	3	2	1	0.588[b]
Elementary	1	0	1	
High school	28	17	11	
Higher	18	9	9	
Occupation				
Homemakers	33	22	11	0.044[b]*
Farmer	12	3	9	
Other	5	3	2	
Religion				
Catholic	28	19	9	0.053[c]
Other	22	9	13	
Household wealth[1]				
Mean (SD)	2.5 (1.4)	2.3 (1.3)	2.9 (1.5)	0.107[a]
Duration of work as microscopist (months)				
Mean (SD)	94.8 (45.9)	111.9 (41.4)	73.1 (42.9)	0.002[a]**
Distance from home to health center (min)				
Mean (SD)	22.7 (30.0)	21.4 (23.2)	24.3 (37.5)	0.736[a]

*Significant place of assignment difference ($0.01 < p < 0.05$)
**Significant place of assignment difference ($0.001 < p < 0.01$)
***Significant place of assignment difference ($p < 0.001$)
[a]ANOVA
[b]Fisher's exact test
[c]Chi-square test was used to clarify the place of assignment difference
[1]This scale scores from 1 to 8 points, with 1 point each for the following: electricity, radio, television, refrigerator, bicycle, motorcycle, bike-car, and tin or cement wall

been possible with one-to-one interviews, especially when there is little prior information on the participants [14, 15].

The FGDs were conducted in the local language (Tagalog) by facilitators who were local malaria experts with extensive experience with FGDs. During the discussions, the following open-ended questions were used to gather the broad viewpoints of the microscopists: microscopists' perceptions of the past situation (motivation for applying), the present situation (job satisfaction, roles, problems, saddest and happiest experiences working as microscopists), and the future situation (willingness towards task shifting) (Table 3).

Audio recordings were transcribed with supervision of the FGD facilitators and analyzed by the framework analysis method using the NVivo 10 software program (QSR International Pty Ltd., Doncaster, Australia) [16]. First, each focus group discussion (FGD) session was recorded and transcribed verbatim (*transcription*). Local malaria experts translated each verbatim transcription from Tagalog into English. These transcribed discussions and field notes served as the primary text documents. All of the translated verbatim transcriptions were read thoroughly and repeatedly to become familiar with the key ideas and recurrent themes (*familiarization*). Then, the transcription was systematically coded multiple times

Table 3 Focus group topics and key questions

Topic			Key questions
Past	Motivation	Q1	Why did you become microscopists?
Present	Job satisfaction	Q2	Are you satisfied with your job as microscopists? Why?
	Role	Q3	How many patients do you see per week in both dry and wet seasons?
		Q4	How many of your patients were diagnosed as having malaria per week in both dry and wet seasons?
	Problems	Q5	What kind of problems did you face while performing your job as microscopists?
		Q6	Do you think there are specific ethnic groups, age groups, sexes, or any kinds of people who are likely to receive your treatment? Are there any people who are not likely to receive it?
	Experience	Q7	Please tell me about your saddest experience working as microscopists.
		Q8	Please tell me about your happiest experience working as microscopists.
Future	Task shifting	Q9	Do you want to expand your job as microscopists? If yes, in which way and how if it is not for malaria?

(*coding*). Using this primal set of codes, the initial thematic framework was developed to structure, label, and define data (*identifying a thematic framework*). Based on this thematic framework, the whole transcription was re-coded (*applying the thematic framework*), and the data were charted into the appropriate parts of the framework matrix to which they related (*charting*). Finally, conclusions were drawn by using charts to define concepts, map the range and nature of the phenomena, create typologies, and find associations between themes with a view to providing explanations for the findings (*interpretation*).

Results

The final results of the analytical framework of the microscopists' perceptions of the past, present, and future are listed in Tables 4, 5, and 6, respectively. In these tables, themes, codes, and descriptions are listed by topic. Figure 1 illustrates the association of all results and the proposed strategies based on these results.

Motivation

Under this theme, participants in the present study indicated that their motivation was based on three themes.

The first was the motivation based on facts, which were the high malaria incidence in their village, limited health care resources in their village, and to have suffered from malaria. The second theme was the motivation based on hope towards the future, the contents of which were devotion to help their village, to eliminate malaria, and inquisitiveness to learn about malaria. The third theme of motivation was that they were nominated by the village captain or midwife because of their job experience as a Barangay Health Worker (BHW) and/or because no one was available (Table 4).

Devotion was mentioned in all FGDs and was the most frequently appearing motivation. It was often mentioned along with the hope to eliminate malaria in their village where limited health service is available.

Our areas are far from the hospital, and we know that Palawan is known for malaria. So I wanted to help my fellow villagers, they (the village inhabitants) will not go to the town (where there is the hospital) just to have malaria smear to know if they have malaria or not. (Code: high malaria incidence, limited health care resources, and devotion)

Table 4 Analytical framework of perception of the past (motivation)

Topic	Theme	Code	Description
Motivation	Fact	High incidence of malaria	High incidence of malaria in the villages and in Palawan.
		Limited health care resources	The health care resource is far away, and it is difficult to commute.
		Suffered from malaria	Experience of having suffered from malaria.
	Hope	Devotion	To help the community, village, and people.
		Eliminate malaria	To prevent, control, and reduce the incidence of malaria
		Inquisitive	To increase knowledge about malaria
	Nominated	Job experience	Experience to be barangay health worker
		No one available	No one was available

Table 5 Analytical framework of perception of the present (job satisfaction, role, problems, and experience)

Topic	Theme	Code	Description
Job satisfaction	Satisfied	Satisfied	Satisfied to be working as a microscopist.
	Achievement of the motivation (hope)	Devotion	To help the community, village, and people.
		Case reduction*	Malaria incidence is decreasing.*
		Inquisitiveness	To increase knowledge about malaria.
Role	Case reduction*	Case reduction*	Malaria incidence is decreasing.*
	More in rainy season	More in rainy season	More patients in the rainy season.
Problems	Working conditions	Supply	Shortage of materials and/or medicine.
		Setting	No electricity, broken equipment,* and/or narrowness of working space.**
		Finances	Incentives differ per municipality and are often delayed. No travel budget for home visits or official trips.
		Working hours	Patients want to be diagnosed any time, no replacement exists,* and no maternal leave was thought to be available.
		Employment	Strict recruitment policy.
		Health damage	Health problems caused by microscopy such as eye problem and headache.
		Limitations	Cannot treat other health problem.
		Politics	After election, policies often change.
	Recipients	Patient	Recurring malaria,** inappropriate intake of medicine,** and/or difficult personality.
		Community	Distrust by villagers, belief in certain religions, and/or belief in traditional medicine (indigenous residents).*
	No/fewer problems	No problems	No problems
		Fewer problems*	Along with reduction in malaria, fewer problems occur.*
Experience	Sad	Community distrust	Difficulty in being trusted by the community.
		Patient death	Patient died because the patient or their family did not trust microscopists and did not seek treatment from microscopists.
		Disagreement in diagnosis*	Diagnoses of medical technologists or private hospitals do not match with those of microscopists.*
		Politics	Autocratic behavior of politically strong persons.
		Working hours	Patient wants to be diagnosed any time, and no maternal leave was thought to be available.
	Happy	Devotion	Could help the patients and community.
		Meeting	Gather with other microscopists in meetings, training, and yearly malaria congress.

*Only mentioned in the FGDs in the northern regions
**Only mentioned in the FGDs in the southern regions

Some applied because they or their family had suffered from malaria and had difficulty in getting appropriate treatment in the hospital or any health care resources, which are far from their village.

Table 6 Analytical framework of perception of the future (task shifting)

Topic	Theme	Code	Description
Task shifting	Willing	Willing	Willing to task shift
	Task	Other samples	Stool, urine, and sputum
		Other diseases	Parasitic disease and tuberculosis

Way back in 1999, 4 of us in our family got sick, me and 3 children. During that time our *barangay* (Tagalog: village) captain was looking for someone to be trained by KLM (the administrating organization of this community-based intervention). I applied and was accepted, thinking to help our barangay. Not only us who got sick but many, that is why I applied.

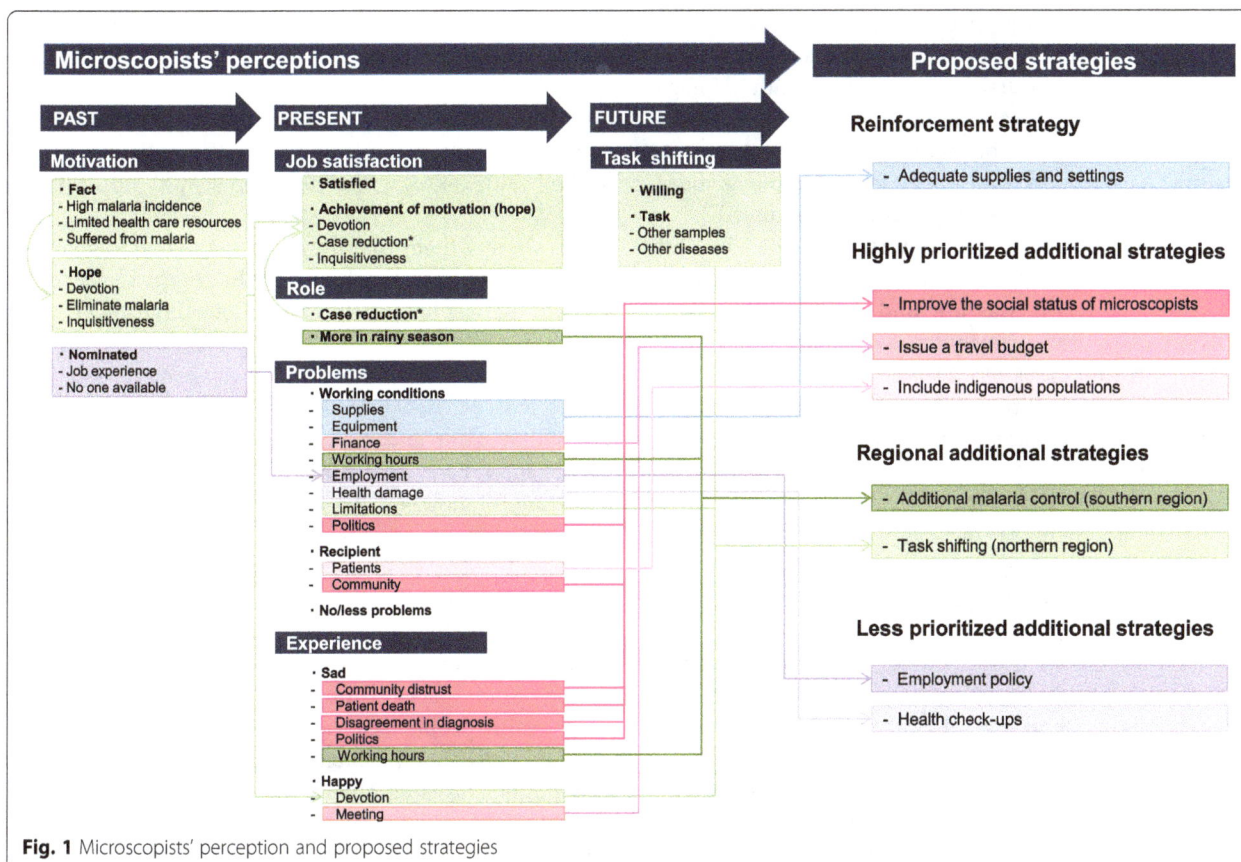

Fig. 1 Microscopists' perception and proposed strategies

My child was given dextrose at RHU (rural health unit). We went home with my child with dextrose, and back again in RHU in the following day because we were not allowed to sleep at the RHU (even it is far from our village). So when I heard of the training I applied to be experienced and to give medicine. There are a lot of cases and it is difficult to commute (to the health care resource). (Code: high malaria incidence, limited health care resources, suffered from malaria, and devotion)

When no one was applying, it seems that the village captain and/or midwife nominated one of their BHW to be a microscopist. Few were forced to be microscopists but ultimately, they were pleased to be one because they were able to help their villages.

Job satisfaction

Participants were satisfied because they could realize their motivation towards the future (hope) (Table 5). They were satisfied because they were able to help the community (devotion) and increase their knowledge about malaria (inquisitive). Some were satisfied because they could learn not only about malaria but also about other medical aspects such as immunization, taking blood pressure, measuring body weight, and assisting in

feeding. This additional knowledge was related by midwifes working in the health centers where the microscopists work. Moreover, the decrease in the incidence of malaria was also an aspect that increased their satisfaction, but it was only mentioned in the northern region (less malaria).

Role

Microscopists from the southern region where the incidence of malaria is high had many more duties and responsibilities than those from the northern region. Moreover, only the FGDs in the northern regions recognized the yearly decrease in malaria patients, whereas none in the southern regions mentioned a decrease (Table 5). The participants from both regions recognized that there were more malaria patients in the rainy season because of the increased number of insect vectors.

Problems

Although the job satisfaction of the participants was high, it was in this section discussing their problems that they most warmed up, and it was the longest section among all of the questions. The problems mentioned in the discussions were classified into three groups: working conditions, recipients, and no/few problems (Table 5).

The most frequently appearing problem was that of working conditions, which consisted of supply, setting, finances, working hours, employment, health damage, limitations, and politics. Among these components, the delay in the purchase or supply of essential materials (mainly Giemsa stain, with a very few mentioning slides, cotton, alcohol, medicine, etc.) was most discussed.

The delay in medical supply was mentioned in both regions, but only in the northern region, in which the incidence of malaria was low and decreasing, was the problem of limited primaquine availability mentioned. If there were no cases of *Plasmodium vivax* in the previous year, then the provision of primaquine is stopped, and if there are cases of *P. vivax*, they have to transport the patient.

> Last January there was one case of *vivax* but we did not have primaquine, because we did not have any *vivax* case the previous year. (Code: supply)

Several limitations of the setting were also mentioned. Electricity is not yet or only partly supplied in rural villages in Palawan, and limited light was causing difficulty in examining malaria especially in bad weather or at nighttime. Some participants were conducting microscopic examination in the open air under the sun. Broken microscopes and solar energy system equipment, and narrowness of the workplace were also mentioned.

> In our case, we have no electricity during the day, only during the night. Yes, our place is very island (very far from the main island), sometimes those from the island will ask for examination in the night, and we need to examine right away. (Code: setting)

Among working conditions, problems related with finances were also often mentioned. The problem of incentives, which differs by municipality and which sometime causes delays, and that of the travel budget were frequently discussed, although some participants said that they were volunteers and were not interested in incentives. A travel budget was needed for official trips to make reports or attend meetings and to make home visits in households scattered about the village. Some microscopists were budgeting their own money for these trips.

> With supplies, I have no problem, even in the *barangay* (Tagalog: village). My problem is the financial. I have incentive. The problem is for travel. We have monthly meeting, if we have report and the expenses in attending meeting is at our own expense. Also if there is urgent call, you have no allowance for that. If we have to refer to other hospital, we use our own money. Those patient who do not have money

for the fare, it is the microscopist who will shoulder the expenses. (Code: finances)

For this travel budget problem, one microscopist had a countermeasure, which was to ask the patient to come to the health center where the microscopist works.

> Yes we told them that they will be the one to come to us and then come back to give the result. So we told them that we help each other. (Code: finances)

Other problems relating to working condition were also discussed. Because patients want to be diagnosed when they want and no backup personnel exist, some participants had to examine the patient during the nighttime or holidays (working hours). Some criticized the employment conditions because of the strict recruitment policy (less than 35 years old with no foster children). Maternal leave was also thought to be not possible. Health damage, especially eye problems and headaches from using the microscope, were also mentioned. Some faced limitations because they cannot treat health problems other than malaria. Politics was also a continuing problem because after an election, new politicians often change the policies and sometime the new head tries to change the microscopist.

Problems of the recipients (patient and community) were also discussed. In the southern region where the incidence of malaria is high, recurring malaria and inappropriate intake of medicine were discussed.

> In my case mam, for example the patient is positive this month then the following month positive again, then next month positive again, always coming back. (Code: patient)

> There was a patient who did not take all the medicine and went back to work, and later that night he have attack of malaria and later he died. I don't know if he had relapse or he is well according to him, but he did not finish the medication. He went back to work, but he was brought to the hospital and later he died. (Code: patient)

Community acceptance of microscopists was also a problem. Some villagers living in the mountains, mainly indigenous people, did not or continued not to trust treatment from a microscopist and were seeking treatment from an *albularyo* (Tagalog: traditional healer). Microscopists inferred that this was because they believed in traditional medicine. Some community members who believed in certain religions also refused to accept treatment from the microscopist and were treating themselves with hand-made medicine.

First, the highest number of cases in San Vicente is Karuray, no. 1, the highest and many cases of malaria, and most of them are not inform because it is difficult to go to them because they believe that malaria is for the *Albularyo* (Tagalog: traditional healer) only. Mam if we come to them they will fight against us. Now we are trying to explain until some are convinced. We started at 2002 and the barangay officials are difficult to work with. (Code: community)

Several participants explained how they had changed the health-seeking behavior of these indigenous residents by teaching about malaria and the microscopist's role. In their villages, indigenous residents come down from the mountains where they live to get a diagnosis and treatment from the microscopist.

In my area of assignment, there are some indigenous residents. They come down from the mountain. Before not and they were afraid. Now they are afraid to die in the forest. We tell them that malaria can cause death, and we can check their smear if they come down. They are still afraid of immunization. They believe that they will not be able to walk after the injection. (Code: patient)

Some participants said that they had no problems or fewer problems. The participants from the northern region said that along with the reduction in malaria, there are fewer problems occurring in relation to their work as microscopists.

In the long run mam, little by little malaria cases became lesser. And our problem is also lesser and other community members understand us, they want us to stay there. (Code: fewer problems)

Experience

The majority of sad experiences of microscopists were related to community distrust. In the beginning of the KLM project, some microscopists faced difficulty in gaining the trust of the community (Table 5). Little by little, the community started to trust microscopists and started to get diagnosed by them. Some blamed microscopists because the patients collapsed after being pricked in the finger for blood sampling. Some patients, especially relatives of politically strong persons, blamed, and sometime tried to sue, the microscopists for misdiagnosis. However, microscopists could face these problems

with confidence because they had proof of blood smears and knowledge about the diagnosis.

One day a patient came from mountain area where malaria was once epidemic but now not too much. The patient was a boy. I made a smear and was positive for *Plasmodium falciparum* 4 (high parasetemia). The father did not believe because the boy was still playing. But later the boy had convulsion. They brought him to private hospital after I diagnosed him as falciparum 4, and I have told the father to give this medicine and bring him to the hospital. Good that the boy is in good health and was also diagnosed falciparum 4 (at the private hospital). I also thought I was wrong but when he was diagnosed as falciparum 4 (at the private hospital), the father said that the microscopist knew that. Then later people started to believe my diagnosis. (Code: community distrust)

Sadly and frustratingly, some microscopists experienced the death of their malaria patients, who were not being diagnosed and treated by microscopists because the family did not trust them (patient death).

In my case, there was a patient positive with malaria who died but was brought to the hospital. I did not diagnose because they said the child is in good health but later had convulsion. They brought the child to the hospital. It was falciparum 4. Need to transfuse blood but it will come from Puerto Princesa City. When it arrived, the boy was already dead. (Code: community distrust, and patient death)

The microscopists from the northern regions sometimes had the frustrating experience of not being believed by the patient that he or she was malaria negative or positive because a medtech or private hospital provided an opposing diagnosis (disagreement in diagnosis). This disagreement was thought to occur because when microscopists first made blood smears, the parasitemia was too low to be examined; because the medicine described by microscopist had worked and the patient had no malaria when he or she received treatment from a medtech/private hospital; or because in the northern region malaria is less endemic than in the southern regions, the medtech/private hospital diagnosed the patient only from their symptoms without also checking blood smears.

Another sad experience was related to politics. Some microscopists had to resign unwillingly because the newly elected person in power wanted to change the microscopist or because there is no system for maternal leave.

Sad experiences relating to working hours were also mentioned. As basically only one microscopist is active per village and works only few days per week, some patients complained about the inconvenience. Patients want to be diagnosed and treated as soon as possible, even at nighttime or on holidays. Even though microscopists have high motivation to devote themselves to their community, it is a difficult burden to accept patients at all hours. Some microscopists found a solution by asking the BHW or midwife to take and store blood smears of the patients when the microscopist is not at the health center, and then they examined the smear later. Even with this solution, other problems occurred because of miscommunication.

Many microscopists mentioned the fact that their ability to help the patients was the happiest experience of their work as a microscopist (devotion). The following statement made by one microscopist describes her happiest experience of being able to help a person suffering from a relapse of malaria and also the fact she could better diagnose and treat malaria patients than the hospital could.

> I have one patient who was always in the hospital. He was always malaria positive. One time, he approached me because he knew that I am a microscopist. Then I found out that he had *Plasmodium vivax* (which is the kind known to relapse without specific treatment). He was treated for 14 days. One month after treatment he came back and gave me chicken because it has been one month that his illness did not occur. (Code: devotion)

Microscopists also were very happy to gather with other microscopists from different municipalities during meetings, training, and the yearly malaria congress. Still, some complained because they had to spend their own money to participate in such occasions.

Task shifting
Microscopists were willing to extend their task and to be trained to examine other samples (stool, urine, sputum) and other disease such as parasites (worms) and tuberculosis (Table 6). The motivation for this task shifting was inspired by their inquisitiveness and devotion. These were also the main motivations to become microscopists, which were related to job satisfaction.

Discussion
In summarizing these results of the microscopists' perceptions (Fig. 1), the present study proposed the following strategies: reinforcement strategy (adequate supplies and settings), highly prioritized additional strategies (improving social status of microscopists, issuing a travel budget, and including indigenous populations), regional additional strategies (additional malaria control in the southern region and task shifting in the northern region), and less prioritized additional strategies (employment policy and health checkups).

Proposed strategies
Reinforcement strategy
First of all, as a key operation, a reinforcement strategy was suggested to avoid the occasional lack of adequate supplies and inadequate settings, which was pointed out by the microscopists. To fulfill the microscopists' tasks, the supply of necessary materials and maintenance of the setting should be well secured. Particularly, microscopists in Palawan frequently mentioned the shortage of Giemsa stain solution because it is the only reagent being charged to the village. In fact, some microscopists had difficulty in asking the village head to purchase Giemsa stain solution. KLM should consider and find solutions to resolve this problem.

Primaquine is an essential drug for the radical cure of *P. vivax* patients by preventing relapses [17] and is also indispensable to the elimination of malaria in Palawan [1]. In 2015, about 4% of estimated cases globally were due to *P. vivax*, but outside the African continent, the proportion of *P. vivax* was 41% [18]. Despite relatively low prevalence measurements and parasetemia levels than *P. falciparum*, along with high proportions of asymptomatic cases, this *P. vivax* is not benign [19]. Without strategies regarding *P. vivax*-specific characteristics, progress toward world malaria elimination will not be realized. Thus, primaquine should be supplied in sufficient amounts by the KLM even in villages where *P. vivax* cases are not common.

In addition, in rural areas of Palawan where the electricity supply is limited, practical implementation of measures allowing the microscopists to fully perform their tasks to diagnose malaria even in bad weather or at nighttime should also be provided.

Highly prioritized additional strategies
Second, as a prioritized additional strategy, improvement of the microscopists' position in society should be required. Many microscopists faced distrust by the community when they started to work. Overcoming this distrust solely through the microscopists' quiet dedication to malaria diagnosis and treatment will not be enough. Public awareness activities to recognize the importance of the microscopic diagnosis or, indeed, the microscopists themselves are needed. Creditable microscopists in the neighborhood enabling free access of villagers to appropriate treatment will eventually acquire the trust among the local communities.

Issuing a travel budget including food allowance and travel insurance to microscopists was also proposed to help find active cases in scattered households and for other official trips. In some municipalities, microscopists were given financial incentives mainly to cover the cost of transportation, but most microscopists in other municipalities were using their own money for their travels. Most of the health centers were basically in the middle of the villages; microscopists sometimes had to cross several mountains to reach scattered households. They said that malaria in such settlements was often times a big problem because of the higher density of malaria mosquitoes. This problem of insufficient travel budget was also mentioned in our previous paper as a problem to be solved [4]. While at the same time, a study that examined different remuneration models of CHWs showed that if payment or incentives are perceived inadequately, then this can demotivate CHWs [20]. Issuing a travel budget should be carefully considered and implemented.

Moreover, many microscopists said that their happy experiences were meeting other microscopists from different municipalities in yearly malaria congresses or other meetings. Therefore, a travel budget for such purposes should be considered to maintain their job satisfaction and consequently maintain or improve the quality of their work.

The other highly prioritized additional strategy was to include indigenous people as a key target population in the KLM activities. As was found in a previous study, some indigenous people were not likely to seek diagnosis and treatment by microscopists in Palawan, and, in fact, they preferred to be treated by traditional healers, or *albularyo* in Tagalog [6]. *Albularyo* were still present in Palawan in 2015 and continued to play a salient role in the health care of some community members in the Philippines. These indigenous populations were vulnerable/at high risk for malaria infection due to the remoteness of their villages, language (Tagalog) barrier, their lack of education and persistently poor health and nutritional status, and, most importantly, their socio-cultural isolation from current government service delivery. A previous study in Palawan reported that community awareness-raising activities by microscopists for indigenous people could strengthen their ability to practice effective malaria prevention and seek appropriate treatment [5, 6]. Precisely, awareness of knowledge on malaria transmission, about which indigenous populations happen to have low knowledge, would strengthen effective prevention [5], and improving their knowledge of malaria symptoms would encourage them to seek appropriate treatment [6].

Malaria control among indigenous populations should be the key to eliminating malaria in Palawan, Philippines, as in other malaria-endemic Asian Pacific countries [11, 21]. Especially in these countries, malaria burden have been significantly reduced [18]. Moving towards malaria elimination, interventions now try to target populations at higher risk of malaria, including indigenous populations, migrants, and forest workers, who are frequently not reached by health services [22, 23].

Regional additional strategies

Third, additional malaria control strategies are required. In the southern region, appropriate diagnosis and treatment by the microscopists alone might not be sufficient to achieve a decrease in the incidence of malaria. Reduction of the number of malaria mosquito breeding sites [24, 25] or the use of long-lasting insecticide-treated nets or indoor residual spraying is needed [26, 27].

In the northern region, task shifting of the microscopists is proposed as a regional additional strategy because microscopists in the present study had high motivation to extend their tasks in a province in which critical shortages of highly educated health professionals are recognized. Epidemiological data also indicate a changing pattern of disease in Palawan [28], for which microscopists can play additional significant roles. With the support of midwives, it will be possible to employ highly motivated microscopists to work on several health problems other than malaria. Several studies have proved that task shifting of community health workers can contribute to addressing the insufficient health workforce worldwide [29, 30].

Less prioritized additional strategies

Finally, as less prioritized additional strategies, the following two items were suggested: an employment policy and the need for health checkups for them.

There might be a need to reconsider the recruitment policy. Although a "strict" policy may easily balance cost-effectiveness, a more appropriate recruitment method will make the present community-based strategy more sustainable. Although microscopic examination exposes to few health hazards, regular health checkups and/or precautions that should be taken to reduce any health problems should be prioritized at malaria congresses or yearly meetings.

Possibility of sympathetic motivation

Along with the proposition of the four strategies as discussed above, the present results represent the general possibility that health service delivery can be strengthened and/or sustainably maintained by CHWs' sympathetic motivation, and not by financial incentives, in resource-poor settings. The success of this community-based malaria control project was suspected to be partly because the project could satisfy the motivation of the microscopists. This led to high job satisfaction, which enhanced their work performance. Their motivation was the simple hope of devoting their work to their malarious villages. Most microscopists became microscopists because they hoped to change the reality (high incidence of malaria, limited health care resources) in their villages and gained high job satisfaction because they could contribute by diagnosing and treating malaria by themselves in their villages. The results of the present study might have been due to the microscopists' characteristics, such as subsistence status (mainly homemakers), religion, and a stable household financial status, and therefore might not be applicable to all resource-poor settings. However, for example, a previous study targeting the same microscopists supports the impact of job satisfaction on work performance [4]. Job satisfaction of the microscopists and other CHWs should be the subject of greater attention and emphasis in order to strengthen sustainable health service delivery.

Limitation

Although the FGD method can provide rich data especially when there is little prior information on the participants, there are some methodological limitations. Unsuitable topics and views exist for the FGD methods. Therefore, it is difficult to suggest a strong recommendation. However, it is also true that the discussions in the FGDs highlighted some dimensions among CHWs' perceptions. Therefore, the proposed strategies are expected to be certainly practical and effective to strengthen the community-based malaria control.

Moreover, the participants of each FGD were around 12. This number was almost the upper limit of the number of participants that were conventionally involved in productive FGDs. To decrease the risk of respondents' being hidden in the crowd and dropping their inputs, the facilitators conducted the FGDs very carefully to get sufficient replies from all the participants.

Conclusion

This qualitative study was based on the bottom-up approach using CHWs' (microscopists) perceptions about their past, present, and future to propose practical and effective additional strategies. It was proven important to understand profound data such as realities or barriers that would help to strengthen the community-based malaria control.

Acknowledgements
Sincere appreciation is expressed to Ms. Imelda Pates who transcribed the audio recording of the focus group discussion.

Funding
The present study was supported by a grant from the Japanese Ministry of Health, Labour and Welfare (H21-Chikyukibo-Ippan-006) and by a grant from the National Center for Global Health and Medicine (25A2). The funders had no role in the study design, data collection and analysis, decision to publish, or preparation of this manuscript.

Authors' contributions
ELAM-T, MJ, and SK designed the present study. ELAM-T, PTR, EAV, and SK conducted the fieldwork and collected the data on the province island. RUA helped to get the information on-site. ELAM-T analyzed the data in discussions with PTR, EAV, and SK, and ELAM-T wrote this paper under the supervision of MJ and SK. All authors read and approved the final manuscript.

Competing interests
The authors declare that they have no competing interests.

Author details
[1]Department of Tropical Medicine and Malaria, Research Institute, National Center for Global Health and Medicine, 1-21-1 Toyama, Shinjuku-ku, Tokyo 162-8655, Japan. [2]Department of Community and Global Health, Graduate School of Medicine, The University of Tokyo, 7-3-1 Hongo, Bunkyo-ku, Tokyo 113-8654, Japan. [3]Department of Parasitology, College of Public Health, University of the Philippines Manila, 625 Pedro Gil Street, Ermita, Manila, Philippines. [4]Pilipinas Shell Foundation, Inc., 5300 Puerto Princesa City, Palawan, Philippines.

References
1. Provincial Health Office of Palawan. Provincial health report, 2012. Palawan: Provincial Health Office of Palawan; 2012.
2. Angluben RU, Trudeau MR, Kano S, Tongol-Rivera P. Kilusan Ligtas Malaria: advancing social mobilization towards sustainable malaria control in the province of Palawan, the Philippines. Trop Med Heal. 2008;36:45–9.
3. Sunguya BF, Mlunde LB, Ayer R, Jimba M. Towards eliminating malaria in high endemic countries: the roles of community health workers and related cadres and their challenges in integrated community case management for malaria: a systematic review. Malar J. 2017;16:10. Available from: http://www.ncbi.nlm.nih.gov/pubmed/28049486. Cited 8 Mar 2018.
4. Matsumoto-Takahashi ELA, Tongol-Rivera P, Villacorte EA, Angluben RU, Yasuoka J, Kano S, et al. Determining the active role of microscopists in community awareness-raising activities for malaria prevention: a cross-sectional study in Palawan, the Philippines. Malar J. 2013;12:384. Available from: http://www.ncbi.nlm.nih.gov/pubmed/24175934
5. Matsumoto-Takahashi ELA, Tongol-Rivera P, Villacorte EA, Angluben RU, Yasuoka J, Kano S, et al. Determining the impact of community awareness-raising activities on the prevention of malaria transmission in Palawan, the Philippines. Parasitol Int. 2014;63:519–26.
6. Matsumoto-Takahashi ELA, Tongol-Rivera P, Villacorte EA, Angluben RU, Jimba M, Kano S. Patient knowledge on malaria symptoms is a key to promoting universal access of patients to effective malaria treatment in Palawan, the Philippines. PLoS One. 2015;10:e0127858. Available from: http://journals.plos.org/plosone/article?id=10.1371/journal.pone.0127858. Cited 22 June 2015.
7. "The Harvard Interfaculty Program on Health Systems". A strategy for health care reform: catalyzing change from the bottom up [Internet]. 2006. Available from: http://www.phsi.harvard.edu/pdfs/reform.pdf. Cited 23 Feb 2015
8. Carrin G, Buse K, Heggenhougen K, Quah SR. Health systems policy, finance, and organization [Internet]. San Diego: Elsevier publications; 2010. Available from: https://books.google.com/books?id=lEXUrc0tr1wC&pgis=1. Cited 23 Feb 2015.
9. Glenton C, Scheel IB, Pradhan S, Lewin S, Hodgins S, Shrestha V. The female community health volunteer programme in Nepal: decision makers' perceptions of volunteerism, payment and other incentives. Soc Sci Med. 2010;70:1920–7. Available from: http://linkinghub.elsevier.com/retrieve/pii/S027795361000198X. Cited 1 Sept 2017
10. King M, King L, Willis E, Munt R, Semmens F. The experiences of remote and rural Aboriginal Health Workers and registered nurses who undertook a postgraduate diabetes course to improve the health of Indigenous Australians. Contemp Nurse. 2012;42:107–17. Available from: http://www.tandfonline.com/doi/abs/10.5172/conu.2012.42.1.107. Cited 1 Sept 2017
11. Sundararajan R, Kalkonde Y, Gokhale C, Greenough PG, Bang A. Barriers to malaria control among marginalized tribal communities: a qualitative study. PLoS One. 2013;8:e81966. Available from: http://www.pubmedcentral.nih.gov/articlerender.fcgi?artid=3869659&tool=pmcentrez&rendertype=abstract. Cited 3 Mar 2015

12. Kim SS, Ali D, Kennedy A, Tesfaye R, Tadesse AW, Abrha TH, et al. Assessing implementation fidelity of a community-based infant and young child feeding intervention in Ethiopia identifies delivery challenges that limit reach to communities: a mixed-method process evaluation study. BMC Public Health. 2015;15:316. Available from: http://bmcpublichealth.biomedcentral.com/articles/10.1186/s12889-015-1650-4. Cited 1 Sept 2017

13. National Statistical Coordination Board. Population of the Philippines census years 1799 to 2010. Manila: National Statistical Coorfinaion Board; 2012.

14. Kitzinger J. Qualitative research. Introducing focus groups. BMJ. 1995;311: 299–302.

15. Rabiee F. Focus-group interview and data analysis. Proc Nutr Soc. 2004;63: 655–60.

16. Pope C, Ziebland S, Mays N. Qualitative research in health care. Analysing qualitative data. BMJ. 2000;320:114–6.

17. World Health Organization. WHO model list of essential medicines 18th list. 2013. Available from: http://www.who.int/medicines/publications/essentialmedicines/en/index.html. Cited 1 Sept 2017

18. World Health Organization. World malaria report 2016: World Health Organization; 2016.

19. Howes RE, Battle KE, Mendis KN, Smith DL, Cibulskis RE, Baird JK, et al. Global epidemiology of Plasmodium vivax. Am J Trop Med Hyg. 2016;95: 15–34. Available from: http://www.ncbi.nlm.nih.gov/pubmed/27402513. Cited 1 Sept 2017.

20. Singh D, Negin J, Otim M, Orach CG, Cumming R. The effect of payment and incentives on motivation and focus of community health workers: five case studies from low- and middle-income countries. Hum Resour Health. 2015;13:58. Available from: http://www.ncbi.nlm.nih.gov/pubmed/26169179. Cited 5 Sept 2017.

21. Xu J-W, Xu Q-Z, Liu H, Zeng Y-R. Malaria treatment-seeking behaviour and related factors of Wa ethnic minority in Myanmar: a cross-sectional study. Malar J. 2012;11:417. Available from: http://www.pubmedcentral.nih.gov/articlerender.fcgi?artid=3529692&tool=pmcentrez&rendertype=abstract. Cited 13 Feb 2015.

22. Wen S, Harvard KE, Gueye CS, Canavati SE, Chancellor A, Ahmed B-N, et al. Targeting populations at higher risk for malaria: a survey of national malaria elimination programmes in the Asia Pacific. Malar J. 2016;15:271. Available from: http://www.ncbi.nlm.nih.gov/pubmed/27165296. Cited 1 Sept 2017.

23. Chuquiyauri R, Paredes M, Peñataro P, Torres S, Marin S, Tenorio A, et al. Socio-demographics and the development of malaria elimination strategies in the low transmission setting. Acta Trop. 2012;121:292–302. Available from: http://www.ncbi.nlm.nih.gov/pubmed/22100446. Cited 1 Sept 2017.

24. Ng'ang'a PN, Shililu J, Jayasinghe G, Kimani V, Kabutha C, Kabuage L, et al. Malaria vector control practices in an irrigated rice agro-ecosystem in central Kenya and implications for malaria control. Malar J. 2008;7:146. Available from: http://www.malariajournal.com/content/7/1/146. Cited 3 Mar 2015.

25. Raghavendra K, Barik TK, Reddy BPN, Sharma P, Dash AP. Malaria vector control: from past to future. Parasitol Res. 2011;108:757–79. Available from: http://www.ncbi.nlm.nih.gov/pubmed/21229263. Cited 3 Mar 2015.

26. World Health Organization. Malaria vector control and personal protection. World Health Organ. Tech Rep Ser. 2006;936:1–62. Available from: http://www.ncbi.nlm.nih.gov/pubmed/16623084. Cited 13 Feb 2015.

27. Killeen GF, Smith TA, Ferguson HM, Mshinda H, Abdulla S, Lengeler C, et al. Preventing childhood malaria in Africa by protecting adults from mosquitoes with insecticide-treated nets. PLoS Med. 2007;4:e229. Available from: http://www.pubmedcentral.nih.gov/articlerender.fcgi?artid=1904465&tool=pmcentrez&rendertype=abstract. Cited 13 Feb 2015.

28. Matsumoto-Takahashi ELA, Kano S. Evaluating active roles of community health workers in accelerating universal access to health services for malaria in Palawan, the Philippines. Trop Med Health. 2016;44:10. Available from: http://tropmedhealth.biomedcentral.com/articles/10.1186/s41182-016-0008-7. Cited 15 Apr 2016.

29. Okyere E, Mwanri L, Ward P. Is task-shifting a solution to the health workers' shortage in Northern Ghana? Kumar S, editor. PLoS One. 2017;12:e0174631. Available from: http://www.ncbi.nlm.nih.gov/pubmed/28358841. Cited 1 Sept 2017.

30. Tsolekile LP, Abrahams-Gessel S, Puoane T. Healthcare professional shortage and task-shifting to prevent cardiovascular disease: implications for low- and middle-income countries. Curr Cardiol Rep. 2015;17:115. Available from: http://link.springer.com/10.1007/s11886-015-0672-y. Cited 1 Sept 2017.

Permissions

List of Contributors

Lenneke Vaandrager and Maria Koelen
Health and Society (HSO) group, Wageningen University, 6700 EW Wageningen, The Netherlands

Valerie Makoge
Health and Society (HSO) group, Wageningen University, 6700 EW Wageningen, The Netherlands
Institute of Medical Research and Medicinal Plant studies (IMPM), Yaoundé, Cameroon

Harro Maat
Knowledge Technology and Innovation (KTI) group, Wageningen University, Hollandseweg 1, 6708 KN Wageningen, The Netherlands

Md. Manirul Islam
Training Unit, icddr, b, 68, Shaheed Tajuddin Ahmed Sarani, Mohakhali, Dhaka 1212, Bangladesh

Nasim Jahan
Department of Psychiatry, BIRDEM General Hospital and IMC, Dhaka, Bangladesh

Md. Delwar Hossain
National Institute of Mental Health, Sher-e-bangla Nagar, Dhaka 1207, Bangladesh

Lisa Waddell, Judy Greig and Mariola Mascarenhas
Public Health Risk Sciences Division, National Microbiology Laboratory, Public Health Agency of Canada, Guelph, ON, Canada

Tricia Corrin and Catherine Hierlihy
Public Health Risk Sciences Division, National Microbiology Laboratory, Public Health Agency of Canada, Guelph, ON, Canada
Department of Population Medicine, University of Guelph, Guelph, ON, Canada

Ian Young
School of Occupational and Public Health, Ryerson University, Toronto, ON, Canada

Calvin Bisong Ebai, Irene Ule Ngole Sumbele and Jude Ebah Yunga
Department of Zoology and Animal Physiology, Faculty of Science, University of Buea, Buea, SWR, Cameroon

Helen Kuokuo Kimbi
Department of Zoology and Animal Physiology, Faculty of Science, University of Buea, Buea, SWR, Cameroon

Department of Medical Laboratory Sciences, Faculty of Health Sciences, University of Bamenda, Bambili, NWR, Cameroon

Leopold Gustave Lehman
Department of Animal Biology, Faculty of Science, University of Douala, Douala, Cameroon

Daisuke Nonaka and Jun Kobayashi
Department of Global Health, Graduate School of Health Sciences, University of the Ryukyus, Uehara 207, Nishihara-cho, Okinawa 903-0215, Japan
SATREPS Project for Parasitic Diseases, Vientiane, Lao People's Democratic Republic

Nouhak Inthavong
Department of Global Health, Graduate School of Health Sciences, University of the Ryukyus, Uehara 207, Nishihara-cho, Okinawa 903-0215, Japan
SATREPS Project for Parasitic Diseases, Vientiane, Lao People's Democratic Republic
National Institute of Public Health, Ministry of Health, Ban Kaognot, Samsenthai Road, Sisattanak District, Vientiane, Lao People's Democratic Republic

Shigeyuki Kano
SATREPS Project for Parasitic Diseases, Vientiane, Lao People's Democratic Republic
Department of Tropical Medicine and Malaria, Research Institute, National Center for Global Health and Medicine, 1-21-1 Toyama, Shinjuku-ku, Tokyo 162-8655, Japan

Paul T. Brey
SATREPS Project for Parasitic Diseases, Vientiane, Lao People's Democratic Republic
Institut Pasteur du Laos, Ministry of Health, Sisattanak District, Vientiane, Lao People's Democratic Republic

Moritoshi Iwagami
SATREPS Project for Parasitic Diseases, Vientiane, Lao People's Democratic Republic
Department of Tropical Medicine and Malaria, Research Institute, National Center for Global Health and Medicine, 1-21-1 Toyama, Shinjuku-ku, Tokyo 162-8655, Japan
Institut Pasteur du Laos, Ministry of Health, Sisattanak District, Vientiane, Lao People's Democratic Republic

Bouasy Hongvanthong
SATREPS Project for Parasitic Diseases, Vientiane, Lao People's Democratic Republic

Center of Malariology, Parasitology and Entomology, Ministry of Health, Vientiane, Lao People's Democratic Republic

Tiengkham Pongvongsa
SATREPS Project for Parasitic Diseases, Vientiane, Lao People's Democratic Republic
Savannakhet Provincial Health Department, Thahea village, Kaysone-Phomvihan District, Savannakhet, Lao People's Democratic Republic

Sengchanh Kounnavong and Souraxay Phommala
National Institute of Public Health, Ministry of Health, Ban Kaognot, Samsenthai Road, Sisattanak District, Vientiane, Lao People's Democratic Republic

Abu Yousuf Md Abdullah, Md Rakibul Islam Shogib, Md Masudur Rahman and Md Faruk Hossain
Department of Geography and Environment, University of Dhaka, University Road, Dhaka 1000, Bangladesh

Ashraf Dewan
Department of Spatial Sciences, Curtin University, Perth, Australia

Choolwe Muzyamba
Maastricht Graduate School of Governance/UNU-Merit, Maastricht University, Maastricht, Netherlands
Lusaka, Zambia

Sonila M. Tomini
Maastricht Graduate School of Governance/UNU-Merit, Maastricht University, Maastricht, Netherlands
Department of Economics, University of Liege, Liège, Belgium

Milena Pavlova
Department of Health Services Research, CAPHRI, Maastricht University Medical Center, Faculty of Health, Medicine and Life Sciences, Maastricht University, Maastricht, Netherlands

Wim Groot
Department of Health Services Research, CAPHRI, Maastricht University Medical Center, Faculty of Health, Medicine and Life Sciences, Maastricht University, Maastricht, Netherlands
Top Institute for Evidence-Based Education Research (TIER), Maastricht University, Maastricht, Netherlands

Iryna Rud
Top Institute for Evidence-Based Education Research (TIER), Maastricht University, Maastricht, Netherlands

Pwint Mon Oo, Aung Thi and Zaw Lin
Central Vector Borne Disease Control Programme, Department of Public Health, Ministry of Health and Sport, Nay Pyi Taw, Myanmar

Khin Thet Wai and Tin Oo
Department of Medical Research, Yangon, Myanmar

Anthony D. Harries
International Union against Tuberculosis and Lung Disease, Paris, France
London School of Hygiene and Tropical Medicine, London, UK

Hemant Deepak Shewade
International Union against Tuberculosis and Lung Disease (The Union), South-East Asia Office, New Delhi, India

Kidanemariam G/Michael Beyene
Ethiopian Food, Medicine and Healthcare Administration and Control Authority, Addis Ababa, Ethiopia

Solomon Worku Beza
GAMBY College of Medical Sciences, Addis Ababa, Ethiopia

Andrea Rivera-Sepulveda
Division of Pediatric Emergency Medicine, Department of Pediatrics, Saint Louis University School of Medicine, 1402 S. Grand Boulevard – Glennon Hall, Room 2717, 63104 Saint Louis, MO, USA
School of Health Professions, University of Puerto Rico Medical Sciences Campus, and School of Medicine, San Juan, Puerto Rico

Enid J.Garcia-Rivera
School of Health Professions, University of Puerto Rico Medical Sciences Campus, and School of Medicine, San Juan, Puerto Rico
Endowed Health Services, University of Puerto Rico School of Medicine, Medical Sciences Campus, San Juan, Puerto Rico

G. Glenn Wilson and Darren Ryder
Ecosystem Management, School of Environmental and Rural Science, University of New England, Armidale, NSW 2351, Australia

Solomon Kibret
Ecosystem Management, School of Environmental and Rural Science, University of New England, Armidale, NSW 2351, Australia
Program in Public Health, University of California, Irvine, CA 92697, USA

Habte Tekie
Department of Zoological Sciences, Addis Ababa University, Addis Ababa, Ethiopia

Beyene Petros
Department of Microbial, Cellular and Molecular Biology, Addis Ababa University, Addis Ababa, Ethiopia

Aye Mon Mon Kyaw, Nay Yi Yi Linn, Zaw Lin and Aung Thi
National Malaria Control Programme/Vector Borne Disease Control, Department of Public Health, Ministry of Health and Sports, Nay Pyi Taw, Myanmar

Soundappan Kathirvel
International Union Against Tuberculosis and Lung Disease, Southeast Asia, New Delhi, India
Department of Community Medicine, School of Public Health, Postgraduate Institute of Medical Education and Research, Chandigarh, India

Mrinalini Das
Médecins Sans Frontières (MSF) OCB, New Delhi, India

Badri Thapa
World Health Organization Country Office for Myanmar, Yangon, Myanmar

Thae Maung Maung
Department of Medical Research, Ministry of Health and Sports, Nay Pyi Taw, Myanmar

Phyo Aung Naing, Thae Maung Maung, Tin Oo and Khin Thet Wai
Department of Medical Research, Ministry of Health and Sports, No. 5, Ziwaka Road Dagon Township, Yangon 11191, Myanmar

Jaya Prasad Tripathy
International Union Against Tuberculosis and Lung Disease, The Union South-East Asia Regional Office, New Delhi, India

Aung Thi
National Malaria Control Program, Ministry of Health and Sports, Naypyitaw, Myanmar

Shishi Wu and Imara Roychowdhury
Saw Swee Hock School of Public Health, National University of Singapore, 12 Science Drive 2 #10-01, Singapore, 117549, Singapore

Mishal Khan
Saw Swee Hock School of Public Health, National University of Singapore, 12 Science Drive 2 #10-01, Singapore, 117549, Singapore
Communicable Diseases Policy Research Group, London School of Hygiene and Tropical Medicine, Keppel St, London WC1E 7HT, United Kingdom

Katsumi Maezawa, Rieko Furushima-Shimogawara, and Shiro Iwanaga
Department of Environmental Parasitology, Tokyo Medical and Dental University Graduate School of Medical and Dental Sciences, 1-5-45 Yushima, Bunkyo-ku, Tokyo 113–8519, Japan

Nobuo Ohta
Department of Environmental Parasitology, Tokyo Medical and Dental University Graduate School of Medical and Dental Sciences, 1-5-45 Yushima, Bunkyo-ku, Tokyo 113–8519, Japan
Depertment of Clinical Nutrition, Faculty of Health Science, Suzuka University of Medical Science, 1001-1, Kishioka-cyo, Suzuka-shi, Mie 510-0293, Japan

Akio Yasukawa
Nishiogi Veterinary Medical Hospital, 4-9-2 Nishiogikita, Suginami-ku, Tokyo 167–0042, Japan

Emmanuel Igwaro Odongo-Aginya and Alex Olia
Department of Microbiology and Immunology, Faculty of Medicine, Gulu University, Gulu, Uganda

Kilama Justin Luwa
Department of Biology, Faculty of Science, Gulu University, Gulu, Uganda

Eiji Nagayasu
Division of Parasitology, Department of Infectious Diseases, Faculty of Medicine, University of Miyazaki, Miyazaki 889-1692, Japan

Anna Mary Auma, Geoffrey Egitat and Gerald Mwesigwa
Vector Control Division, Ministry of Health, Kampala, Uganda

Yoshitaka Ogino
Department of Parasitology, Kochi Medical School, Kochi University, Nankoku, Kochi 783-8505, Japan
Department of Haematology and Respiratory Medicine, Kochi Medical School, Kochi University, Nankoku, Kochi 783-8505, Japan

Eisaku Kimura and Toshihiro Horii
Department of Molecular Protozoology, Research Institute for Microbial Diseases, Osaka University, Suita, Osaka 565-0871, Japan

Yukiko Higa, Kyoko Futami and Noboru Minakawa
Department of Vector Ecology and Environment, Institute of Tropical Medicine, Nagasaki University, 1-12-4 Sakamoto, Nagasaki 852-8523, Japan

Hanako Iwashita
Department of Vector Ecology and Environment, Institute of Tropical Medicine, Nagasaki University, 1-12-4 Sakamoto, Nagasaki 852-8523, Japan
Department of Bacteriology, Graduate School of Medicine, University of the Ryukyus, 207 Uehara, Nishiharacho, Okinawa 903-0125, Japan

Peter A. Lutiali
NUITM-KEMRI Project, Kenya Medical Research Institute, Nairobi, Kenya

Sammy M. Njenga
Eastern and Southern Africa Centre of International Parasite Control (ESACIPAC), Kenya Medical Research Institute, Nairobi, Kenya

Takeshi Nabeshima
Department of Virology, Institute of Tropical Medicine, Nagasaki University, Nagasaki, Japan

Andrew Page
Translational Health Research Institute, School of Medicine, Western Sydney University, Penrith, New South Wales, Australia

Felix Akpojene Ogbo
Translational Health Research Institute, School of Medicine, Western Sydney University, Penrith, New South Wales, Australia
Prescot Specialist Medical Centre, Welfare Quarters, Makurdi, Benue State, Nigeria

Pascal Ogeleka, Ifegwu K. Ifegwu and Akorede O. Awosemo
Prescot Specialist Medical Centre, Welfare Quarters, Makurdi, Benue State, Nigeria

Anselm Okoro
Society for Family Health, Justice Ifeyinwa Nzeako House, 8 Port Harcourt Crescent Area 11, Garki, Abuja, Nigeria

Bolajoko O. Olusanya and Jacob Olusanya
Centre for Healthy Start Initiative, 286A Corporation Drive, Dolphin Estate, Ikoyi, Lagos, Nigeria

John Eastwood
Ingham Institute for Applied Medical Research, 1 Campbell Street, Liverpool, New South Wales 2170, Australia
School of Women's and Children's Health, The University of New South Wales, Kensington, Sydney, New South Wales 2052, Australia
School of Public Health, The University of Sydney, Sydney, New South Wales 2006, Australia
School of Public Health, Griffith University, Queensland, Gold Coast 4222, Australia
Department of Community Paediatrics, Sydney Local Health District, Croydon Community Health Centre, 24 Liverpool Rd, Croydon, New South Wales 2132, Australia

Farzana Ferdous
Graduate School of Comprehensive Human Sciences, University of Tsukuba, Tsukuba, Japan

Shahnawaz Ahmed, Mohammod Jobayer Chisti and Tahmeed Ahmed
International Centre for Diarrhoeal Disease Research, Bangladesh (icddr, b), Dhaka, Bangladesh

Sumon Kumar Das
International Centre for Diarrhoeal Disease Research, Bangladesh (icddr, b), Dhaka, Bangladesh
School of Public Health, The University of Queensland, Brisbane, Australia

Abu Syed Golam Faruque
International Centre for Diarrhoeal Disease Research, Bangladesh (icddr, b), Dhaka, Bangladesh
Nutrition and Clinical Services Division, icddr, b, 68 Shaheed Tajuddin Ahmed Sarani, Mohakhali, Dhaka 1212, Bangladesh

Dilruba Nasrin
Center for Vaccine Development and Department of Medicine, University of Maryland School of Medicine, Baltimore, MD, USA

Karen L. Kotloff and Myron M. Levine
Center for Vaccine Development, Department of Pediatrics and Medicine, University of Maryland School of Medicine, Baltimore, MD, USA

James P. Nataro
Center for Vaccine Development, Department of Pediatrics and Medicine, University of Maryland School of Medicine, Baltimore, MD, USA
Department of Pediatrics, University of Virginia School of Medicine, Charlottesville, VA, USA

Enbo Ma
Health Promotion Center, Fukushima Medical University, Fukushima, Japan
Department of Clinical Trial and Clinical Epidemiology, Faculty of Medicine, University of Tsukuba, Tsukuba, Japan

Khitam Muhsen
Department of Epidemiology and Prevention Medicine, School of Public Health, Sackler Faculty of Medicine, Tel Aviv, Israel

Yukiko Wagatsuma
Department of Clinical Trial and Clinical Epidemiology, Faculty of Medicine, University of Tsukuba, Tsukuba, Japan

Hunachew Beyene
College of Health Sciences, Hawassa University, Hawassa, Ethiopia
School of Public Health, Addis Ababa University, Addis Ababa, Ethiopia

Wakgari Deressa and Abera Kumie
School of Public Health, Addis Ababa University, Addis Ababa, Ethiopia

Delia Grace
International Livestock Research Institute, Nairobi, Kenya

Shigeyuki Kano
Department of Tropical Medicine and Malaria, Research Institute, National Center for Global Health and Medicine, 1-21-1 Toyama, Shinjuku-ku, Tokyo 162-8655, Japan

Emilie Louise Akiko Matsumoto-Takahashi
Department of Tropical Medicine and Malaria, Research Institute, National Center for Global Health and Medicine, 1-21-1 Toyama, Shinjuku-ku, Tokyo 162-8655, Japan

Department of Community and Global Health, Graduate School of Medicine, The University of Tokyo, 7-3-1 Hongo, Bunkyo-ku, Tokyo 113-8654, Japan

Masamine Jimba
Department of Community and Global Health, Graduate School of Medicine, The University of Tokyo, 7-3-1 Hongo, Bunkyo-ku, Tokyo 113-8654, Japan

Pilarita Tongol-Rivera and Elena Andino Villacorte
Department of Parasitology, College of Public Health, University of the Philippines Manila, 625 Pedro Gil Street, Ermita, Manila, Philippines

Ray Uyaan Angluben
Pilipinas Shell Foundation, Inc., 5300 Puerto Princesa City, Palawan, Philippines

Index